A Physician's Guide to
Health Care Management

To my parents Maurice and Flora Albert and my aunt and uncle Philip and Ella Mandelbaum

A Physician's Guide to Health Care Management

Edited by

Daniel M. Albert, MD
Professor and Chairman
Department of Ophthalmology and Visual Sciences
University of Wisconsin
Madison, Wisconsin

©2002 by Blackwell Science, Inc.
a Blackwell Publishing Company

Editorial Offices:
Commerce Place, 350 Main Street, Malden, Massachusetts 02148, USA
Osney Mead, Oxford OX2 0EL, England
25 John Street, London WC1N 2BS, England
23 Ainslie Place, Edinburgh EH3 6AJ, Scotland
54 University Street, Carlton, Victoria 3053, Australia
Other Editorial Offices:
Blackwell Wissenschafts-Verlag GmbH, Kurfürstendamm 57, 10707 Berlin, Germany
Blackwell Science KK, MG Kodenmacho Building, 7–10 Kodenmacho Nihombashi, Chuo-ku, Tokyo 104, Japan
Iowa State University Press, A Blackwell Science Company, 2121 S. State Avenue, Ames, Iowa 50014-8300, USA

Distributors:
The Americas
Blackwell Publishing
c/o AIDC
PO Box 20
50 Winter Sport Lane
Williston, VT 05495-0020
(Telephone orders: 800-216-2522; fax orders: 802-864-7626)

Australia
Blackwell Science Pty, Ltd.
54 University Street
Carlton, Victoria 3053
(Telephone orders: 03-9347-0300; fax orders: 03-9349-3016)

Outside The Americas and Australia
Blackwell Science, Ltd.
c/o Marston Book Services, Ltd.
PO Box 269
Abingdon
Oxon OX14 4YN
England
(Telephone orders: 44-(0)1235-465500; fax orders: 44-(0)1235-465555)

Acquisitions: Laura DeYoung
Development: Angela Gagliano
Production: Jonathan Rowley
Manufacturing: Lisa Flanagan
Marketing Manager: Toni Fournier
Cover design by Cambridge Communication Design
Typeset in $9^{1}/_{2}$ /12pt Palatino by Graphicraft Ltd, Hong Kong
Printed and bound by Sheridan Books, Michigan, USA

Printed in the United States of America
02 03 04 05 5 4 3 2 1

Library of Congress Cataloging-in-Publication Data

A physician's guide to health care management/edited by Daniel M. Albert.
    p. ; cm.
  ISBN 0-632-04581-7 (pbk.)
    1. Medicine—Practice.   2. Managed care plans (Medical care)—United States.   3. Medical care—United States.
    [DNLM: 1. Delivery of Health Care—organization & administration—United States.   2. Managed Care
Programs—economics—United States.   3. Practice Management—United States. W 84 AA1 P4995 2002]
  I. Albert, Daniel M.
  R728. P496 2002
  362.1'068—dc21   2001003057

Contents

v

List of Contributors

Daniel M. Albert, MD, MS
Professor and Chairman, Department of
    Ophthalmology and Visual Sciences
University of Wisconsin Medical School
Madison, WI

Michael E. Bernstein, JD
Senior Vice President
United Wisconsin Services, Inc.
Milwaukee, WI

Lawton R. Burns, PhD, MBA
Professor of Health Care Systems and
    Management
University of Pennsylvania, PA

Mark A. Covaleski, PhD, CPA
School of Business
University of Wisconsin, Madison, WI

Karen J. Cruickshanks, PhD
Department of Ophthalmology and Visual
    Sciences
Department of Preventive Medicine
University of Wisconsin, Madison, WI

James E. Davis, MD, MS
Department of Family Medicine
University of Wisconsin, Madison, WI

David L. DeMets
Department of Biostatistics and Medical
    Informatics
University of Wisconsin, Madison, WI

Gordon Derzon, BA, MHA
University of Wisconsin and Clinical Hospital
    Superintendent Emeritus
Clinical Professor, Department of Preventive
    Medicine
University of Wisconsin, Madison, WI

Esther R. Dyer, DLS
Executive Director
American-Italian Cancer Foundation

Alan C. Filley, PhD
Professor Emeritus, Department of Management
    and Human Resources
University of Wisconsin, Madison, WI

Marian R. Fisher, PhD
Department of Biostatistics and Informatics
University of Wisconsin, Madison, WI

Richard Friedman, MD
Vice President, Medical Affairs
Queen's Medical Center
Honolulu, HI

Dennis G. Fryback, PhD
Professor of Population Health Sciences and
    Industrial Engineering
University of Wisconsin, Madison, WI

Louis Gapenski, PhD
Department of Health Services Administration
University of Florida, FL

Charles C. Lobeck, MD
Professor Emeritus of Pediatrics and Preventive
    Medicine
University of Wisconsin, Madison Medical
    School, Madison, WI

Timothy D. McBride, PhD
Associate Professor of Economics, Public Policy,
    and Gerontology
University of Missouri, St Louis, MO

Monte D. Mills, MD
The Children's Hospital of Philadelphia and
    University of Pennsylvania
Department of Ophthalmology, PA

Larry E. Pate, PhD
Visiting Professor of Management and Human
  Resources
University of Illinois, Urbana-Champaign, IL

Bruce E. Spivey, MD
Clinical Professor of Ophthalmology
Cornell and Columbia Universities, NY

Burton Wagner, MAB, JD
Health Care Department
Reinhart, Boerner, Van Deuren, Norris, and
  Rieselbach, SC
Madison, WI

Elizabeth M. Zaher, BSN, MS
Vice President of Marketing
University of Wisconsin Medical Foundation
Madison, WI

David R. Zimmerman, PhD
Professor of Industrial Engineering
Director of the Center for Health Systems
  Research and Analysis
University of Wisconsin, Madison, WI

Foreword

It is an honor for me to introduce this timely, unique book that adds significantly to medical practice literature and to the extraordinary publication record of Dr Daniel Albert. The uniqueness of this contribution stems from the integrated, comprehensive treatment of the topic, and from the collection of authors who wrote their chapters as an extension of their graduate studies in health management. The cohesiveness of the book reflects the well organized leadership of Dr Albert and his dedication to bringing information on the business of medicine into a form comprehensible to medical students, residents, and fellows. In commenting on the book, I would like to offer my personal perspectives first and then describe the contents and how the knowledge herein can be used by an emerging generation of physicians in need of this knowledge.

"Good medicine and good business don't always mix," said my father to me on many occasions when I had the pleasure of accompanying him as he practiced general medicine in St Louis and made hospital rounds and house calls on Sundays. This experienced and very successful primary care practitioner frequently emphasized the difficulty of mixing these two aspects of his professional life because of his health care convictions and his limited knowledge of the world of business. Indeed, Dr Robert J. Farrell was similar to most general practitioners of 1933–76 in that he cared for patients who paid his fee for service with cash or a variety of payment-in-kind methods (e.g., food, household work, etc.). It wasn't until 1965, when Medicare appeared, that he really needed business acumen. As with most doctors, however, he had to learn business practices on the job as he struggled with third-party payor mechanisms. In fact, he seemed reluctant to accept Medicare until the financial advantages became evident. He would have benefited greatly from Dr Albert's book. Indeed, the third generation of physicians in the Farrell family (my son Michael) emphasized upon reading the manuscript that "times have changed . . . with the expansion of managed care, an entire generation (or two) of physicians have grown up with little or no business acumen." Having been exposed to both generations, I think it is remarkable that the medical profession has experienced a 180 degree shift and changed so profoundly in only a quarter-century.

Consequently, it seems ideal that this book begins with a description of the "Forces Shaping Health Care Delivery." The chapter by Monte Mills sets the stage for understanding the emergence of managed care as a force that overcame many other forces. Section One also provides the economic and political context that has shaped the current delivery systems. I particularly enjoyed the recommendations of Bruce Spivey and Esther Dyer on the role of the individual physician as an advocate. Their philosophy is similar to mine [1], but as my son said, "the tradition has been that the medical community leaves activism/advocacy to groups such as the AMA, all the while bemoaning the situation or ignoring it at its own (and our) peril." I believe that the opportunities for advocacy and methods for achieving success ("avenues"[1]) are so well delineated that every physician should be committed to serving this role whenever appropriate for both individuals and populations of patients. In the 21st century, nothing less is needed to deal effectively with the challenges of managed care and preventive medicine.

Section Two, on "Physician Management Skills," is superb. All practising physicians are managers—whether they want to admit it or not. David Zimmerman's chapter emphasizes the value of human resource management. He is correct in his simple but profound statement that "the ultimate human resource goal is *retention*" because "the costs of staff turnover...are often underestimated." This section also describes the added value of strategic management and appropriate personal behavior. One of my mentors, Charles Lobeck, summarizes the ABCs of managerial conduct and warns us all that "perhaps being a physician desensitizes executives to the need for professional behavior."

Section Three provides an excellent description of health care economics, particularly as related to managed care. Mark Covaleski's chapter is the core element of *A Physician's Guide to Health Care Management*. His fundamental, lucid description of "Health Care Accounting and Finance" is the most concisely informative communication I've read on this topic. It is a "must read" component for medical students and residents, as well as for practicing physicians who want to be enlightened. The next section discusses scientific, ethical and legal aspects of medical practice. Tracing the evolution of Western medicine, Dan Albert's chapter, "Medical Ethics," captures history and destiny very effectively as he describes "The Transition from Individual to Population Medicine." As a new kind of duty emerges for each physician to function in part as a "resource allocator," a responsibility for "dual stewardship" [2] forces attention to evidence-based medicine that is in the best interest of our patients. This consideration *per se* rationalizes the scope of *A Physician's Guide to Health Care Management*. Indeed, the "dual stewardship" arguments of Brendan Minogue [2] provide a strong impetus for readers to learn well the business practices needed to complement medical practice activities so that they can fulfill the duty Minogue emphasizes to "balance the interests and wishes of the patient with the welfare of the health care system."

Dr Albert will find it gratifying to know that this book—the 21st in his career, in addition to over 500 original articles—has succeeded in filling a void. His graduate training in health management, leading recently to a M.S. degree, has been translated very effectively into a book that also reflects Dan's passion for enhancing patient care. It could certainly make a difference for the next generation of physicians as they strive to overcome the deficiencies of the past and accept the "dual stewardship" duty of the new millennium.

In closing I must say, despite my father's warning, that this book convinced me that good medicine and good business can, and should, mix well. Congratulations, Dan, on a job well done.

Philip M. Farrell, MD, PhD
Alfred Dorrance Daniels Professor
on Diseases of Children
Dean, University of Wisconsin Medical School
Vice Chancellor for Medical Affairs

1. Farrell PM. Avenues for child advocacy. *The Pharos of Alpha Omega Alpha* 1997; **61**: 38–42.
2. Minogue B. The two fundamental duties of the physician. *Acad Med* 2000; **75**: 431–42.

Preface

It is the goal of every medical student, resident, and fellow to complete the formal medical training and to launch his or her medical career as a competent physician. Each has been thoroughly trained to listen, question, examine, think, diagnose, and treat—and to carry out all of these functions by drawing on a broad base of knowledge and experience. As their practice commences, it comes as a shock to many, however, to find that the effectiveness of individual physicians is dependent on the health care system in which they work.

The American health care system is in a state of flux without precedent in our history. The reasons for this are multiple and complex. They include:

- New and expensive medical technologies
- Restructured contractual arrangements between patients and doctors
- The altered relationships between doctors and hospitals
- Cost shifting to pay for care rendered to patients
- New demographics as our population ages
- High patient expectations for a long and healthy life
- A wide range of regulatory interventions in the health market
- A hostile legal environment which has led to defensive medicine
- Mounting administrative costs related to delivery of care
- An emphasis on efficiencies and quality of care by managed-care organizations.

This is only a partial list of the stresses related to managing the triad of quality care, access to care, and cost of care. To deal effectively with these complexities physicians must be knowledgeable in matters outside the traditional clinical realm. The physician entering practice must be well-informed in areas such as cost containment, health care delivery management, patient satisfaction, reimbursement, compliance, health law, and ethics.

It is our goal to have *A Physician's Guide to Health Care Management* serve as a primer for medical students and house staff who will shortly need to meet the challenges of a changing health care market. The book provides practical advice and information necessary to understand the complex aspects of current medical care. This book will also be useful to more senior physicians who are faced with the same challenges.

A Physician's Guide to Health Care Management is divided into four sections. This first deals with the forces shaping health care delivery, and explains how we have arrived at the present juncture. The second section provides information regarding basic physician-management skills. This is followed by a consideration of the economic aspects of managed care. The concluding section addresses the medical, scientific, and legal considerations in health care delivery.

This work draws its inspiration from the nonresident Masters Program in Health Administration at the University of Wisconsin-Madison. Many of the authors of the ensuing chapters are from the faculty of that outstanding program. They are augmented by selected experts and leaders in the field from other institutions and organizations. The editor is greatly indebted to these authors for recognizing the need for *A Physician's Guide to Health Care Management* and generously giving their time and talent to this effort. Their acceptance of the editing necessary to keep this book concise and affordable is appreciated. Michelle Chizek managed the manuscript, oversaw communications among all contributors, and coordinated the final editorial changes. Kevin Campbell assisted with the editing. Jim Krosschell, Chris Davis, and Laura DeYoung at Blackwell Science provided the necessary support on the part of the publisher to make this book a reality. I thank our Dean, Philip Farrell, MD, PhD and his son Michael Farrell, MD for their careful reading of the manuscript and the gracious introduction. As always my wife, Eleanor Albert, remains my best and most exacting editor.

Daniel M. Albert

Notice: The indications and dosages of all drugs in this book have been recommended in the medical literature and conform to the practices of the general community. The medications described do not necessarily have specific approval by the Food and Drug Administration (FDA) for use in the diseases and dosages for which they are recommended. The package insert for each drug should be consulted for use and dosage as approved by the FDA. As standards for usage change, it is advisable to keep abreast of revised recommendations, particularly those concerning new drugs.

1

Historical Aspects of Managed Care

Monte D. Mills

Managed care is the systematic coordination and control of the use of health care services, in order to contain health costs, improve quality, or both [1]. In the context of today's health care delivery system, managed care includes both the organizations designed to provide this care and the techniques used to manage health care delivery and control costs.

Propelled by the demands of payers (primarily government and employers) for accountability and cost controls in health care [2–5], the percentage of workers in private companies who are enrolled in some form of managed care program increased from less than 30% in 1988 to 70% in 1995 [2,6], and it was expected to exceed 80% in 2000 [7]. To many physicians and other health providers, managed care appears to be a recent phenomenon, without historic precedent. Despite their recent rapid evolution, however, managed care organizations and techniques originated decades ago.

History and Development of Managed Care Organizations

Physician Groups, Prepaid Physician Services, and Staff Model HMOs

Through the early twentieth century, physician practice was dominated by independent practitioners and small partnerships, financed directly by patients' fees. There were few restrictions on prices or quality, and both varied widely. State licensing requirements were varied and poorly enforced, and proprietary medical schools awarded medical degrees with the most mar-

ginal training. It was not until after the Flexner report described the poor state of medical training in 1910 that a degree from a medical school became a uniform requirement for licensure in most states [8].

Despite the predominance of independent, fee-for-service practice at that time, some forms of group practice and prepayments for medical services existed. Railroads, mining companies, steel mills, and the military were among the large organizations that had physicians on contract to provide services to employees. Social organizations, such as mutual benefit societies, unions, and fraternal organizations, also occasionally had contracted arrangements with physicians to provide services to members [9–12]. These contractual, prepaid arrangements were denounced as unethical by the American Medical Association (AMA) as early as 1907, and were never widely used [8].

Some of the earliest large-group physician practices involved in prepaid service contracts included the Western Clinic in Tacoma, Washington, the Bridge Clinic in Washington and Oregon, and the Ross-Loos Clinic in Los Angeles. At the Western Clinic, employers (large lumber operations) paid 50 cents per member per month for physician services [13]. Services were later extended to employees' families as well. The Ross-Loos Clinic developed a prepaid, contracted service for employees of the Los Angeles Water Department in the 1920s [11].

Unlike the earlier prepaid programs run by clinics that accepted both fee-based and prepaid patients, the Group Health Association in Washington, DC and the Kaiser Permanente Clinics

1

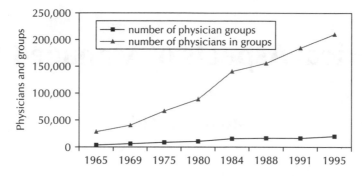

Figure 1-1. Number of physicians in group practice and number of groups, 1965–95. (Modified from Havlicek PL. *Medical Groups in the US: A survey of practice characteristics.* Chicago: American Medical Association, 1996: 45, Chapter 8, Table 8.1.)

in California were founded in the late 1930s to provide exclusively prepaid physician services to members on the basis of a capitation fee. Kaiser-Permanente developed to serve the employees and dependents of the Kaiser construction and shipbuilding organizations. Group Health Association was an offspring of a mortgage insurer, which recognized health care expenses as a cause of mortgage foreclosures. Individuals rather than employers paid monthly membership fees [11,14,15].

The term "health maintenance organization" (HMO) was first used to describe these prepaid medical plans in the 1970s. It was not until the Health Maintenance Organization Act of 1973, which gave financial incentives to the development of this type of physician group, that the model became widespread. The rapid growth of HMOs after 1973 has paralleled the integration of physicians into group practices (Figs 1-1 and 1-2). Currently, the term "HMO" describes both physician groups that directly accept risk contracts (usually capitation) for patient care and insurers and other organizations who contract with providers on a similar basis. Although the original HMO provider model was the group practice staff model, network, independent practice association (IPA), and mixed-model HMOs are currently more common (Fig. 1-3). About 25% of individuals with health insurance in the US are HMO members (Fig. 1-4). In the late 1990s, about 25% of individuals with health insurance in the US are HMO members [7].

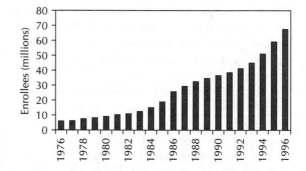

Figure 1-2. Health maintenance organization enrollees, 1976–96. (Modified from American Association of Health Plans, www.aahp.org)

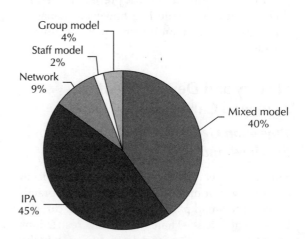

Figure 1-3. Health maintenance organization by plan type. (Modified from American Association of Health Plans, Managed Care Facts January 1998, www.aahp.org)

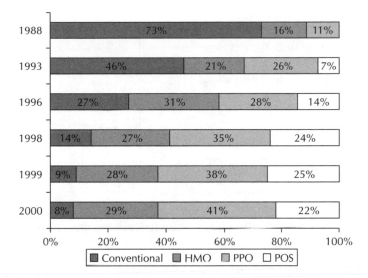

Figure 1-4. Health plan enrollment for covered workers, by plan type, 1988–2000. (From Employee Health Benefits 2000 Annual Survey. Henry J. Kaiser Family Foundation [Menlo Park, CA] and Health Research and Educational Trust [Chicago, IL], Exhibit 6.1, 2000: 81. This information was reprinted with permission of the Henry J Kaiser Family Foundation of Menlo Park, California. The Kaiser Family Foundation is an independent health care philanthropy and is not associated with Kaiser-Permanente or Kaiser Industries.)

Network and IPA Model HMOs

An IPA is a group of physicians who contract collectively for managed care patients, while practicing independently. This physician organization type traces its origin to 1954, when the San Joaquin County Medical Society in California formed a group as a foundation, partly in response to competition from Kaiser [13]. It negotiated contracts on behalf of the physicians, accepted risk for the health care services, and provided quality-of-care management. Physician members continued to operate their own practices independently. The San Joaquin Medical Foundation was the first IPA model HMO, a structure that was copied by medical societies and other physician groups across the US [16].

The network model HMO was pioneered by the Health Insurance Plan of the greater New York City area (HIP), in the 1940s, as a health insurance provider for the employees of New York City. Rather than employing physicians, HIP contracted with providers on a capitation basis, passing the risk for health services on to the physicians. The network model HMO has been reproduced widely by both for-profit and not-for-profit insurers throughout the country [12].

Preferred Provider Organizations

Groups of independent physicians, sometimes in collaboration with hospitals and other providers, have organized to offer discounted services on a fee-for-service basis in preferred provider organizations (PPOs). Similar to an IPA model HMO, a PPO negotiates and contracts on behalf of multiple independent practitioners. Unlike an HMO, a PPO does not accept risk for health services, and physicians are usually reimbursed on a discounted fee-for-service basis, although other managed-care strategies such as utilization management are often used. This organizational structure originated in the 1970s, and it is currently the most common type of managed care.

Insurance for Physician and Hospital Services

Despite the existence of managed-care organizations, indemnity (fee for service) health insurance developed rapidly in the post-Second World War period to become the dominant form of health insurance in the US. Separate from the development of prepaid group practices, and partly in reaction to it, groups of independent physicians organized to offer insurance for their services in the 1930s and 1940s. In 1939, the California Medical Society organized California Physician Services, which evolved into the Blue Shield physician insurance [17]. Unlike the prepaid groups and HMOs, Blue Shield and other "traditional" indemnity health insurers reimburse members or pay providers directly on a fee-for-service basis, without limitations on providers or utilization. By the 1950s, indemnity was the predominant form of medical coverage in the US [8].

Over time, the utilization control techniques of managed care, including utilization review, disease management programs, and other cost control mechanisms, have been applied to indemnity programs. Few "pure" indemnity insurance programs without any utilization or cost-controlling mechanisms remain.

Early Health Care Reform and the Expansion of HMOs

In the 1970s, a surge in health care inflation (see Fig. 1-3) led to growing interest in prepaid health plans. The Health Maintenance Act of 1973, amended in 1976, created incentives for the formation of HMOs and provided federal grants and loans, and it prompted steady growth in the number and size of managed-care organizations. Between 1970 and the mid-1980s, HMO enrollment quadrupled [18]. This growth continued into the 1990s (see Fig. 1-2), with 67.5 million enrollees in HMOs in 1997.

The two largest government health insurance programs, Medicare and Medicaid, also developed managed-care programs to contain costs. In 1983, Medicare began paying hospitals prospectively based on diagnosis, followed in 1992 by a reform of physician payments using a resource-based relative value scale. The number of Medicare beneficiaries enrolled in HMOs more than doubled from 1992 to 1997, with more than 15% of program members using HMOs (Figs 1-5 & 1-6). Medicaid had similar growth in

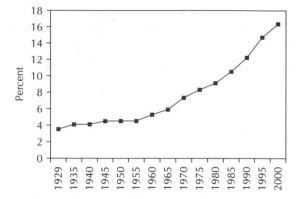

Figure 1-5. Percentage gross domestic product spent on health care, 1929–2000. (Modified from Folland S, Goodman AC, Stano M. *The Economics of Health and Healthcare*, 2nd edn. Upper Saddle River, NJ: Prentice Hall, 1997: 3. Reprinted by permission of Prentice-Hall, Inc., Upper Saddle River, NJ.)

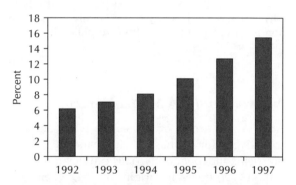

Figure 1-6. Proportion of Medicare beneficiaries in managed care plans, 1992–97 (as a percentage). (Adapted from American Association of Healthplans, Managed Care Facts January 1998, www.aahp.org)

managed care with two-thirds of all recipients in an HMO, PPO, or other managed-care program [18].

The History of Managed Care Strategies and Techniques

In addition to institutional structure, managed care includes strategies and techniques to control costs. These include limiting payments to providers and restricting patients' access to providers, influencing clinical decisions through utilization management and quality assurance, and shifting financial risks from payers and insurers to providers.

Reimbursement of Providers and Shifting Financial Risks

Under traditional fee-for-service, providers are paid for services, with all risks for financial losses borne by the insurer. Physicians have no incentive to reduce costs; in fact, they have the financial incentive to increase services.

Most forms of managed care shift financial risk to the providers and offer incentives to the providers to reduce costs. In the staff model HMO, physicians are paid by salary or other mechanism that is not linked to utilization of services. In this way, managed-care organizations avoid giving physicians incentives to increase utilization. Increasing the integration of providers with the insurance function has also been used to align the financial incentives of physicians with those of the managed-care organization. IPA and network model HMOs achieve this by paying providers per individual covered (capitation) or by setting aside a "withhold" to cover excess medical losses.

Channeling Patients and Access Controls

Under traditional indemnity insurance, patients are free to see any provider. Managed-care organizations channel patients to a limited number of providers, either exclusively (closed-panel HMO) or through a system of financial and logistical barriers (PPO, point of service [POS, etc.]). Patients agree in advance to a limited choice of providers in exchange for reduced costs, expanded coverage, or both.

Providers under managed-care agreements accept reduced payment (discounted fee-for-service) or financial risks (capitation and withholds) in exchange for the preferential channeling of patients into their practice. Providers usually also agree in advance to limitations in covered service and to utilization controls. Managed-care organizations select providers on the basis of alignment with the cost and quality goals of

the organization. They try to exclude high-cost providers.

Management of Clinical Decisions: Utilization Management, Health Promotion and Preventive Services, and Disease Management

Under traditional fee-for-service health care, patients and providers make clinical decisions without influence by payers or insurers. Providers have no financial incentive to reduce costs or restrict services. Managed-care organizations review member services to determine whether they are medically necessary and delivered at an appropriate level and cost. This is called utilization management.

Utilization management is ubiquitous today, although it was not a part of most indemnity health insurance plans until the 1970s. Indemnity insurers first developed precertification of admissions and procedures, concurrent review of hospitalizations, and case management, and limited the use of high-cost health services [12]. These techniques are now almost synonymous with managed care.

Fee-for-service insurance provided no incentive to patients or providers for preventive health care services. Innovative managed-care organizations have developed strategies to provide health screening, preventive services, and other wellness programs. As the organization is at risk for services needed by members, any strategy to avoid illness and reduce the use of services members will help control costs. These activities were a major argument in support of the HMO Act of 1973.

Unfortunately, few health-promotion activities have rapid, measurable effects on the use of services. The tendency of members to change plans, and the costs and complexity of preventive services have limited the effectiveness of this strategy, although it remains a part of most managed-care plans.

HMOs and other managed-care organizations have also developed preferred patterns for the treatment of common conditions. Lower costs, improved quality, and increased efficiency are the goals of the predetermined care paradigms generated by these organizations for frequent and chronic diseases.

Conclusions

Managed-care systems have become the dominant form of health care financing in the US over the last decade in response to payers' demands for cost containment. Despite this relatively recent shift away from fee for service, the organizations and techniques of managed care have evolved gradually over the past century. Market-driven health care reform, along with the reform of government health care programs and legislative changes, are the primary forces responsible for this transformation of the US health care finance and delivery system.

References

1. Fox PD. An overview of managed care. In: Kongstvedt PR, ed. *The Managed Health Care Handbook*, 3rd edn. Gaithersburg, MD: Aspen Publishers, 1996: 4–5.
2. Consumerism in health care new voices. Washington, DC: KPMG. January 1998: www.us.kpmg.com/ps/hcls/publications/ Accessed 1/28/00.
3. Bodenheimer T, Sullivan K. How large employers are shaping the health care marketplace, Part 1. *N Engl J Med* 1998; **338**: 1003–7.
4. Bodenheimer T, Sullivan K. How large employers are shaping the health care marketplace, Part 2. *N Engl J Med* 1998; **338**: 1084–7.
5. Roth BE. The current health care environment and stages of market development. *Gastroenterol Clin North Am* 1997; **26**: 715–25.
6. Frakes JT. Managed care. Evolution and distinguishing features. *Gastroenterol Clin North Am* 1997; **26**: 703–14.
7. Health Insurance Association of America. *The Source book of Health Insurance Data*. Washington, DC: Health Insurance Association of America, 1999.
8. Starr P. *The Social Transformation of American Medicine*. New York: Perseus Books, 1982.
9. Burnstein SS. Prepaid health care in the United States. *Illinois Med J* 1981; **160**(2): 83–5.
10. Kearney PR, Engh CA. History of the American health care system: Its cost control programs and incremental reform. *Orthopedics* 1997; **20**: 237–47.
11. O'Connor K. Pioneers in patient care. *Healthplan* 1997; **38**(3): 70–5.
12. Shapiro S. An historical perspective on the roots of managed care. *Curr Opin Pediatr* 1996; **8**: 159–663.
13. Mayer TR, Mayer GG. HMOs: Origins and development. *N Engl J Med* 1985; **312**: 590–4.
14. Fawley IL. A historical perspective on health reform. *Medical Group Management Journal* 1992; **39**(2): 44–9.
15. Mayer TR, Mayer GG. HMOs: Origins and development. *Topics Health Record Management* 1986; **6**(4): 5–12.
16. Fox PD. An overview of managed care. In: Kongstvedt PR, ed. *The Managed Health Care Handbook*, 3rd edn. Gaithersburg, MD: Aspen Publishers, 1996: 5.
17. Raffel MW, Raffel NK. *The US Health System. Origins and Functions*, 3rd edn. New York: John Wiley & Sons, 1989.
18. American Association of Health Plans. *Number of People Enrolled in HMOs, 1976–96*. Washington DC: American Association of Health Plans (www.aahp.org) accessed 1/28/00.

2

Changing Health Care Economics: The Impact of Managed Care on Academic Medical Centers

Gordon Derzon

Over the past decade, extraordinarily rapid changes have occurred in health care economics, presenting a significant challenge to academic medical centers. The challenge is to adapt to these changes and continue to provide excellence in the delivery of health care, education and research—the three missions embraced by the 118 academic medical centers in the US. These organizations typically include a medical school, several other health disciplinary schools such as nursing and pharmacy, and a teaching and research hospital.

Academic medical centers have expanded dramatically over the past 50 years, largely as a result of increasing university support, significant federal research funding, and the availability of clinical revenues. Government support increased exponentially in the 1960s with the inception of the federally funded Medicare and Medicaid programs. Academic medical centers have both contributed and gained from the enormous scientific and technology advances that have fueled additional governmental and private support for biomedical research. These gains have led to significant cost reductions in some areas of medical care and significant cost increases in others.

Over the 30 years of somewhat uncontrolled growth, expansion occurred with relatively little regard or concern for costs. Reimbursement for the most part was based on charges and governmental reimbursement took into consideration the significant costs of education. Very little premium was placed on cost containment, and extensive care was provided on an inpatient basis. Education for health professionals was geared to the inpatient setting.

The funding of academic medical centers has changed significantly over the past 30 years. In 1970, research revenues to medical schools were twice the amount of patient revenues. Now, revenues generated by faculty for professional services are two and a half times greater than research revenues. At least 30% of clinical income is "contributed" to defray the costs of educational activities within the academic medical center. There has been significant overall growth of the health care workforce, especially in the number of physician subspecialists within academic medical centers. In fact, medical school faculty personnel increased by 50,000 from 1970 to 1992 whereas the number of medical students grew by just 10,000.

Academic medical centers face major new challenges. Profound economic pressures from employers and government to contain costs have significantly affected medical practice. Academic medical centers are being challenged to preserve their critical elements in an economy that has largely changed course. This new market-driven environment needs to be cost competitive and accessible, having high service standards, effectively assuming and managing financial risk for all segments of the payer market, and providing innovative service design as a result of the clinical research and teaching that is at the heart of the academic medical center.

The growth in managed care, which was gradual through most of the 1970s and 1980s, accelerated during the 1990s. A very rapid shift from traditional indemnity plans to health maintenance organizations (HMOs) has taken place in both large and small businesses. The proportion of employees in large firms enrolled in managed-care plans grew from 5% in 1984 to 50% in 1993. Similarly, in firms employing fewer than 50 workers, it grew from 22% in 1993 to 69% in 1995. By 1998, only 14% of employees in large firms (over 200 employees) were enrolled in conventional plans [1].

Much of this growth could be attributed to large employers providing financial incentives to employees selecting the managed care option. These incentives generally provided for full employer payment or minimal employee funding of comprehensive health benefits. In Wisconsin, for example, the state covered the full cost of health insurance for state employees enrolling in HMOs as opposed to a significant required co-payment by employees who wished to continue traditional indemnity coverage. Within 2 years, over 90% of all state employees converted from indemnity to HMO coverage.

Health care cost growth slowed during the late 1980s and 1990s. It is not clear whether the growth of HMOs influenced this trend. In many cases, employers offering HMOs have lower premiums, but in others HMO premiums are not significantly lower than other insurance premiums. New reimbursement arrangements at the federal and state government levels have had a definite impact on containing health care cost increases. The traditional HMO concept of limiting provider options and choice of providers has created significant backlash. Consequently, HMO point-of-service plans that provide employees freedom to choose their providers are experiencing the greatest growth increases. They generally require an additional premium, and from the employee's perspective are very similar to indemnity plans because they permit individuals to select their own providers.

Academic medical centers have been forced to accept new reimbursement arrangements resulting from managed care, and they have done so with mixed success. Initially, a number of institutions developed their own HMOs. Others entered into contracts with established insurance plans, and some developed joint venture arrangements. Several decided that there was no need to accommodate new reimbursement arrangements, and they have suffered the consequences of that decision. The level and rapidity of managed care penetration varied greatly throughout the country, as did responses from academic medical centers.

Most academic medical centers were unprepared and not properly organized to respond to the profound and extremely rapid changes. Many were and still are burdened with cumbersome decision-making and inadequate internal communication processes. Medical schools and their teaching hospitals have been traditionally inward and departmentally focused, and have not been organized to function as fully integrated health care systems [1].

The clinical departments are generally very autonomous. Departmental practice plans with their own financial structures, compensation plans, and decision-making processes generally focus on maintaining the department's fiscal and academic viability. In this context, funds are allocated within departments to support research and departmental overhead. There is also in most instances a "dean's tax" that is forwarded to the medical school dean for the overall support of the medical school.

This financial structure contrasts greatly with the fully integrated clinical enterprise, in which the clinical departments and hospital collectively pool and allocate funds with the overall objective of delivering high-quality care in the most efficient manner. Each academic medical center has been faced with the challenge of the transition from the traditional departmental structure into the integrated clinical enterprise, while at the same time maintaining departmental education and research excellence. Success has varied greatly as our academic medical centers struggle to integrate clinically, thereby more effectively positioning themselves to compete successfully in the new environment where a premium is placed on price, accessibility, quality, and assumption of financial risk.

A further challenge to academic medical centers is that they are generally burdened by higher costs as a result of their serving large numbers of medically indigent patients, providing both a higher acuity level of care and significant financial support to the academic enterprise. These factors have traditionally been recognized by Medicare and to a limited extent by Medicaid. However, managed-care insurers for the most part have not been willing to reimburse academic medical centers at higher levels.

With governmental and managed-care reimbursement strongly influencing reduced inpatient stays, academic medical centers have been forced to shift a much greater portion of clinical activities into ambulatory care settings. This has required major program modifications and in many instances major capital expenditures, because historically most academic medical centers had somewhat limited ambulatory care capabilities. In some instances, the location of academic medical centers created major logistical problems for patient access.

Academic medical centers, with their major focus on high-tech tertiary care, have had to allocate substantial new financial resources to the development and ongoing operation of primary care programs. Some have recruited new faculty, whereas others have acquired, or affiliated with, established practices. This has proven to be a major additional expense and in most cases has required substantial continuing subsidization. The sources of these subsidies—the higher revenue-generating clinical departments and the hospitals—have not all adapted to this new funding requirement, thereby creating significant levels of tension and discomfort in most academic medical centers. The blending of cultures traditionally focused on the provision of highly specialized tertiary care with that of primary care providers, who increasingly control the flow of referrals to specialists, has been very difficult.

Transferring major components of teaching to the ambulatory settings has created further difficulties. Clinical productivity in the ambulatory setting decreases as practitioners spend time teaching trainees. Those objectives espoused by supporters of managed care—namely, development of treatment protocols, patient education, prevention, and problem-based learning—are all of great virtue. However, they also require an educational time commitment that must be funded. This funding has not been forthcoming from health maintenance plans, all of which have been faced with serious price competition and have not been willing to support educational costs.

Pitfalls Encountered in Rapidly Changing Reimbursement Mechanisms

With the major shifts in reimbursement from indemnity plans in which usual and customary charges were the determinant of reimbursement to the negotiated reimbursement arrangements between managed-care insurers or self-insured employers, academic medical centers have had to develop the ability to negotiate effectively on their own behalf. This has stimulated most academic medical centers to reorganize their individual departmental practice plans into an integrated group practice, which would then be in a position to represent the entire faculty physician group. Taking it one step further, a number of centers integrated their practice plans with their hospitals and, in some instances, other care venues such as home health providers. The newly developed contracting function forced providers to develop accurate cost information that could be used as a basis for determining acceptable reimbursement. It also required them to determine equitable formulas for the distribution of revenues emanating from managed-care contracts.

In the late 1980s and throughout the 1990s, most academic medical centers negotiated contracts in which they accepted payments from health plans that were lower than their actual costs. The concept of marginal pricing—establishing pricing below total costs but above variable costs—has been embraced in the health care industry, where considerable under-utilized capacity exists. It is assumed that incremental clinical activity will generate additional revenue that will partially offset fixed costs and improve financial performance.

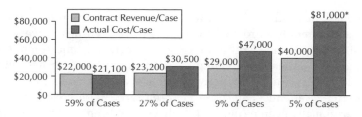

Figure 2-1. Risks associated with prospective payment "bump hunting." When to say "no." The graph shows contract revenue versus actual cost per commercial coronary artery bypass graft (CABG)[†]. (From University Health Consortium. The 10 highest-cost cases generated a total loss of $400,000. [*]Highest cost case: $134,000. [†]Data from actual contracts, midwest member.)

This assumption works only if volumes actually do increase and if the amount of revenue that exceeds variable costs is sufficient to cover fixed costs. Competitive marketplace pressures throughout the country placed academic medical centers in the untenable position of agreeing to contracts that would not deliver desired results, but would retain and it is hoped increase clinical volumes in order to make fuller use of excess capacity while reducing unit costs. As costs increased as a result of the introduction of new technology and inflationary increases in variable costs, excess capacity continued to provide managed-care organizations with enough leverage to threaten academic medical centers with nonrenewal of contracts.

Academic medical centers attract a large percentage of the most acutely ill patients. This factor must be taken into consideration when negotiating contracts. A 1999 study conducted by the University HealthSystem Consortium (UHC) illustrates the problem by noting that the costliest 5% of all cases of coronary artery bygrass grafts exceeded revenue by an average of $40,000 per case (Fig. 2-1).

Virtually identical results were noted at other centers, the cardiovascular surgery volumes in which are among the highest and the managed-care contracts of which are among the top performers in terms of per-case revenue generated. What this example illustrates is that, at a minimum, it is critically important to build adequate outlier reimbursement into future managed-care contracts.

Another predictor of higher-than-average costs is transfer of cases to academic medical centers. A recently competed analysis by the UHC highlights the greatly contrasting costs of patients admitted to university hospitals via transfers from other institutions compared with those admitted directly. It concludes the following:

- Approximately 85% of all patients transferred between hospitals are transferred to an academic health center (AHC).
- Average UHC member's transfer cases account for 11% of total discharges.
- Transfer patients cost 55% more than nontransfer patients with the same diagnosis; their case mix index is 49% higher.
- For the six highest-volume transfer diagnoses, the mortality rate for transfer patients was three to six times that of nontransfer patients who had the same diagnosis; average length of stay for transfer patients was 2.5–5.0 times that for nontransfer patients with the same diagnosis.

The increased cost of transfer cases is illustrated in Fig. 2-2. Within the six most common transfer diagnoses for the member shown, the ratios of transfer costs to nontransfer costs range from 1.5 to 4.4. Unless managed-care contracts specify otherwise, AHCs are paid identically for transfer and nontransfer cases.

The outlier factor and transfer data help to confirm that academic medical centers do indeed serve patients at higher-acuity levels. Reimbursement from managed-care organizations must take this into consideration.

To protect themselves from patient channeling by their competitors, a number of academic medical centers have taken on the responsibility for total provision of health. They have assumed

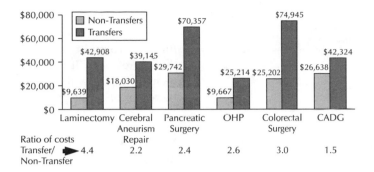
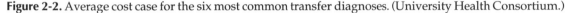

Figure 2-2. Average cost case for the six most common transfer diagnoses. (University Health Consortium.)

ownership of managed-care organizations or partnered in ways that assumed total or very significant financial risk. Instead of becoming profit centers, most of these arrangements have resulted in substantial financial losses. Some centers have successfully extricated themselves through a transfer of ownership or sale to another entity. Others, fearing substantial loss of clinical activity with its adverse educational and financial implications, have remained in the business even though, in some cases, revenue generated through their own plans is less than revenue received from other managed-care organizations.

The difficulties experienced in managed care contracting will continue. This requires academic medical centers to focus inwardly and take major initiatives to be as cost-efficient as possible without compromising access or patient care. The high degree of variability in costs among academic medical centers suggests that adaptation of "best practices" and careful internal monitoring of costs must be implemented. Organizational inefficiencies must be corrected and unnecessary expenditures eliminated. The use of high-cost services must be controlled. Pharmaceutical costs have risen dramatically, making it necessary to control the use of high-cost medications. Physicians must assume the leadership in the introduction and successful implementation of practice guidelines and protocols. Health care practitioners need to be enlisted and familiarized with the high costs of medical care. Their compensation must be correlated with their ability to care in a cost-efficient manner. This requires the introduction of productivity targets and responsibility for controlling costs through efficient

practice management and appropriate use of resources.

Future Reimbursement Trends and Implications

Two major trends evolved during the 1980s and 1990s that are anticipated to continue in the twenty-first century. These are a significant increase in the elderly population and the increase in the population aged under 65 with partial or no health insurance coverage. These trends have significant implications for academic medical centers as well as all other health care providers. The percentage of the population aged over 65 is estimated to rise from 13% of the total population in 1985 to 21% in 2030. In the 20-year period from 2010 to 2030, the portion of the population aged over 65 is expected to grow by as much as it has increased in the preceding 80 years.

As the population aged over 85 years approaches 20 million, compared with the current 3 million, health care providers will be faced with greatly increased demands. This growth in numbers of elderly people will create increased pressure to finance unavoidable health care needs for the projected 80 million Medicare recipients. It is questionable whether Medicare is currently structured to provide the projected level of financial support needed. There will continue to be inflationary cost increases. Expensive new technology and pharmaceuticals will further exacerbate the financial situation. Inevitably, health care premiums will rise at least as fast as they

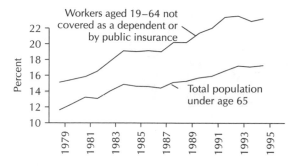

Figure 2-3. Percentage of uninsured persons, workers, and total population under age 65, 1979–95. (From Kronick R, Gilmer T. Explaining the decline in health insurance coverage, 1975–99. *Health Affairs* 1999; **18**(2): 30–47.)

have in the 1990s. There is also a good possibility that Medicare's eligibility age will be raised to 67. Employers will gradually reduce financial support for health insurance for retirees, and some may also reduce financial support for current employees. The successful implementation of new therapies and drugs may moderate current cost increases, but will over the long term increase costs, as patients who previously may not have survived their acute illnesses live for extended periods of time. They will then be burdened with long-term chronic care costs.

As the costs of health care continue to increase, fueled by the demographic changes in the population, another event is occurring that will have major impact on providers, particularly academic health centers that serve a disproportionate share of the medically indigent population. The percentage of uninsured workers between the ages of 19 and 64 rose from 15.1% in 1979 to 23.5% in 1995, and it is expected to continue to increase (Fig. 2-3).

An explanation for this phenomenon is that as health care per capita spending increased more rapidly than income per capita, the percentage of workers not provided with health insurance increased. This disparity is expected to continue. An ever-increasing percentage of the under-65 population will not have health insurance. This can be avoided only through a combination of increased employer and government contributions. At this time, when the economy is

as strong as it ever has been, there is substantial resistance from employers to increasing their financial commitments to health coverage for their employees. It is also unlikely that governmental support will substantially increase unless there is a concerted public effort.

Future Organization of Managed Care

In response to widespread consumer dissatisfaction, health care plans are now responding by offering more provider choice and a greater variety of benefits and options. There is considerable diversification occurring in health plans with respect to provider networks, benefits, and geographic markets. In response to consumers' demand for choice, point-of-service products are overtaking traditional plans for single-network structures. Within the network, most plans are reducing gatekeeping functions and loosening or eliminating prior authorization requirements. Health plans that previously offered one type of plan are now offering a full menu of plans such as point-of-service option, preferred provider organizations (PPOs), and Medicare HMO and supplement products. Benefit arrangements are also becoming more flexible. Deductibles and coinsurance, prevention services, inclusion or exclusion of drugs, mental health services, long-term care, and, even more recently, holistic medicine such as acupuncture and massage are now offered.

Managed-care plans are beginning to branch out. Instead of limited marketing to large employers and government entities, small employers or even individuals are now the focus of many managed-care marketing efforts.

All of these activities make it clear that managed-care organizations will continue to have a major impact on academic medical centers. They will continue to place emphasis on cost containment, access, patient satisfaction, and quality. In each of these areas, academic medical centers will be challenged to improve their performance. Many centers have begun to tackle each of these areas and have made significant progress in controlling costs. Despite progress to date, efforts must continue to be made on this front because managed-care providers facing pressure from employers will continue to favor low-cost providers, assuming that access, patient satisfaction, and quality are all satisfactory.

In the future, managed-care patients will have a larger role in choosing their own health care providers. The challenge will be to create measurable value to help patients and health care plans to make their decisions.

Reference

1. Marquis S, Long S. Trends in managed care and managed competition 1993–97. *Health Affairs* 1999; **18**(6): 75–89.

3

Managing Medicine: Health Care Politics and Policy

Bruce E. Spivey and Esther R. Dyer

Physicians are in a prime position to influence political action to the benefit of the health care delivery system. Being involved in the political process can be time-consuming, but there are ways to target your involvement to maximize your investment. Physicians are compelling advocates and their voice should be heard. Young physicians should take an interest in the political process because they will develop opportunities to be influential in a more meaningful way.

Advocacy for health care policy requires tenacity, knowledge, and participation with others. To affect the political process requires experience, contacts, and hard work, as well as timely and accurate information. This chapter is intended as a primer to introduce the young physician to involvement in health care politics and policies.

Political involvement is a long-term endeavour. Physicians may become agitated about specific legislative acts and become all consumed by them, and then they may wonder why their efforts have little effect. It is only through a continuous investment of time, energy, and money —primarily for patients and secondarily for your self-interests—that political advocacy becomes most effective. It is not easy, and generally not very productive, to work on a one-time basis. It is the long-term "care and feeding" of the political process that yields the most impact for patients and physicians.

Influencing health care politics and policy is a complex task. Yet, to leave the political arena to others, and to avoid positive advocacy simply because it is difficult and frustrating, is no reason to forsake it. The first organ transplantations, the first dialysis, and the first understanding of diabetic care were difficult and frustrating topics, and yet of critical importance to medicine. There is no way for a primer of this sort to substitute for the reality of personal involvement. This must be accompanied by a clear understanding of the issues and a consistent involvement with legislators and the legislative process.

Involvement in a political arena is like that portion of medicine in which a role model or mentor can be of immense help. Find someone you trust and respect and wish to emulate, who is active in this area, and he or she will be more than pleased to help you to become involved. It is intended to be a starting point for physicians who wish to become involved in affecting the political processes that impact their practices and their ability to provide quality care for patients, and provides a rationale for physicians to become involved.

Physicians, from the time they enter their undergraduate training through medical school and beyond, are taught to deal in a process that involves a hypothesis, research, data, and conclusions. The legislative process includes many other factors, based less on hard data than on interpretations and public opinion. Shifting coalitions, advocacy, compromise, trade-offs, personal/social relationships, history, regional interests, and tradition all may become factors in the legislative process. Physicians must be involved in the process in order to affect the outcome in a positive way. It is important to keep in mind that politics is art, not science!

At the heart of politics is the art of compromise. Compromise is the way that most contentious debates between relatively equal advocate positions balance out. In the long run, those who are viewed as being more in control are likely to lose some of that control rather than gain additional control. This phenomenon is a familiar and recurring one, particularly in health care politics. Nonphysician providers wanting to increase their scope of practice by legislative means have succeeded over time by creating and continuing an advocacy, and thus pressure on legislators to compromise. These efforts of nonphysicians have encroached on physicians' control of medical practice over a multidecade process. This type of compromise often offends physicians new to the political process.

The political neophyte is often very distraught, because experience would dictate that compromise should not occur. In politics, however, balanced, well-grounded positions do not always prevail over publicly popular, well-funded contrary arguments. Medicine may lose out to organized persistent counterforces if rational and unified arguments are not presented in a persuasive manner.

Definitions

The New Oxford Dictionary defines politics as the activities associated with the governance of a country or area, especially the debate or conflict among individuals hoping to achieve power. Health care politics are played out among professional organizations, nonprofit-making groups, and public and private sector interest groups at many different levels. The end result of the political process is legislation based on policy, which is defined as "a course of action adopted or proposed by a government, party, business or individual" (*The New Oxford Dictionary*). Influencing the political process to affect a desired outcome or stop an undesirable one is called advocacy, the process of speaking out in favor of a belief or political position to influence public support and persuade policy-makers.

The Political Process or "All Politics Is Local"

Tip O'Neill, a former Speaker of the US House of Representatives, once said: "All politics is local." To say that all politics occurs locally is a vast oversimplification, but it is true that "grassroots" advocacy is effective and that all politics is grounded locally. Each physician can have an impact. Knowing, supporting, and being in touch with legislators are critical. At the same time, it is likely that those of opposing viewpoints are similarly in touch with the same legislator.

In theory, the legislator balances the impact of proposed legislation on his or her district with its impact on the nation, state, or city, and its conformity with his or her party's platform. In fact, many legislators are concerned mainly with the interests of their constituents.

In other words, the abiding concern of most legislators is to be re-elected. National legislators have to spend an inordinate amount of time raising money. However, many things besides money count in the election process: support, visibility, and assistance in large and small ways. Physicians must contribute both time and money to their legislators, developing continuing relationships, and recruit others who can influence, contribute, or similarly support them.

The National Perspective

Although legislation is usually emphasized in the political process, two other extremely important activities deserve consideration: the annual federal budget and the regulatory actions of federal and state agencies. *Legislation* forms the framework for public policies and programs. *Regulations* must be written to implement the legislation. In addition to classic legislation and authorizing programs, which are known as authorization bills, the annual federal budget process has huge implications for health care and physicians' practices. It now establishes payment levels for physicians, hospitals, and other providers. An example is legislation known as the Balanced Budget Act of 1997. This bill, which was designed to create a check on the federal budget, had serious negative financial implications for hospitals and physicians. Some legislators admit that many of the ramifications of the legislation were unintended. An annual budget resolution brings multiple House and Senate committees into play (often in conflict) in balancing out federal spending limitations.

Regulations implementing Congressional content are developed by agencies such as the Health Care Financing Administration (HCFA), Food and Drug Administration (FDA) and state health departments. Such regulations evolve through a process that includes an opportunity for public comment. These often have immense impact on the daily practice of medicine (e.g., Medicare payment schedules for each procedure or hospital discharge), and even the approved drugs that can be used (FDA). Communication with the management and staff of these agencies is critical in the ongoing process of advocacy. Mention should also be made of the opportunity to participate on provider advisory councils at the state and local level for Medicare and Medicaid programs.

Other Public Participation Issues

Physicians have long felt they do not have a "level playing field" when it comes to negotiations with managed-care companies. Physicians in independent private practice are viewed by the Federal Trade Commission (FTC) as competitors and thus cannot jointly negotiate. Physicians who are employed (e.g., by a medical school or in a single corporation from which they receive their income) can bargain together. An independent practice association (IPA) that contains individual or small group practices cannot "bargain." It must operate on what is called the "messenger model," and thus its physicians cannot act in economic concert. During the 1990s, physicians began to explore unionization (separately or as a part of an established national union) to advance their negotiating capabilities. This movement, small at the early part of the twenty-first century, is an unknown factor in the future of physician advocacy.

Physicians, when well informed, courteous, and articulate, have stature that can create influence beyond their numbers in the political process. Physicians can have major influence with legislators and regulators. Advocacy for a particular viewpoint requires focus, constancy, and tenacity, as well as a balanced and rational presentation of the issues.

Organizational Medicine

When the issues are contentious, it may appear that "who knows whom" is often the deciding factor in victory or defeat. In actuality, influence is augmented by better arguments and greater support more than by loyal friendships. Allies are important in moving a political agenda ahead.

Knowledge of the system, organization, strength in numbers, coalitions created, persistence, and timeliness will help any political efforts. Some physicians never achieve it, and never want to. Fortunately, we have colleagues who find this process stimulating and engaging. It is important for those who are not engaged in the struggle to support our colleagues who are, and for those who are involved in advocacy to do everything possible to educate our colleagues to assist them. It is also important to become involved with the lay community in garnering support or creating coalitions to promote a legislative agenda.

Historically, the American Medical Association (AMA) has been identified by the public as an advocate for all of medicine. As medicine has become increasingly fragmented, primarily on grounds of reimbursement, the AMA appeared to advocate for one specialty over another, with the result that each specialty now has lobbying groups at the national and state level. This began in the 1970s, and was increasingly obvious because essentially every specialty society and every nonphysician group that wished a more independent practice status also developed federal and state legislative organizations. Examples include the American College of Surgery (ACS), American Society of Internal Medicine (ASIM), American College of Physicians (ACP), and the American Academy of Ophthalmology

(AAO). These national organizations have been in the forefront of analyzing and reviewing the potential impact of legislation and impending regulation on physicians' practices. Examples of nonphysician groups include the nurse midwives, the nurse practitioners, and the optometrists, among many. Many also provide advocacy training.

Advocacy is serious business and one that requires skill and commitment. The AMA operates a "Campaign School" and has committed other resources to develop physicians' advocacy skills. Many professional associations and nonprofit organizations provide advocacy training and legislative analysis.

Coalition Building

The ever-changing legislative environment provides many opportunities for physicians, their professional organizations, and others to work together for a common cause. Coalition building was a critical factor in the successful passage of the Children's Health Insurance Act. Physician groups, insurers, and nonprofit organizations worked together to pass federal legislation successfully that funded improved access to health insurance for children. The publications and websites of many organizations, such as those of the AAO, contain excellent information on federal legislation and regulations. Another example is the ACS, which through its socioeconomic affairs department tracks socioeconomic, legislative, and regulatory issues affecting the field of surgery.

There are other organizations within and related to medicine that have been important for various spheres of influence. Among these are the Association of American Medical Colleges (AAMC), the American Hospital Association (AHA), the pharmaceutical industry, the instrument manufacturers, the graduates of foreign medical schools, and the advance practice nurses and midwives. A website with information pertaining to many aspects of medicine is that of the AAMC. It provides timely access to pending legislation through the publication of *Washington Highlights*, an update on the previous week's legislative activity.

Influencing Health Care Politics and Policy: The Role of the Individual Physician

What can individuals do to advocate successfully in the political arena? Only rarely can an individual have the same impact as a coalition. It is usually the case that a thoughtfully orchestrated group effort, first with the individual legislator and then involving multiple legislators, develops a certain momentum and results in the desired type of outcome.

A consternation for reformers at all levels of health care politics is that health care policy is diffuse and often uncoordinated. It is difficult to identify what interventions will result in the desired change or lack of change. The AMA and other sophisticated physician groups are adept at mobilizing support at all levels of the spectrum of health care politics.

Physicians and lay people working together through nonprofit organizations can have a major impact on health care policy and funding. The AMA, for example, provides a basic introduction to political action for physicians through its campaign school. It is important to note that legislation is not often proposed unless need has been well established and long advocated, and many bills are introduced that never become law.

Cultivating strong relationships with new legislators can be an important strategy to maximize your influence. If you can be involved at the outset in a legislator's first campaign, and continue that involvement as he or she moves to seniority and perhaps to national office, your personal contact, the legitimacy and fairness of your arguments, and the availability and access that you can create can be an enormously powerful tool going forward. Therefore, the importance of advocacy and involvement at the state level cannot be underestimated.

State Legislative Advocacy

At the present time, the existence of multiple sources of financing for the delivery of health care services results in multiple targets of opportunity for identifying intervention strategies at various levels of government and collaboration with other organizations. Although information about specific state legislation can be found through state medical societies or directly from the legislative bodies at the state level, there are some general protocols that generally apply to the legislative process.

In general, a bill to enact a law is proposed by a legislator in committee. Many comprehensive pieces of legislation are the product of collaboration. The scope of state legislation is broad—that which affects physicians directly and deals with issues such as managed-care reform, medical malpractice, licensure, and continuing medical education requirements, Medicaid, and public health and safety. State legislators introduce bills on behalf of their constituents as well as of interest groups.

Typically, bills affecting the practice of medicine are referred to a health committee for review. A fiscal committee may also review health legislation to assess the cost aspect. Traditionally, chairs of committees are very influential, and their position is based in part on seniority and party affiliation. Committees typically decide on bills by a majority vote, often along party lines. If a committee rejects a bill, it does not normally proceed further. On the other hand, if all the committees to which it was assigned approve it, the bill is usually brought to the floor of the chamber for debate, possibly amendment and voting by the body sitting as a committee of the whole. Although a bill may be amended on the floor of a legislature, points of view are often crystallized by the time legislation leaves the committee. Thus it is preferable to exert influence as early as possible in the process. If the bill receives a majority vote in the first house, it must then proceed through much the same process in the second house (the exception is Nebraska, which has only one house). The bill can be amended or voted down at any time during this process.

The presiding officers of the committees or the chambers are key influences on a bill's outcomes. The first chamber must approve amendments from the second chamber. If the bill survives the legislative process, it is then presented to the Governor for a signature. If the Governor fails to sign the bill into law, the legislature can override that veto by a two-thirds vote of both chambers [1].

Federal Legislative Examples
Patients' Bill of Rights

The current Patients' Bill of Rights debate is instructive for physicians to consider. As managed care has become dominant in the American health care system, many individual physicians feel that they have lost control of their practices and believe that they are being dictated to by the insurance companies. Legislation touted as "patients' rights" developed in several states (Texas, New York, and California) before being pursued at a national level. Physicians and patients joined together to create a potent force at the local level and decry policies preventing patients from seeing their regular family physician. State medical societies lobbied hard and effectively to enact legislation requiring insurance companies to share accountability for making medical decisions and regulate medical practices, once the provenance only of physicians, such as how long a patient should stay in a hospital after surgery (popularly known as "drive-by deliveries" and "drive-by mastectomies").

Now the battle for patients' rights has taken center stage at the national level where the political stakes are particularly high. In addition to the specific policies, each party wants to claim the mantle of protecting patients while, at the same time, responding to their own special interests. Veterans from the states are leading the national effort on both sides and physicians are being employed in the debate as never before. In fact, physicians are one reason the debate has been as successful as it has been on the national level: physician members of Congress from the majority party have forced the leadership to address patients' rights despite resistance as a result of concerns about allowing health maintenance organizations (HMOs) to be sued.

A variety of coalitions have propelled the patients' rights movement forward. Many of the professional organizations have combined to endorse one piece of legislation, making it much more compelling, e.g., one coalition under the aegis of the National Partnership for Women and Families contains the AMA, the American Academy of Pediatricians, the American College of Obstetricians and Gynecologists, the American Lung Association, American Nurses Association, American Psychological Association, the American College of Physicians/American Society of Internal Medicine, and the American Society of Plastic and Reconstructive Surgery as participants, in addition to other members. Other coalitions such as the Patients' Access to Care coalition consist of the provider and specialty organizations focused on more narrow principles in several pieces of patients' rights legislation rather than endorsing one comprehensive piece of legislation. Although it is clear from the state actions that legislation in this area is necessary, determining federal legislation requires lengthy negotiations on issues that may not be medical at all, e.g., one ongoing debate is the Democrat's desire to have a patients' rights campaign issue and an equally strong desire on the Republican front to deny that issue by enacting some form of legislation.

Medicare Cancer Clinical Trials

Although the Patients' Bill of Rights fight has been high profile, it is likely to be the first in a series applying legislation to medical decisions. Another example of physicians influencing the legislative arena is with cancer clinical trials. Patients participating in clinical trials must pay for all routine hospital costs out of pocket because insurance companies will not pay for experimental therapies. However, in many cases new therapies often offer the best hope to patients dying of cancer. Currently, only 3% of eligible patients participate in cancer clinical trials (National Cancer Institute), in part because of the cost, delaying and slowing progress against cancer. Physicians with the Association of American Cancer Institutes (AACI) and the American Society of Clinical Oncologists (ASCO), as well as patient advisory groups such as the National Breast Cancer Coalition, are at the forefront advocating reimbursement of routine hospital costs for people participating in cancer clinical trials. As the drugs are provided by the investigator or the maker (by law, patients cannot be charged for therapies used in clinical trials),

the only associated costs are the routine ones such as blood pressure monitoring, etc. The AACI and ASCO have both published studies demonstrating the low costs of routine care and the high impact on providing reimbursement, and their scientific contribution to the cause has been extremely helpful. Maryland has passed state legislation requiring reimbursement and the issue has been introduced at the national level. There are even attempts to ensure that this issue is addressed by the patients' rights legislation.

Sources of Public Policy Information for Health Care Issues

State medical societies provide useful information about grassroots lobbying and current information on pending legislation. Much of this information is presented on their websites. Access to legislative information is readily accessible via the National Conference of State Legislatures (NCSL) website.

Although this information is interesting, and indeed helpful if the physician knows what to look for, it does not enable users easily to understand the implications of new bills for their practices or specialties. Thus, the legislative analysis undertaken by the AMA and state practitioner societies, or by specialty organizations such as the AAO, is important.

The Medical Society of the State of New York (MSSNY) has a well-developed government relations program. Its website provides information on current bills, links to the legislature, and a guide to grassroots advocacy that includes a mechanism to contact legislators. Another example of the type of information provided by state medical societies can be found in the "Government Center" on the website of the California Medical Association (CMANET). CMANET provides information on legislative priorities, bill tracking, and interaction with regulatory agencies about physician practice issues such as managed care and licensure.

In summary, at both the state and national level, there is a complex legislation process. It is based on a system of referral to Committee where the amendment process occurs in detail. It is generally too late to affect many bills—with the exception of stopping some—if they are adopted in a bipartisan committee effort. Committee chairs, both majority and minority, and their staff have a huge influence over the legislative developments in their early phases. Special energy needs to be placed in advocacy early on, because early intervention shapes policy outcomes.

After a bill is enacted, it must be implemented through funding, regulation, and administration. This is the provenance of state and federal agencies charged with writing rules and regulations to carry out these laws. The state departments of health and insurance, medical licensing boards, consumer protection, and many other state bodies can issue rules and regulations that have an impact on the practice of medicine, and potentially on the physician's ability to deliver quality patient care. Opportunities to be heard occur in the rule-making process.

Collaboration Beyond the Physician Community

It is important that physicians become involved not just with other physicians, but also with organizations that are involved in issues affecting physicians and their practices. Many national organizations have local chapters that would welcome physician participation, e.g., a pulmonary specialist can make an important contribution and gain political influence by participating in the American Lung Association (ALA). The website of the ALA is extremely well organized and provides an excellent guide to issues on the national and state levels relating to lung disease, tobacco control, and legislation. *Capitol Hill Basics* is an excellent guide to communicating and visiting Capitol Hill, as well as understanding the legislative process and decoding staff titles.

Another nonprofit organization that involves physicians, health professionals, and lay people in advocacy issues is the March of Dimes (MOD). A pediatrician or obstetrician/gynecologist would gain influence by serving on the public affairs committee of a local MOD chapter. MOD has an impressive Government Relations Office in Washington, DC. A great deal of information about legislation affecting prenatal care, health research policy, and children's health insurance, is contained on its website. Not all nonprofit health- or disease-oriented organizations are active in advocacy. Some organizations such as the Alzheimer's Association provide excellent information to access social services and research but do not emphasize advocacy or legislative efforts.

Reference

1. Adapted from *The Eye MD Advocate: A primer*, a text by the Secretariat for State Affairs of the American Academy of Ophthalmology. Based on the American Medical Association, *Representing Medicine: Developing constituent skills—Participant's handbook*, Grassroots Training Seminar, Participant's Handbook.

4

Leadership and Decision-making in Medicine

Larry E. Pate and Alan C. Filley

Guiding an organization through major change requires leadership based on moral courage, trust, respect, and service to others.
James O'Toole

Few, if any, topics have received as much attention in the management literature as leadership. When the first edition of Ralph Stogdill's long-awaited *Handbook of Leadership* was published in 1974, it contained a listing of 3000 books and articles on leadership. By 1990 with the publication of the third edition of what had become *Bass & Stogdill's Handbook of Leadership* [1], that number had grown to 7500. Conservative estimates suggest that the number has doubled to 15,000 over the past decade.

Thus, with so much written, it is perhaps not surprising for us to note at the outset that there are a number of conflicting themes concerning leadership. Perhaps this is why leadership guru Warren Bennis [2] quips that, "Leadership is like beauty; it's hard to describe, but you know it when you see it." According to leadership scholar Bernard Bass, "there are almost as many different definitions of leadership as there are persons who have attempted to define the concept" [1, p. 11]. Indeed, researchers have variously regarded leadership as:

1. a focus of group process
2. the art of inducing compliance
3. the exercise of influence
4. an act or behavior
5. a form of persuasion
6. a power relationship

7. an instrument of goal achievement
8. an emerging effect of social interaction
9. a differentiated role
10. the initiation of structure
11. some combination of elements.

Some studies [3–6] have examined the role of leadership in hospitals and health care settings. However, most such research has been from the perspective of hospital administrators or head nurses rather than physicians [7]. Studies involving physicians [6,8] have been less concerned with leadership itself, and more concerned with resource-allocation decisions made by physicians—or with the relative power of physicians, nurses, and administrative personnel.

For example, Wilson and McLaughlin [6], in a study of 26 decision-making issues within a university hospital, found that the relative influence of medical school faculty and senior administrators depended on the issue raised (e.g., selecting a dean of medicine vs financial and budgetary concerns).

The purpose of this chapter is briefly to review key points from this large body of literature on leadership, and then recommend a few useful frameworks for physicians to use when faced with critical leadership decisions. We take the contemporary position that the process of *managing* a system is quite different from the process of *leading* within that system [2,9–11], and that both of these processes are desired and necessary for effective health care systems. We also take the position that the primary challenge of leadership is not limited to the act of leading, but to doing so with integrity, moral courage, and high ethical standards [12]. Finally, we take the position that the dual processes of leadership and decision-making are inherently connected, such that the careful application of decision-making models and techniques can help physicians to make difficult leadership decisions.

To understand leadership we first need to consider its context. As observed by Warren Bennis, founding chairman of the Leadership Institute at the University of Southern California, and former President of the University of Cincinnati, "Any text without context is pretext" (W Bennis, personal communication). By this, Bennis means that the context of events is critical for understanding and interpreting those events, and that as the context changes so will our interpretation of both the events and the outcomes (see also Pate *et al.* [12]).

In the case of leadership, the primary context is the arena of the organization itself. Thus, we start with a brief overview of the literature on organizations as complex systems and discuss four key interacting components—structure, technology, tasks, and people—that define such systems. We consider the role of leadership as a critical integrating factor in the management of an organizational system. Next, we review the various historical approaches—trait, behavioral style, contingency—that have been taken by leadership researchers and theorists over the past 80 years, and we identify an emerging new frame approach. Finally, we draw primarily from the decision-making literature to suggest three simple frameworks—ACES, RAID, and SWOT (see below)—that physicians can use when faced with difficult leadership decisions.

Organizations as Complex Systems

Although leadership is clearly an essential ingredient to the smooth functioning of any organizational system (compare Bass [1] for a review), it is by no means the only factor of importance. Organizations have long been conceptualized as *systems* [13–15] that interact with their environments. Inputs (I) to a system are processed (P), transformed into outputs (O), and then returned

to the organization's environment (E), which then generates new inputs, and the cycle repeats itself. A health care system, for example, admits patients (inputs) who are diagnosed and treated by the medical staff (processed) before they are later released (outputs) to return to the local community (environment), where they may refer others to the system (new inputs).

However, not all systems are of the same variety or involve the same levels of complexity or uncertainty, as nicely delineated by Kenneth Boulding [16]. The *open systems* model—level 4 within Boulding's hierarchy of nine levels—has been used most often to characterize organizations (compare Pondy and Mitroff [15] for a review). The primary distinguishing feature of open systems thinking is the extent to which inputs are able to penetrate the boundary of the system and affect how the system operates.

A convenient illustration of systems thinking can be seen in the problem–intervention–evaluation (PIE) notes from patient charting, typical of health care systems. From the patient's perspective, the initial interaction with the patient's external environment (hospital staff) leads to a preliminary diagnosis and statement of the problem (P). The resulting intervention (I) represents new inputs to the system (patient). These new inputs are processed by the patient, resulting in new outputs to the environment (changes in behavior), which are evaluated (E) by the medical staff to determine the potential need for additional intervention. When applying the PIE note to an organizational system, one simply substitutes the organization for the individual patient—the processes remain quite similar.

The internal system of the organization contains at least four core interacting components:

1. structure
2. technology
3. tasks
4. people.

Structure as a Core System Component

The structure of an organization, defined as "how job tasks are formally divided, grouped, and coordinated" [17], can facilitate or undermine efforts to manage the system and accomplish organizational objectives.

Factors that are generally considered when management tries to design an appropriate structure include the following:

- Specialization: to what degree are tasks subdivided into separate jobs?
- Departmentalization: on what basis are jobs grouped together?
- Chain of command: to whom do individuals and groups report?
- Span of control: how many individuals can a manager efficiently and effectively direct?
- Centralization and decentralization: where does decision-making authority lie?
- Formalization: to what degree will there be rules and regulations to direct employees and managers?

Typically, a tightly controlled or *mechanistic* structure (characterized by extensive work specialization, rigid departmentalization, narrow spans of control, a clear chain of command, high formalization, and high centralization) is used when the primary strategy is to minimize costs. In contrast, a loosely controlled or *organic* structure (characterized by low specialization, low formalization, wide spans of control, free flow of information, cross-functional teams, and high decentralization) is used when the primary strategy is to introduce new products and services.

Technology as a Core System Component

Technology refers to "how an organization transfers its inputs into outputs" [17], and research has found technology to differ in such factors as intensity, complexity, and level of routine, e.g., the technology used in genetic research, a nonroutine activity, is radically different from the technology used in admitting patients, a routine activity. It has long been held that technology becomes more sophisticated and routinized as an organization grows in both size and complexity (compare Filley [18]), and that an organization should protect its core technology for survival [14].

Various recent approaches to organizational effectiveness in industry, such as total quality management (TQM) and continuous improvement processes, flexible manufacturing systems, and re-engineering (compare Luthans [19] for a review), have resulted from the use of innovative new technologies, e.g., flexible manufacturing systems have been used effectively to reduce the cost of mass production through the integration of computer-aided design, engineering, and manufacturing. Such approaches, in turn, place new demands on other components of the system and on other forms of technology, such as mediating and long-linked technology [14].

Tasks as a Core System Component

The tasks that employees perform have also been found to differ in complexity, significance, uncertainty, and level of routine. Further, an individual's perceptions of the tasks to be performed —particularly perceptions of task significance, task identity, and skill variety—have consistently been found to affect the individual's judgment of the meaningfulness of the task, which in turn affects motivation and performance [19,20]. By increasing an employee's perception of task significance and other core job characteristics, such as autonomy and feedback, supervisors can achieve substantial improvements in such factors as employee motivation, commitment, performance, and job satisfaction. The leadership and management literature has devoted considerable attention over the years to understanding the tasks performed by both leaders and followers, with primary emphasis on the extent to which the structuring of subordinate tasks represents a key element of effective leadership [1,10]. Perhaps not surprisingly, leaders tend to give more freedom to highly competent and cooperative subordinates than to less competent or less cooperative subordinates [21]. Groundbreaking research by Henry Mintzberg [22,23] shows leadership to be one of 10 critical roles that managers perform.*

---

* These 10 managerial roles are figurehead, leader, liaison (interpersonal roles); monitor, disseminator, spokesperson (informational roles); and entrepreneur, disturbance handler, resource allocator, and negotiator.

People as a Core System Component

Nothing would happen within an organization without skilled people to perform the work, to do so within the existing structure and with existing technology, and to push the boundaries and vision of the organization to new levels (compare Nanus [24]). Thus, it should not be at all surprising, particularly within a chapter on leadership and decision-making, for *people* to be regarded as a core component of an organizational system.

Hundreds of research studies in industrial–organizational psychology, managerial psychology, and organizational behavior have found people to differ in such factors as attitudes, motives, emotions, tolerance for uncertainty, and cognitive skills (compare the literature [19,25,26]). Further, some leaders, such as Winston Churchill and Martin Luther King, have been able to exert strong influence through personal characteristics such as eloquence and charisma [10].

Leaders as key people represent a critical integrating mechanism whereby organizational systems can accomplish both long-run and short-run objectives. But what *is* leadership and what do we know about it? What approaches to leadership have been taken in the past, what is the evidence for and against them, and are these approaches useful for the twenty-first century? If some or all of the earlier approaches no longer hold, what advice can be given to a new generation of leaders, particularly physician leaders, who face the continual challenges and opportunities of leading others?

A Brief History of Leadership Theory and Research

The earliest writings and advice on leadership can be traced to the Chinese classics of the sixth century BC, Egyptian hieroglyphics of 5000 years ago, and Greek heroes in Homer's *Iliad* (compare Bass [1]), although most management books consider Machiavelli's *The Prince* [27] to be an early starting point. Machiavelli proposed that "there is nothing more difficult to take in hand, more perilous to conduct, or more uncertain in its success, than to take the lead in the introduction of a new order of things," and he advocated a highly authoritarian approach to leadership.

Most recent leadership and management books [10,17,19] classify leadership theory and research into three broad categories:

1. trait approach
2. behavioral style approach
3. contingency approach.

In retrospect, each of these approaches has probably told us more about what leadership is *not* than what it is. We briefly discuss each of these approaches, characterized here as leadership "dead ends," and then address an emerging new fourth approach, which we refer to as a frame approach.

Leadership Dead End No. 1: Trait Approach

The first systematic theorizing on leadership, popular until the mid-1940s, has come to be known as the trait approach. Trait theorists took the position that some people had superior qualities, mostly innate, that set them apart from others and determined their capacity to lead. Traits such as height, weight, appearance, physique, energy, age, and education were all used to classify individuals into "leader" or "follower" categories. Bird [28], for example, lists 79 such traits that were used in 20 of these early leadership studies (see, for a review, Bass [1]).

The underlying premise of the trait approach was that physical characteristics and personality traits could be used to identify those who had "the right stuff" to serve as leaders. Once identified, these people could then be placed into leadership positions, e.g., if a Pennsylvania coal mine in the early 1900s needed a new foreman, they might pick the biggest, meanest, strongest, ugliest worker with the most self-confidence—all traits—and then make that person the new boss.

Unfortunately, trait researchers rarely addressed the issue of leader effectiveness or considered the role that environmental factors played in shaping leader behavior. In time, it was eventually recognized that the trait approach did not tell us much at all about leadership. We now know, as succinctly stated by Pate [29], that "[t]here are no innate 'traits' that someone else has that will make that person a better leader than you" (p. 63).

Leadership Dead End No. 2: Behavioral Style Approach

The second major systematic approach to the study of leadership, generally known as the behavioral or behavioral style approach, recognized important differences in leader behavior but still tried to find the "one best way" to lead (compare the literature [10,19]). Here the premise was that leadership did not rest with the traits or characteristics of the leader, but with his or her *style* of behavior (e.g., concern for people vs concern for task). Further, the belief was that leadership style could be taught if research could simply confirm which of the various styles of leader behavior was always "best." This approach began to take root with the research of Lewin *et al.* [30] on autocratic, democratic, and laissez-faire styles of leader behavior. Their findings, although crude in retrospect and not particularly surprising in light of what is now known of other historical events preceding the Second World War, suggested that a democratic style of leadership was the "best" style.

However, it was not until the end of the Second World War, prompted by widespread concern over the poor training that had been provided throughout the war to American junior military officers, that serious attention was paid to this new behavioral-style approach to leadership. By the late 1940s, funded research on employee-centered and organizational-centered styles of leadership had begun at the University of Michigan, and funded research on considera-tion (C) and initiating structure (IS) styles of leadership was being conducted at Ohio State University.

Over the past 50 years there has been a huge amount of research in this area, particularly research using revisions of the initial Ohio State instruments,* and we refer the interested reader to the 1200-page volume by Bass [1] for fur-

ther information. None the less, this behavioral approach also proved to be a "dead end" in fur-thering our understanding of leadership because it did not take into account the several other factors that were known to influence leader behavior. As recently summarized, "there is no 'best' style of behavior that someone else has learned—and that you haven't—that will make that person a better leader than you" [29].

Leadership Dead End No. 3: Contingency Approach

By the mid-1960s, leadership researchers had be-gun to consider situational factors and other con-straints that were thought to influence a leader's effectiveness, resulting in what is now known as the contingency approach. The first of sev-eral contingency theories was proposed by Fred Fiedler [31], who argued strongly that leader behavior (LB) was a function of the leader's per-sonality (LP), subordinate group characteristics (GC), and the situation (S), such that $LB = f(LP, GC, S)$.

The primary theoretical advantage to the contingency approach was that leadership was no longer seen as fixed or that a "one best way" of leading could be identified for all situations and circumstances. Instead, this approach tried to identify the various situational contexts (by spe-cifying "if-then" relationships) wherein one style of leader behavior would be expected to be more effective than another, e.g., in Fiedler's highly controversial contingency theory,[†] he advocated assigning a *task-focused* leader to situations that were either highly favorable or highly unfavor-able to the leader, whereas he would assign a *human relations-focused* leader to situations that were moderately favorable to the leader.

Later contingency theories emphasized the unique relationship shared between a leader and each subordinate (Graen's vertical dyad linkage model), the extent to which leaders are able to motivate and guide subordinate behavior toward

---

* The Leader Behavior Description Questionnaire (LBDQ) that was given to subordinates, and the Leader Opinion Questionnaire (LOQ) that was given to leaders (see [44,45]).

[†] One scathing review of Fiedler's approach, published in *Administrative Science Quarterly*, by leadership scholar Chester A. Schriescheim, ended with the suggestion that a label should be affixed to all copies of Fiedler's book to warn readers that "Use of this book may be hazardous to your leader effectiveness."

accomplishing objectives (House's path-goal theory), and decisions about the level of employee involvement (Vroom–Yetton and Vroom–Jago models). However, the bottom line is much the same for all of them, namely that research has been unable to specify all of the relevant contingencies to be able to say precisely what the leader should do in a given situation.

An Emerging New Frame Approach

Over the past 10 years or so, as a result of the writings of respected leadership scholars and practitioners such as Warren Bennis [2], Max DePree [32], Jim Kouzes and Barry Posner [33], and Burt Nanus [24], a promising new approach has been emerging. As recently noted by Larry Pate [29, p. 63]:

> When management gurus like Tom Peters or Warren Bennis talk about leaders "doing the right thing" and managers "doing things right", they are being more than just clever. They are reminding us of the essential ingredients of character and integrity and high ethical standards inherent to good leadership. They are confirming what most of us have known all along, but failed to fully recognize—that the previous views of leadership may have been all wrong.

There is, as yet, no agreed-upon name for this new approach, although most anyone who has been following the trends will recognize that contemporary thinking about leadership has shifted. Indeed, contemporary thinking about organizations themselves has also been changing (compare the literature [34,35]). Some of the recent talk has been about *charismatic* leadership, some is about *visionary* leadership, some about *transformational* leadership vs *transactional* leadership, and still other about *spiritual* leadership. Although there are subtle differences between each of these approaches, there is also a common element having to do with redefining leadership as something that is rooted deep within the individual, not as a trait, but as a result of the leader's own personal growth. It reflects a more seasoned, sensitive, caring, ethical, and humane way of doing things.

For example, a recent[†] postcard from the Center for Creative Leadership in Greensboro, North Carolina shows a photo of an Asian businessman on one side of the card with the caption: "What I learned not only changed the way I lead, it changed the way I live." On the reverse, they write:

> At the Center for Creative Leadership, we focus on self-awareness as the first step in leadership development. So managers leave our programs with a deeper understanding of themselves and how they relate to others, not only in their careers, but in their lives as well. It's what makes our approach unique. . . .

Perhaps it is thinking like this that prompted Bennis [2] to suggest that leadership could not be taught, but it *could* be learned.

We refer here to this new approach as a frame approach, because the focus generally has been on the "frame" or "lens" that leaders use for viewing the world and their powerful influence on others around them. As recently observed by Gareth Morgan [35, p. 189]:

> Leadership ultimately involves an ability to define the reality of others. . . . In managing the meanings and interpretations assigned to a situation, the leader in effect wields a form of symbolic power that exerts a decisive influence on how people perceive their realities and hence the way they act. Charismatic leaders seem to have a natural ability to shape meaning in this way.

It is because of this new perspective that several writers have made the important distinction between *managing* and *leading* [11]. To some extent, the notion of alternative ways of viewing things is not at all new. Indeed, it was 20 years ago that Charles Hampton-Turner [36], then at the London Business School, identified 60 such alternative perspectives which he referred to as "maps of the mind." But what *is* new in leadership theory is a heightened awareness of the importance of human decency, integrity, and moral courage.

---

† May 2000.

Let us now turn our attention to a few practical tools that can help physicians change their own frames about what it means to lead.

Alternative Techniques for Changing the Frame

We now briefly discuss three techniques that can help physician leaders to see things differently, to change their own frames about what to do and how to do it, and to make the tough choices that leaders often have to make. Each of these techniques is simple, portable, practical, and easy to use. They are also easy to remember by their four-letter acronyms—ACES, RAID, and SWOT.

Technique No. 1: ACES Decision-making Technique

Leaders often have to make the tough choices, the ones with no obvious "best" answer, the sort where you feel that whatever you do you're "damned if you do, damned if you don't." Research shows that, in such cases, the natural tendency is to want to avoid the decision, pass the responsibility to someone else, or try to find reasons to justify an inferior course of action [37].

The ACES technique, developed over the past 15 years by Pate [38,39], is intended precisely for those tough leadership decisions where the decision-maker is "stuck," where there is no clear alternative, and where procrastination and other methods of avoiding the decision have probably already done some damage. ACES is an acronym that stands for:

Assumptions
Criteria
Evoked set
Strategy.

The essence of the ACES technique is that often the assumptions we make are flawed, or we have not adequately clarified what we want, or we have not considered relevant options that could lead to a superior solution. ACES provides a simple structure for challenging assumptions, assigning weights to various criteria, and expanding the set of options for making the deci-

sion. Although research on the ACES technique thus far is limited (compare Pate and Nielson [40] for a brief review), the anecdotal evidence on the value of the technique has been overwhelmingly positive. Further information on the technique or its use in changing the leader's frame can be found in both academic [38] and practitioner [39] journals, or by contacting the authors of this chapter directly.

Technique No. 2: RAID Backward Planning Technique

The second technique that physicians and other medical professionals may find useful in their roles as leaders is the RAID backward planning technique (compare the literature [26,41]). The RAID technique starts not with the current situation, but with the leader's vision or "dream" of the future, and then provides a simple framework for managing that dream (see also Bennis [42]).

RAID asks the individual first to focus on the outcomes desired, and then to identify the key actions necessary to achieve them. The technique also compels the leader to establish appropriate milestones to indicate successful progress toward these desired outcomes. As recently noted by Pate and Chesteen [26, p 59], "... rather than start with the decision itself, RAID starts with where we want to get to, which determines the decisions that must be made, along with priorities for each of them."

The sequential planning stages of the RAID technique are:

Results desired
Actions necessary to produce the results
Indicators to watch
Decisions that remain.

As it turns out, medicine provides us with a convenient mechanism, the clinical pathway, for illustrating these planning stages. Therefore, we examine each of the RAID steps in the context of the clinical pathway.

Results Desired
The RAID backward planning technique places primary focus on determining the desired outcomes for any situation or new initiative. The

leader first considers what measure and what value are most likely to lead to a successful outcome. This result is understandably dependent on any specific challenges faced by the leader at the time. To be most useful to the leader, desired results should be phrased in clearly measurable terms. Examples of possible results-oriented goals might be:

- Medical staff turnover reduced by 30% within 6 months
- Patient satisfaction measurements improved by 20% in 3 months
- Patient after coronary artery bypass graft (CABG) discharged 5 days postoperatively without incident
- Patient post-Total Knee Replacement (TKR) discharged 3 days postoperatively without incident
- Patient complications post-thrombolytic therapy decreased by 40% in 3 months.

The last three examples come directly from clinical pathway goals. Note that the pathways begin with a goal, a desired outcome. Note also that the results desired are clear and measurable—thus easily communicated to others in the multidisciplinary team. The leader is likely to find ease of communication an essential element in the formation of these goals. The level of involvement and commitment by team members is dependent to a large extent on understanding the goals.

Actions Necessary to Produce the Results

The second step in applying the RAID technique is to identify the actions necessary to achieve the results that were listed in the first step. It is essential for the leader to consider relevant inputs that contribute to successful outcomes, as measured by the parameters established in the first step. Of these inputs, the leader should determine the essential activities that drive the results desired. One method is to provide a list of priority and secondary activities that have a causal and then a supportive relationship to the desired responses. In the example of the post-CABG clinical pathway patient, actions might include the following:

- Provide intravenous analgesic therapy as needed every 15–30 min in recovery

- Monitor mixed venous saturation readings every 30 min × 4 h in intensive care unit (ICU)
- Obtain pulmonary artery catheter measurements every 1 h × 6 h in ICU
- Dangle postoperative day 0
- Ambulate 30 feet postoperative day 1
- Remove sternal dressing and all drains postoperative day 2.

Note, again, that these actions are clear and measurable. In addition, there is a clear and logical progression in chronological sequence (immediate postoperative through subsequent days). If actions are not understood, we have no reason to expect the desired results to be achieved. Using the clinical pathway example, a calendar of activities could be established, whereby each activity carefully builds on each preceding intervention, ultimately leading to the successful attainment of the desired outcome.

Indicators to Watch

Each action that is identified in the second step should be expected to lead to one or more of the desired results. Therefore, these actions represent milestones that should be monitored. Just as a loving parent might carefully watch for developmental milestones in his or her children as an indication of progress toward the desired outcome of a healthy and "normal" child, so the dedicated manager will monitor key indicators of progress inherent to any new project or intervention.

The challenge to the leader is to establish appropriate indices and a reasonable timetable for attaining each milestone. As with the prior step of determining necessary actions, the determination of appropriate indicators can often be accomplished through cross-functional or interdisciplinary teams. Carefully guided by the leader, the resulting lists of interventions and expected milestones can be far superior to compilations made by individuals working alone—even individuals who are regarded as experts in their respective fields.

To continue with the CABG example, a typical clinical pathway might identify clinical milestones for successful progress similar to the following:

- Extubated within 6 h postprocedure
- Chest tube drainage <100 ml/h within 6 h postoperatively
- Chest tubes removed postoperative day 1
- Patient ambulating in hall >40 feet postoperative day 1
- Chest radiograph within normal limits (WNL) on postoperative day 2.

Each indicator follows the same chronological form as the prescribed actions of the second step in the RAID planning sequence. In fact, the indicators at times may be more closely related to individual actions than the actions themselves are related to the ultimate desired result. The importance of this step for the leader is that it can establish an effective means by which to measure incremental progress toward the ultimate goal of the plan.

Decisions that Remain

Several decisions generally need to be made after the initial implementation of a strategic plan. This final step in the RAID planning sequence recognizes that variances can and do occur with any plan. Indeed, as observed by the ancient Chinese proverb: "We make plans to throw them away." The strategic plan developed by the RAID technique is a dynamic and adaptive plan—subject to change as the external environment and progress toward the plan's goals dictate. Where possible, the leader should try to identify not only the decisions that remain, but also even the order in which they will be taken.

A familiar part of a clinical pathway form is the area to record variances from the plan on any specific variable and/or day. The practitioner is aware of the need to apply additional critical thought and decision-making to the patient's condition as a result of the variance away from one or more of the indicators/milestones that were established in the third stage of the backward planning process. Identification of possible plan variances, and the key decisions that apply to these potential disruptions, is often referred to as contingency planning.

Whatever we call it, the anticipation of the need for further decision-making helps the prudent leader to mitigate risk and minimize any negative impact on achieving the desired results.

This final step represents an ongoing evaluation that is essential in any therapeutic intervention process. Prudent application of all stages of the RAID technique, including this continuing process of evaluation, provides the leader with a powerful tool for creating results-oriented action plans.

Technique No. 3: SWOT Strategy Analysis

This third technique, SWOT analysis, is especially useful in helping the leader to consider important variables both inside and outside the organization. Similar to the "prayer" of the popular inspirational quotation, this technique helps the leader to identify those things that can be changed, those that cannot be changed, and provides a practical framework for assessing the difference. The key to this analytical tool is to categorize decision variables into *internal* and *external* domains. Internal variables can be further identified as strengths or weaknesses. External variables are opportunities or threats. This technique provides the leader with a structured mechanism for viewing these critical variables.

Curiously, we have found no one who can tell us the exact origins of SWOT, but it is normally associated with the work on competitive advantage by Professor Michael Porter of the Harvard Business School [43]. SWOT analysis is often applied to the consideration of new projects for an organization. The technique can be especially valuable when used in conjunction with other methods, such as the RAID technique, because SWOT describes the resources to be brought to bear and the potential obstacles to achieving the desired results that are identified by RAID. In addition, by focusing on both the internal and external environments, SWOT presents the leader with a more balanced and realistic assessment of the potential for success.

Strengths

Strengths are those factors within an organizational system that can be viewed as distinctly positive in contributing to the successful outcome of a desired initiative. The strengths may include factors such as:

- specializations
- competencies
- access to resources (internal)
- location
- current funding mix.

A thorough assessment of strengths represents the identification of all the critical resources that exist within the organization to be applied to the challenge, or new focus. Strengths are also the first variables that a leader can exert direct influence over.

Weaknesses

The second grouping of factors is also internal. Weaknesses are those variables that may lead to undesired outcomes. Many of these factors can be seen as either the same as, or the antithesis of, the strengths:

- Lack of specialization (or specialization in the wrong areas)
- Lack of competencies
- Resources (internal) not applicable to the current challenge
- Inappropriate location
- Lack of current funding (or restrictions placed on funding).

A leader is expected to use objective and critical thinking skills. However, the challenge of being objective while being immersed in the politics of the system is a major factor driving the use of outside consulting firms to help with strategic analysis and planning. A large part of the difficulty for leaders is to understand that a particular factor, such as a strong competency, can be both a definite strength and a weakness.

A common medical example of this problem is that of a patient with nonspecific complaints of general malaise, on seeing any number of specialists, receiving an equivalent number of differing diagnoses—each physician attributing the underlying etiology to his or her own area of expertise. Although this anecdote may be a bit of an exaggeration, it none the less illustrates the potential weakness that exists in performing an analysis from exclusively within the system.

Opportunities

The first of the two external variables is opportunities. In all probability, one or more of the opportunities will have already been recognized (either formally or informally), especially if the leader is contemplating some new action. The purpose of developing a list of opportunities is to ensure that all the critical external environmental factors that either directly or indirectly contribute to the potential for a successful outcome have been considered. Opportunities include many variables, such as:

- Regulatory environment and changes (positive)
- Economic environment (such as declining lending rates)
- Local resources (such as area employment pool)
- Lack of competition
- High external demand for services.

Opportunities may also be pre-existing yet unserved, or they may be new, as a result of recent changes in the external environment, e.g., a new form of technology, such as a superior heart monitor or a more portable magnetic resonance imaging (MRI) machine, may become available, or a major competitor may come up for sale or even drop out of the arena.

Opportunities may be primary or secondary to the leader's decision, e.g., primary opportunity might be provided by the new technology of blending computed tomography technology with focused radiotherapy for cancer. A secondary opportunity that the leader might recognize would be the availability of many certified radiology technicians trained to assist in the use of this new technology.

Although environmental changes may account for a significant number of the opportunities that present themselves to leaders, those leaders must diligently monitor the environment to be the first to identify such opportunities. This is one reason why administrators subscribe to the premier periodicals and join the major professional organizations in their fields.

Threats

The second external factor is threats. These variables offer the potential for undesired outcomes in the proposed plan of action. Just as with strengths and weaknesses, threats can often represent the antithesis of the list of opportunities:

- Regulatory environment and changes (negative)
- Economic environment (such as increasing loan rates)
- Local resources (such as area employment pool, or low unemployment rates)
- Lack of competition
- Low demand for current services.

Failure to accurately identify such environmental threats can lead to an overly optimistic and naïve evaluation in the decision-making process. On the other hand, over-estimates of the threats may cause a "paralysis by analysis" and the leadership can lose the opportunity to move first, on the erroneous belief that threats can be mitigated by still further analysis.

SWOT analysis is an organizational tool. As with all other techniques, it can greatly improve the quality of the decisions made by systematically considering the information that is organized within its structure. To the extent that the analysis itself does nothing to alter the variables being analyzed, there is no justification for a repetitive and/or drawn-out SWOT processes. Every effort should be made to conduct a thorough and insightful analysis, with contributions from a full spectrum of functions from within the organization. Once the list of SWOT variables has been identified, however, the leader is likely to have the information needed for making an informed decision. Further study beyond a systematic SWOT analysis rarely contributes to the mitigation of the threats. More commonly it just decreases opportunities as others make the tough decisions based on their own analyses.

Conclusions

This chapter has examined the extensive body of research and theory on leadership and leader behavior in order to provide direction and assistance to physicians as they find themselves in key leadership roles. Much of the work in leadership over the past 80 years has been characterized here

as "dead-ends," on the ground that these previous efforts have told us far more about what leadership is *not* than what leadership is.

However, we have also identified an emerging and promising new frame approach to leadership, an approach solidly based on the premise that leadership comes primarily from within the individual and is not tied to a particular role or formal position within an organization or organizational system. The challenge for leaders today, physicians included, is to make ethical and responsible decisions, even in the face of strong pressure from constituents or the rest of the organization to do otherwise.

Most all of us have seen powerful movies, such as *Patch Adams* or *Dead Poet's Society*, that show the kind of courage that is needed under adverse circumstances. The challenge for leaders is not just to understand the distinction between leading and managing, but to follow through and actually *do* the right thing. Often integrity and principle will go unrewarded and unrecognized. If a physician's primary personal goal is rewards or recognition, ethics and principles may be ignored. However, if the intent is to help build a better world, one that is more decent and humane, and where cooperation and not hatred is the norm, the challenge of ethical leadership for physicians is a very real one.

Finally, we have discussed three very simple, yet practical, techniques—ACES, RAID, and SWOT—that physicians can use in those difficult moments when they need help in seeing things differently or changing their own frames when serving in important leadership positions.

As we began this chapter with an insightful quote from a highly respected and humane leadership researcher, Jim O'Toole of The USC Leadership Institute, we will end with one from a highly respected and humane executive, Max DePree, former chairman and CEO of Herman Miller, Inc., the successful furniture maker:

> Leadership is much more an art, a belief, a condition of the heart, than a set of things to do. The visible signs of artful leadership are expressed, ultimately, in its practice.

References

1. Bass BM. *Bass and Stodgill's Handbook of Leadership: Theory, Research, and Managerial Applications*, 3rd edn. New York: Free Press, 1990.
2. Bennis W. *On Becoming a Leader*. Reading, MA: Addison-Wesley, 1989.
3. Duxbury ML, Armstrong GD, Drew DJ, Henly SJ. Head nurse leadership style with staff nurse burnout and job satisfaction in neonatal intensive care units. *Nursing Res* 1984; **33**(2): 97–104.
4. Nealey SM, Blood MR. Leadership performance of nursing supervisors at two organizational levels. *J Appl Psychol* 1968; **52**: 414–22.
5. Sheridan JE, Vredenburgh DJ. Structural model of leadership influence in a hospital organization. *Acad Manage J* 1979; **22**: 6–21.
6. Wilson MP, McLaughlin CP. *Leadership and Management in Academic Medicine*. San Francisco: Jossey-Bass, 1984.
7. LaMonica EL. *Nursing Leadership and Management: An experiential approach*. Monterey, CA: Wadsworth Health Sciences Division, 1983.
8. Fried KW. Power acquisition in a health care setting. An application of strategic contingencies theory. *Human Relations* 1988; **41**: 915–27.
9. Bennis W, Nanus B. *Leaders: the Strategies for Taking Charge*. New York: Harper & Row, 1985.
10. Daft RL. *Leadership Theory and Practice*. Fort Worth: Harcourt Brace, 1999.
11. Kotter JP. *A Force for Change: How Leadership Differs from Management*. New York: Free Press, 1990.
12. Pate LE, Golembiewski RT, Rahim A. Managing change versus achieving progress. Images of an ethical future. In: Rahim A, Golembiewski R, Pate L, eds. *Current Topics in Management*, Vol. 2. Greenwich, CT: JAI Press, 1997.
13. Leavitt HJ. Applied organizational change in industry. Structural, technological, and humanistic approaches. In: March J, ed. *Handbook of Organizations*. Chicago: Rand McNally, 1965.
14. Thompson JD. *Organizations in Action*. New York: McGraw-Hill, 1967.
15. Pondy LR, Mitroff II. Beyond open systems models of organization. In: Staw B, ed. *Research in Organizational Behavior*, Vol. 1. Greenwich, CT: JAI Press, 1979.
16. Boulding K. General systems theory—the skeleton of science. In: Buckle W, ed. *Modern Systems Research for the Behavioral Scientist*. Chicago: Aldine, 1968.
17. Robbins SP. *Organizational Behavior*, 8th edn. Upper Saddle River, NJ: Prentice Hall, 1998.
18. Filley AC. *The Compleat Manager: What works when*. Champaign, Il: Scott Foresman, 1978.
19. Luthans F. *Organizational Behavior*, 8th edn. Boston: Irwin/McGraw-Hill, 1998.
20. Hackman JR, Oldham GR. Motivation through the design of work: Test of a theory. *Organizational Behavior and Human Performance* 1976; August: 250–79.
21. Pate LE. Laboratory effects of subordinate competence and cooperativeness on managerial behaviour. *Int J Manage* 1988; **5**: 180–7.
22. Mintzberg H. Retrospective commentary on "The managers' job: Folklore and fact". *Harvard Business Review* 1990; **168**(2): 170.
23. Mintzberg H. The managers' job. Folklore and fact. *Harvard Business Review* 1975; **53**(4): 49–61.
24. Nanus B. *Visionary Leadership: Creating a Compelling Sense of Direction for Your Organization*. San Francisco: Jossey-Bass, 1992.
25. Driver MJ, Pate LE. Decision making. In: Luthans F, ed. *Virtual Organizational Behavior*. New York: McGraw-Hill, 1996.
26. Pate LE, Chesteen SA. Decision making and work motivation: Reframing the role of the pharmacist from intervention to direct patient care. In: Nimmo C, ed. *Staff Development for Pharmacy Practice*. Bethesda, MD: American Society of Health-System Pharmacists, 2000.
27. Machiavelli N (1513). *The Prince*. New York: Mentor Press, 1962.
28. Bird C. *Social Psychology*. New York: Appleton-Century, 1940 [cited by Bass, 1990].
29. Pate L. Anyone can manage: But to lead requires a bit more [Guest column for *Your Business* section]. *Madison Magazine* 1999; **41**(7): 63.
30. Lewin K, Lippitt R, White RK. Pattern of aggressive behavior in experimentally created social climates. *J Social Psychol* 1939; **10**: 271–301.
31. Fiedler FE. *A Theory of Leadership Effectiveness*. New York: McGraw-Hill, 1967.
32. DePree M. *Leadership is an Art*. New York: Dell Publishing, 1989.
33. Kouzes JM, Posner BZ. *The Leadership Challenge: How to Get Extraordinary Things Done in Organizations*. San Francisco: Jossey-Bass, 1987.
34. Handy C. *The Age of Unreason*. Boston: Harvard Business School Press, 1989.
35. Morgan G. *Images of Organization*, 2nd edn. Thousand Oaks, CA: Sage, 1997.
36. Hampton-Turner C. *Maps of the Mind*. New York: Macmillan, 1981.
37. Janis IL, Mann L. *Decision Making: a Psychological Analysis of Conflict, Choice, and Commitment*. New York: Free Press, 1977.

38. Pate LE. Improving managerial decision-making. *J Manage Psychol* 1987; **2**(2): 9–15.
39. Pate LE. ACES trump: Try this practical tool for making tough personal or professional decisions [Guest column for *Your Business* section]. *Madison Magazine* 1999; **41**(3): 47.
40. Pate LE, Nielson TR. Empirical findings on the ACES decision-making technique. *Psychol Reports* 1996; **78**: 1049–50.
41. Pate L. All accounting is basically a subtraction problem. RAID a Tool for Feed-Forward Planning, Wisconsin CPA. [Published *Wisconsin Inst Certified Public Accountants*] 1999; **3**(7): 26–7.]

42. Bennis WG. Managing the dream: Leadership in the 21st century. *J Organizational Change Manage* 1989b; **2**(1): 6–10.
43. Porter ME. *Competitive Advantage: Creating and Sustaining Superior Performance*. New York: Free Press, 1985.
44. Stogdill RM. *Handbook of Leadership*. New York: Free Press, 1974.
45. Stogdill RM, Coons AE. *Leader Behavior: its Description and Measurement*. Columbus, OH: College of Administrative Science, Ohio State University, 1957.

5

Human Resource Management

David R. Zimmerman

This chapter focuses on the management of human resources in health care organizations. Human resource issues are pervasive in any service industry, and one can argue that they are particularly important in the health care field, where the performance of those who deliver care can have, quite literally, life-and-death consequences. Human resource management in health care has undergone enormous changes in the last decade, a combined result of fundamental changes in both the health care and human resource environments.

In this chapter, we focus on topics that affect some of the most important human resource functions and issues. Even within topics, our coverage is limited by space constraints, and we try to compensate by offering additional sources for the reader to access more detailed information. There are, of course, general textbooks on human resource management, some of which focus directly on the health care industry. One recent addition to this field is *Essentials of Human Resources Management in Health Services Organizations*, edited by Fottler *et al*. [1].

This chapter is directed at physicians in medical management, rather than at human resource administrators. We focus on what a physician needs to know about human resource management. Also, to the extent that it is possible, we focus on all health care staff, not just physicians, although in some cases the issues as they relate to physicians are quite different from those for other staff. This results partly from the fact that physicians are sometimes not employees but act more as contractors. Often they expect to be treated differently from other staff members. In some cases this is quite legitimate; in others it

may be questioned, and their differential, or deferential, treatment may itself cause problems with other staff members.

A Framework for Studying Human Resource Management

Effective human resource management can best be described as "systematizing and formalizing common sense". The best policies reflect the basic attributes of fairness, respect, and clear communication. No matter what the issue, this simple principle may be the most valuable of all: Does the policy, practice, or solution to a problem pass the test of common sense in dealing with colleagues and co-workers?

To formulate a "system" of health-care human resource management, it is useful to appeal to an overall model. Such a model has been developed by Heneman and his colleagues [2]; we modify it slightly for use in a health care environment. This modified model is shown in Fig. 5-1. The model identifies the primary functions of human resources, as well as the critical outcomes of those functions. It also identifies important internal and external factors that affect human resource functions and outcomes.

Human Resource Outcomes

Figure 5-1 identifies the primary outcomes that human resource policy and management seek to achieve or influence. Perhaps the best way to view these outcomes is chronologically: the health care organization must *recruit* staff members by making itself attractive to them, while at

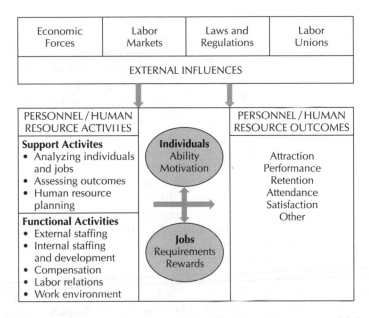

Figure 5-1. Human resource management framework. Modified from Heneman *et al.* [2].

the same time using effective *selection* practices to hire the right people. Once the entrant is on board, human resource attention turns to *performance*. This is typically done by *matching* the incumbent to the position and offering appropriate *rewards* for the desired performance.

The ultimate human resource goal is *retention*, keeping staff members whose performance enables the organization to reach its objectives. The costs of staff turnover, especially in the health care field, are often underestimated.

For staff members, satisfaction with the position and the organization, the reward structure, and relationships with colleagues is paramount to staying and performing well. The relationship between satisfaction and performance is more complicated than conventional wisdom suggests.

The human resource outcomes just described have two important applications. First, they can —and should—contribute to the overall goals of the organization. Second, they can—and should —be used to measure the effectiveness of human resource policies and practices.

Human Resource Functions

The model of Heneman *et al.* [2] identifies necessary human resource functions. In a health care setting, some of these focus mainly on the delivery of care, whereas others focus on attracting, retaining, and generating acceptable performance from staff members. Another way of viewing these functions is in terms of whether they are proactive or reactive. It is useful to think of human resource management as having two overall functions:

1. To develop systems and procedures for various activities, from recruitment and selection through discipline and termination.
2. To respond efficiently to all situations that arise in the production (i.e., health care delivery) system.

Effective human resource management requires careful attention to both functions. The first is important because good systems and procedures can minimize the occurrence of staff problems and inspire confidence in the fairness of the decision-making process. The second function is important because responsiveness to personnel problems is one of the most tangible measures of effectiveness in the eyes of the staff.

Individuals and Jobs

An important part of the model of Heneman *et al.* is the relationship between individuals and jobs.

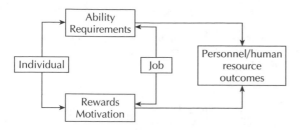

Figure 5-2. The correspondence between individual and job characteristics. (Modified from Heneman *et al.* [2].)

In Fig. 5-1 this role is depicted as intervening in the relationship between human resource functions and outcomes. A more detailed treatment of this critical relationship is found in Fig. 5-2, which shows how one aspect of the job relates to a corresponding aspect in the individual. A person's performance is a function of both ability and motivation. Each of these elements can be directly linked to two attributes of the job—requirements and rewards.

The key to maximizing performance is therefore, on the one hand, to match the person's ability to the requirements of the job and, on the other, to match the rewards of the job to the person's motivation.

External Influences on Human Resource Management

Figure 5-1 also reveals that there are external factors that limit the ability of management to implement human resource policies and practices. This is especially true in the health care field. For health care managers, all of the traditional external constraints exist—legal requirements, technology, economic factors, and institutional factors such as collective bargaining. In addition, several recent developments in health care have had an especially strong effect on human resource policy.

Legal and Public Policy Developments

The following laws and policy developments have placed stringent requirements on managers as they carry out human resource functions.

Antidiscrimination Laws

Federal and state laws prohibit employers from making employment decisions on the basis of certain characteristics, including race, sex, religion, age, disability, and several other factors. The cornerstone of these efforts is Title VII of the Civil Rights Act of 1964 (42 U.S.C. @ 2000e), which prohibits discrimination in employment on the basis of race, color, religion, sex, or national origin. Many of the decisions of the Equal Employment Opportunities Commission (EEOC), which administers the law, have come in discharge cases, although recently potential discrimination in promotion decisions (particularly against women and minorities) has received more attention from the EEOC.

Several other federal statutes expand the antidiscrimination focus, including the Age Discrimination in Employment Act, the Americans with Disabilities Act of 1990, and the Equal Pay Act of 1963. The Age Discrimination in Employment Act has had a profound impact on retirement policies, because, with certain exceptions, no employee can be required to retire. The employer must also take great care, in dismissing an older (typically over 40) worker, that the action is not being taken on the basis of age. The Americans with Disabilities Act (ADA) protects individuals in certain disability classes from discrimination in hiring and promotion. It also imposes obligations on the employer to make certain "accommodations" for disabled workers or applicants.

Sexual Harassment

This policy area addresses "unwelcome sexual conduct", which can take two different forms. The first is known as *quid pro quo,* in which the subordinate must submit to sexual advances from a supervisor in return for employment advancement, or in which failure to submit to such advances might lead to employment harm. The second form of harassment, known as *hostile environment,* involves situations in which, even if there is no sexual favor sought, the behavior of the perpetrator is not welcomed by the individual, is based on the prohibited factor (e.g., sex), was offensive to a reasonable person, and was known by the employer.

Family and Medical Leave law

The federal Family and Medical Leave Act of 1993 (U.S.C. @ 2601) provides broad employee benefits in the area of unpaid leave for such things as childbirth and early child care, an employee's health condition, or the need to care for a family member. Various state laws have been passed as well.

Collective Bargaining Environment

Another important area of public policy in the health care field is the resurgence of unions and collective bargaining. Labor relations in health care, as in most other industries, is primarily governed by two relatively old pieces of legislation: the National Labor Relations Act of 1935 (NLRA) and the Labor Management Relations Act, sometimes called the Taft–Hartley Act, which amended the NLRA. Since 1974, hospital employees and those in other health care settings have had the right to engage in collective bargaining.

For the purposes of collective bargaining, federal law dictates that employees be placed in "bargaining units" based on similar interests, job conditions, working relationships, and other factors. In contrast to its policy toward other industries, the National Labor Relations Board (NLRB) has determined that hospital workers should be placed into one of eight bargaining units. Many experts think that this has enhanced the opportunity for unions to win representation elections, in which case all the employees in that unit are represented by the union.

Health Care Environmental Factors

Many of the external factors previously identified are relevant to all industries, not just health care. However, there are important developments in the health care environment that have shaped and influenced human resource management in that field. First, the decentralization of health care has essentially redefined what one means by the term "health care organization." Health care services are both more centralized, with larger medical clinics, and less "institutional," as care is provided in a variety of settings. The management of human resources is now defined less in terms of care settings and more in terms of care plans.

Internal Factors Affecting Human Resource Management

The major internal factors affecting human resource policy and management include organizational philosophies (values) and market strategy. Sometimes their effects are underestimated.

One philosophical trend that has had an important impact on human resource policy is total quality management (TQM). One of the cornerstones of TQM, for example, is that compensation policy should not be based on performance appraisal, mainly because of the shortcomings of performance appraisal systems. TQM separates individual performance evaluation from the organization's pay structure, although few organizations follow this strictly. A corollary to this is TQM's emphasis on system performance versus individual performance. As one can imagine, a performance evaluation process focused on the system of production as opposed to individual producers would look very different from most processes in use today.

Another example of a philosophy with important implications for human resource management is patient-centered care, which can lead to fundamental changes in the structure, staff roles, and decision-making processes in health care delivery.

Market strategy also plays an important role in human resource management. An aggressive policy of expansion through buyouts and mergers, for example, can wreak havoc on employment policy, turnover, recruitment of new staff, and incumbent staff satisfaction, especially if, as is often the case, these activities are carried out without considering their human resource consequences. Mergers can disrupt existing policies and create a climate of insecurity that can severely damage staff morale.

Performance Evaluation

Performance evaluation is one of the most important functions of human resource managers, and it has been a target of substantial criticism in recent years. Many believe that performance evaluation has fallen short of its potential because of deficiencies in its actual practice [3].

Purposes of Performance Evaluation

Traditionally, the purposes of performance evaluation have been organized around two themes:

1. To provide a basis for administrative decisions, such as promotion/demotion/termination, compensation, or the need for training.
2. To improve employee performance by providing feedback to the employee about strengths and weaknesses.

More recently, a third purpose has begun to emerge, particularly as the tenets of TQM gain acceptance. Performance evaluation is seen as an important way to assess the effectiveness of organizational policies, programs, and systems. In particular, there has been increasing interest in using performance evaluation to determine whether organizational systems or subsystems, such as delivery of care in a particular unit, are operating effectively and efficiently.

Major Issues in Performance Evaluation

Several major issues must be resolved in the development and implementation of an effective performance evaluation system. We discuss some of the most important things to keep in mind rather than providing a detailed analysis of each issue.

Types of Evaluation Methods

Performance evaluation methods can be of two general types—absolute standards and comparative methods. With absolute standards, the employee is evaluated against a common standard, without regard to how he or she performs compared with other workers. Common methods in this category include graphic ratings, forced-choice, and checklists of performance dimensions, which are often weighted for importance. Identification of "critical incidents" is another example of an absolute standard rating method; here the behaviors of the employee as they relate to good or bad performance on critical

matters are identified. Some evaluation experts have sought to provide more standardized reference points for evaluators, which led to the development of the Behaviorally Anchored Rating Scale (BARS), in which the employee is judged on various important dimensions of job performance, but with explicit linkages noted between types of behaviors and how that is translated into specific numerical values.

Comparative methods, as the name implies, involve comparing one employee with another, which in effect *ranks* the employees. Paired comparisons, forced distribution, alternative ranking, and straight ranking are all evaluation methods within this category. Comparative rankings are useful in making decisions about promotion or other administrative action, when limited to the existing employees. However, many consider the methods inadequate in that they force the rater to choose between employees, when in reality the performance of more than one employee may be acceptable or unacceptable.

Who Should Evaluate Whom

There are many views on the efficacy of peer evaluations, supervisor assessment, subordinate review, and combinations of these approaches. Which scheme is best is difficult to answer. Regardless of the scheme, it is important to obtain ratings from more than one person, if possible. Preferably these should come from raters above, below, and at the same level as the person being rated.

Principles of Performance Evaluation

There are two overriding principles of performance evaluation. First, performance evaluation is an issue of *measurement*. Second, it is an issue of *communication*. These two relatively simple concepts are often ignored in developing performance evaluation systems.

Assessing performance carries with it all of the challenges inherent to developing measures of any aspect of health care. The performance measures must be valid (i.e., they must accurately reflect the behavior necessary to perform the job effectively), they must be reliable (i.e., they must be stable across time and across individuals conducting the evaluation), they must be feasible to carry out, and they must be well understood by both the reviewer and the subject of the evaluation. In fact, the most common problems in performance evaluation are all problems that have been identified in measurement generally: problems such as the "halo effect," in which the employee is rated high or low across the board because of a high rating in one area; "central tendency," in which many or all employees are rated about the same [4]; "similarity to me," where the rating is based on how closely the employee resembles the rater on that dimension [5]; and two somewhat conflicting problems— "recency" effect, in which events occurring more recently are given disproportionate weight, and "past performance," in which perceptions about events long ago (e.g., during the previous review period) are carried forward.

Effective performance evaluation is also a matter of communication. In the development of the performance evaluation system, it is critical to have the input of those who will be using it and those who will be its subjects. Involving these parties in development will help them to understand the new system and make them more likely to accept it. Once the system is developed, communication about results and how they will be used will be essential to its ultimate acceptance.

Another principle to keep in mind follows from TQM. In the course of evaluating an employee's performance, it is important to consider to what extent the performance (good or bad) is attributable to the system of operation as opposed to the individual's part in it. Many health care units have improved both system and individual performance by keeping this dual perspective in mind.

A Systematic Framework for Measuring Performance

Perhaps the single most important principle in performance evaluation is to establish a standardized framework for evaluating all employees. To do this, it is necessary to identify the following items:

- The dimensions of performance that are important, such as technical skill, interpersonal relations, administrative effectiveness, etc.

- For each dimension, the criteria that are important in determining how effectively the person has performed the function.
- For each criterion, the measures that will be used to assess performance, as well as the standard used, if any, to judge performance adequacy.
- For each measure, the sources of information that will be tapped.

An example of how this framework can be used to structure the performance evaluation for a specific position—in this example, the chair in a department of pediatric medicine—is provided in Table 5-1, which can be thought of as a matrix for the performance of that position. The matrix shown is for illustrative purposes and is oversimplified and incomplete. However, this approach can provide the necessary standardization to evaluate all positions, even those across occupational groups and organizational units.

Selection: Staffing the Organization

Staffing the health care organization is often viewed, justifiably, as one of the most important human resource functions. Yet this function is frequently treated in a cavalier manner, with little thought given to the principles that can make staffing both a more effective and a more efficient process. In this section we examine some of the principles of good selection policy and practice. Our focus is primarily on selection rather than recruitment. A good discussion of recruitment policies and practices in health care organizations can be found in Landau and Fogel [6]. An excellent, more comprehensive treatment of staffing in organizations is provided in Heneman and Heneman [7].

There are two essential principles that should be kept in mind in the development and implementation of an effective selection policy in any health care organization:

1. Selection and recruitment are complementary, often iterative and simultaneous, functions. Indeed, they can be viewed as the same function from opposite perspectives. Recruitment seeks to attract individuals whom the

Table 5-1. Performance Evaluation Position: Chair, Department of Pediatric Medicine.

Dimension	Criteria	Measure/Standard	Information source

1. Technical competence /ability	Patient care:
	• Diagnosis
	• Referral
	• Treatment
	  –Prevention
	  –Effectiveness
		Complication rate for outpatient procedures $<X\%$
		Accuracy of diagnosis $>X\%$, sample of cases
		Immunization rate $>X\%$
		ALOS within X SDs of means, selected diagnosis
		Readmission rate for asthma $<X\%$	

2. Productivity/Efficiency	Productivity Resource management	Number of office visits (compared with average) Patient care costs $X\%$ less than annualized capitation	
3. Interaction with patients	Responsiveness Attitude toward patients: • Sensitivity • Respect • Listening ability • Honesty Patient education	Response to calls: • Same day call return rate $X\%$ Patient satisfaction $>X\%$: • Staff ratings on patient interaction • Total patients' complaints $<X\%$ Participate in community health education events	Records Patient survey Staff survey
4. Interaction with colleagues and staff	Relationship with colleagues • Taking responsibility • Listening • Respect for colleagues Relationship with subordinates • Respect • Open to suggestions • Sensitivity • Honesty	Percentage of time taking calls Colleagues' opinions on responsibility Colleagues' opinions Subordinate/colleague/ supervisor opinions	Records Colleague questionnaire Questionnaires
5. Administrative duties			

ALOS, average length of stay; SD, standard deviation.

organization believes will be strong performers in the long run, whereas selection seeks to predict accurately whether the potential or actual recruits are likely to be strong performers.

2. Selection must be closely linked to performance evaluation, and it should take its direction from that function. This is a surprising statement to many, yet it represents a simple but critical element in the effective staffing of health care organizations. If the primary goal of selection is to predict accurately strong future performance, the criteria and measures used to select a candidate must closely reflect the criteria and measures that are deemed important in subsequently assessing the performance of that candidate, once he or she becomes an incumbent in the position. Yet, often there is very little correspondence between selection criteria and performance criteria for the same position. This is a critical mistake, and one that is easily correctable. To choose the appropriate selection criteria and

measures, look first to the criteria and measures used to assess performance in the position under consideration.

Selection must be viewed as an investment by the organization. As such, its benefits and costs must be carefully accounted for. The benefits of a correct decision and the costs of an incorrect decision must be well understood. These benefits and costs typically involve two primary elements:

1. The benefits or costs while the person is on the job. These involve the benefits (or costs) of higher (lower) performance, lower (higher) training costs, lower (higher) costs of performance evaluation and disciplinary measures, and higher (lower) morale on the part of the incumbent's co-workers.
2. The costs of turnover. Turnover costs are an ill-understood, often underestimated consequence of management decisions in general, and selection decisions in particular. These costs include the direct costs of recruiting a replacement, the opportunity cost of lost production from the position, and the opportunity cost of lost production from those involved in recruiting and selecting the replacement. (See Landau and Fogel [6] for a more detailed discussion of turnover costs.)

The general principle noted in the previous section, that performance evaluation is essentially an issue of measurement, also holds true for selection. Consequently, the guiding principles of measurement, reliability, and validity of the measures and measurement instruments are central to effective selection practices.

Effective selection is a matter of tapping the most important attributes of job performance, measuring the candidate's potential for strong performance on those attributes, and deciding whether the potential is sufficient to warrant continuing the recruitment process and eventually hiring the candidate. Addressing the selection function in this manner leads to a systematic approach to carrying out the function. First, determine the dimensions of job performance (from your performance evaluation system) that

are most important. Next, determine what measures—and sources of information—you will use to assess each candidate on each of those dimensions. Then, undertake a systematic evaluation of each potential candidate on each dimension and measure.

To implement this strategy effectively, you will need to have a good understanding of what standards you will impose—i.e., on each dimension and measure, what will be considered unacceptable, acceptable, and exemplary "scores"? It is also essential that all people involved in this assessment process have a consistent, uniform understanding of these standards, to ensure that the process is reliable across parties.

Selection Instruments—Simulating the Job

In considering the appropriate selection tools and instruments to use to evaluate a candidate, evaluators often fall back on the old saw, "The best predictor of performance is past performance." For the most part this is true, but it is not always the case. Most people have some memories of excellent teachers who do not make effective administrators, or outstanding physicians who do not make strong department heads, medical directors, or organizational executives. The most reliable way to ensure that the appropriate person is being selected for the position is to identify the critical performance measures of the position being recruited for, not the position a candidate held or currently holds.

This simple principle leads to a corollary principle in selecting the appropriate instrument(s) to evaluate a job candidate: find the selection instrument or method that allows you to predict most closely their performance in the job under consideration. To accomplish this, selection experts are increasingly turning to some form of job simulation. Simulating the demands of the position is hardly a new phenomenon. Many organizations have been using assessment centers and other such techniques to evaluate candidates—especially for internal promotion —for many years. Simulating a future job or employment situation is sometimes thought to be more difficult in the health care field, particularly in high-level clinical positions, but the trend toward "work sampling" is even occurring in this environment. Many organizations will now observe physician and nursing candidates in their current work environment, or engage in peer review of case records, or even invite the candidate to spend some time actually working in the recruiting organization. Although all the important dimensions of job performance cannot be assessed in this manner, it is good general practice to evaluate the candidate in an environment closely simulating their eventual position, if possible.

The Employment Interview

It is probably true that no single method of evaluating job candidates is so roundly criticized and yet so frequently used as the employment interview. The interview, particularly the unstructured interview, has consistently been found to be one of the least reliable and valid predictors of future job performance [7–9]. There are several reasons why it is invalid:

- It often confuses selection and recruitment—because these are often conflicting functions, it leads to a "schizophrenic" situation, for both evaluator and candidate.
- It is often unstructured and unfocused.
- Often the criteria and measures, as well as the standards of predicted performance, are not well or consistently understood across evaluators.

Although these problems are all too frequent, the interview does not have to suffer from them, and it can be a very effective and efficient way of both evaluating candidates and making sure they have a realistic view of the position and the work environment. A few tips can help improve the prospects of an effective interview:

- Make sure that the interview is structured, with specific questions or areas of inquiry clearly formulated and understood.
- Know the purpose of each question and section of the interview. This includes understanding whether the question is designed to evaluate

the candidate or help recruit him or her by providing a positive, realistic view of the job and work environment.
- Determine, a priori, among the various evaluators what is the standard for judgment, i.e., what is a good or bad response.
- Most importantly, make sure that the ultimate validity of the interview items is evaluated by assessing the correlation between future job performance and the candidate's "performance" on the interview.

Compensation

Compensation management has become an increasingly complex and sophisticated function in most health care organizations. Traditionally, the human resource management unit has provided consultation and advice to organizational executives. Although that is still the typical mode of operation, the increasingly complicated and legalistic environment has made it virtually imperative that a strong, sophisticated, compensation management team with considerable authority to review and even veto management decisions be available. As the following discussion documents, compensation management in today's health care environment is no place for amateurs. It is also true that any discussion of compensation within the space constraints of this chapter could not hope to do justice to the topic. Consequently, we offer below a discussion of some of the primary recent trends in compensation policy and management, and exhort the reader to ensure that his or her health care organization develops and maintains access—internally or externally through consultant groups—to a team of compensation experts that can keep pace with the fast-changing environment of health care staff compensation.

Outside Influences

Earlier in the chapter, we noted the importance of external factors and internal management values to effective human resource policy and practice. Nowhere is this truer than in compensation management. Externally, the plethora of laws and regulatory obligations has made the development and implementation of sound compensation policy a challenging, frustrating, but extremely important task. The following are but a sample of the federal laws and regulations that must be carefully understood and heeded in managing compensation:

- Fair Labor Standards Act (29 U.S.C. ~ 203(e)(1))
- Equal Pay Act (29 U.S.C. ~ 206)
- National Labor Relations Act (29 U.S.C. ~~ 151–197)
- Family and Medical Leave Act (Pub. L. no. 103–3)
- Employee Retirement and Income Security Act (29 U.S.C. ~~ 1001–1461)
- Title VII of the Civil Rights Act (42 U.S.C. ~~ 2000e-2000e-17)

In addition to these federal labor requirements, significant events have taken place in the health care world that have had an enormous impact on compensation policy and practice, e.g., the emergence of the Medicare Resource Based Relative Value System (RBRVS) has had as large an impact on physician compensation as the Medicare Diagnostic Related Groups (DRGs) had on overall hospital and medical care reimbursement in the mid-1980s. Inside the organization, the popularity of the TQM movement has posed a fundamental challenge to conventional compensation policy, and it would have had a huge effect on the factors that affect pay if one of its basic tenets—that pay should not be based on performance, but rather on other factors—had been embraced more fully throughout the industry. In sum, the compensation management is hardly the simple, unfettered domain of top management; instead, it is heavily influenced by federal health reimbursement policy, employment law, increasing health care competition, a transfer of risk from payer to deliverer, and a host of other external and management value-driven factors.

Direct Compensation

Compensation management is typically divided into direct and indirect compensation. Direct compensation refers to salary levels and structure, whereas indirect compensation refers to policies concerning benefits and other nonsalary compensation. Salary management in the health care organization, as in other industries, is typically driven by basic elements of the job—job descriptions, job analyses, job evaluation, and the pricing of jobs. For the most part, this job-based model has historically been an internal function, with the relationship between job pay levels set relative to other job sets in the organization. However, increasingly in health care, compensation policy is also driven by "market pricing" considerations, in which the salary levels in the health care organization are set in part by how the specific job in the health care unit relates to similar positions in other organizations in the relevant market, which could be local, regional, or national. This has become especially popular in occupations of high demand, such as some physician specialties, nurses, therapists, etc.). It has, in part, replaced simple "across the board" increases because tightly limited resource dollars must be distributed to ensure that the most difficult to replace human resources are protected. Highly sophisticated market surveys have become an institution in the field of clinician compensation; many health care networks now rely on these surveys as a primary determinant of clinician salary levels.

Another important factor affecting health care compensation is the increasingly fierce competition in the health care field. A corollary to this development has been the still growing popularity of capped reimbursement systems in which the risk has been transferred from payers to deliverers of care. These developments, in combination, have led to a growth in incentive pay mechanisms, especially for upper level clinicians and executives. There are two interesting elements to these incentive systems. First, they incorporate an interesting and more diversified mix of criteria as the basis for the incentives, as well as more creative ways of implementing them, e.g., direct incentives based on cost savings or utilization limits are much more common than they were a decade ago. In terms of methods, many clinics now impose a "set aside" or "hold-back" on physician compensation—and sometimes even revenue distribution to entire departments—with a portion of compensation held until the end of the fiscal year, and doled out on the basis of attainment of cost savings, utilization goals, and productivity objectives. The second interesting element is that more of the incentive systems are now based on group rather than individual performance. Entire departments of multispecialty clinics, for example, will be put on a cost-based incentive system, with internal allocation of the rewards either left to the departments themselves or formulated by central clinic administration. Either way, these systems are yet another example of the movement to distributing risk in a far more decentralizing way than was the case previously.

Benefits

The world of indirect compensation to clinicians has become far more complex over the last decade, with the vast array of legal and regulatory obligations that must be met. Nevertheless, benefits represent a growing area of compensation, even in the health care field which traditionally has ranked behind other industries in the importance of benefits to the total compensation package. Benefits were responsible for 36% of all health care compensation in the late 1990s [10].

A related development over the previous decade has been the increase in choice offered to employees in their benefit packages. "Cafeteria-style" benefit packages have become very popular, as a way of permitting employees to choose the portfolio of benefits of greatest use to them, given their individual situations, while at the same time holding the line on the costs of those benefits. Offering flexibility in medical insurance, in particular, has been a popular approach, given the number of multiple working person families in today's economy.

Still another popular development in benefits management has been the emergence of tax-deferred benefits. To some extent, this has come as a result of increasingly restrictive taxation policy, in which previously nontaxed benefits were challenged on the grounds that some employees were receiving nontaxed benefits that other employees had to pay with "after-tax dollars." Now, however, there are increasing examples of income deferral programs which permit employees to purchase various benefits, such as

health care and/or retirement annuities, with "before tax" dollars, thereby lowering their tax obligations. In the future, we can probably look toward an ongoing tension between a reduction in benefits (relative to direct pay) as more benefits are taxed, and a relative increase in benefits if more of them are offered on a "before-tax basis."

Conclusion

This chapter has documented the significant increase in the complexity of the human resource environment and the consequent need for increasing sophistication in the management of those human resources. Still, two very basic points made at the beginning of the chapter ring true:

1. First and foremost, human resource management is based on *common sense*. The common-sense principles of equity (actual and perceived) and fairness are still the cornerstones of human resource policy and practice.
2. Effective human resource management relies heavily on the development and implementation of *systems*—systems for managing human resources such that there is a consistency in approach, and systems for dealing with human resource problems in a consistent, fair, and timely way.

Many of the most important human resource functions involve measuring performance— current performance, predicting future performance, individual performance, and the performance of groups, such as departments, units (e.g., emergency rooms), or systems such as admissions or lab tests and communication of results. In this respect, they are very similar to other functions of health care organizations, which engage in diagnosis, disease management, and communication of results to highly interested parties.

The relationship between human resource management and other management and organizational goals must be remembered and addressed. Strategic decisions, such as mergers and consolidation, have profound impacts on the human resources of an organization; in turn, human resource decisions can have huge effects on the success of those strategic actions.

References

1. Fottler MD, Hernandez SR, Joiner CL. *Essentials of Human Resources Management in Health Services Organizations*. Albany, NY: Delmar Publishers, 1998.
2. Heneman HG III, Schwab DP, Fossum JA, Dyer LD. *Personnel—Human Resources Management*, 4th edn. Homewood, IL: Irwin Publishers, 1989.
3. Joiner CL, Hyde JC. Performance appraisals. In: Fottler MD, Hernandez SR, Joiner CL, eds. *Essentials of Human Resources Management in Health Services Organizations*. Albany, NY: Delmar Publishers, 1998: 223–47.
4. Lowe TR. Eight ways to run a performance review. *Personnel J* 1986; **65**(1): 60–2.
5. Ivancevich JM, Glueck WF. *Foundations of Personnel/Human Resource Management*, 3rd edn. Plano, TX: Business Publications, 1986.
6. Landau J, Fogel D. Selection and placement. In: Fottler MD, Hernandez SR, Joiner CL, eds. *Essentials of Human Resources Management in Health Services Organizations*. Albany, NY: Delmar Publishers, 1998: 166–96.
7. Heneman HG III, Heneman RL. *Staffing organizations*. Middleton, WI: Mendota House, 1992.
8. Dipoybe RL, Gaugler BB. Cognitive and behavioral processes in the selection interview. In: Schmitt N, Borman WC *et al.*, eds. *Personnel Selection in Organizations*, 1st edn. San Francisco: Jossey-Bass, 1993: 135–70.
9. Dipboye RL. *Selection Interviews: Process Perspectives*. Cincinnati: Southwestern Publishing, 1992: 150–80.
10. Joiner CL, Jones KN, Dye CF. Compensation management. In: Fottler MD, Hernandez SR, Joiner CL, eds. *Essentials of Human Resources Management in Health Services Organizations*. Albany, NY: Delmar Publishers, 1998: 248–70.

6

Competitive Strategy

Lawton R. Burns

Introduction: What is Competitive Strategy?

Competitive strategy is usually defined as a series of steps undertaken to outperform one's competitors in the marketplace or to earn supernormal returns compared with the industry. How the firm gets to this advantageous position is the subject of some debate, however. Many people believe strategy serves as a guide to the *future* direction, initiatives, and programs that the firm will pursue. This definition connotes deliberate, purposive behavior, i.e., the firm can consciously map out the opportunities and threats in its environment, design a course of action that matches these opportunities with its own internal strengths and capabilities, and take concrete steps to implement this course of action. To others, strategy is not so much deliberate as emergent, i.e., strategy represents an explanation of the firm's *past* actions, a post hoc interpretation of the firm's pattern of behavior that represents more incremental responses to environmental changes, serendipitous decisions, learning behavior, and innovation—none of which is specified or conceptualized in advance.

Each of these views has its limitations. On the one hand, the deliberate view of strategy suggests a formalized and somewhat mechanical process of assessing the firm's capabilities (e.g., strengths and weaknesses) and analyzing the firm's environment (e.g., opportunities and threats). This culminates in the well-known SWOT analysis which seeks alternative courses of action that match the former to the latter. However, the SWOT analysis provides no clue about the best course to choose and the best

means to implement it, and offers no opportunity for the firm to learn as it interacts with its environment. Moreover, it presumes that managers are good at assessing their firm's weaknesses as well as their strengths. On the other hand, the emergent view of strategy suggests a lack of central vision in the firm, which may lead to organizational drift at the least and financial disaster in times of crisis. Moreover, the learning approach to strategic decision-making is costly and time-consuming.

Which view of competitive success is correct? Both probably are, as Henry Mintzberg has argued [1,2]. Successful firms are both deliberate and adaptive, engaged in linear as well as nonlinear thinking, "planning to learn" as well as "learning to plan" [3]. Scholars of the organizational innovation process have similarly concluded that successful change requires an "ambidextrous organization" which can flexibly adjust between stable and disruptive routines. Management theorists interested in organizational structure and design have reached the similar conclusion that successful firms must balance the need to be simultaneously both centralized and decentralized, global and local, large and small [4–6].

Given this dual view, it is extremely difficult to teach executives how to "do strategy." The latter part of strategy is an intuitive and incremental process which involves learning, feedback from, and mutual adjustment to a changing market environment. It is in essence a creative process. To be sure, there are new theories of organizational learning and the "learning organization," but these are more concerned with how firms acquire new insights and information from their customers, markets, and fellow employees than with the formulation of competitive strategy. Consequently, the field of competitive strategy focuses more on its deliberate aspects, specifically with two analytic components: an assessment of external competition in the market, and an assessment of the firm's unique resources and capabilities which enable it to gain competitive advantage in this market.

Industry and Market Assessment

The field of competitive strategy owes much of its origin and rigor to the work of Michael Porter at the Harvard Business School [7,8]. An economist, Porter described how the economics of industries and market competition shape business strategy by their effects on industry profitability (and thus industry attractiveness to potential new entrants). The ability to earn excess profits in an industry is a siren song to investors and new entrants; however, new entrants will intensify competition and drive down any excess returns.

Porter classified the economic factors shaping industry profitability into five forces:

1. intensity of rivalry among incumbents in the industry
2. threat of substitute products
3. buyer power
4. supplier power
5. threat of new entrants into the industry.

For each of these forces, Porter asked: "Is it sufficiently strong to reduce or eliminate industry profits?" If the answer is yes, competitive pressures are likely to be quite strong, and thus the industry may be a less attractive arena in which to compete and/or deploy one's capital. If the answer is no (at least for some of the five forces), then industry conditions may confer market power on incumbents and serve as an external source of competitive advantage. Firms gain competitive advantage by exploiting weaknesses in the five forces in their industry structure, or by adopting strategies to modify these forces and reduce competitive pressures.

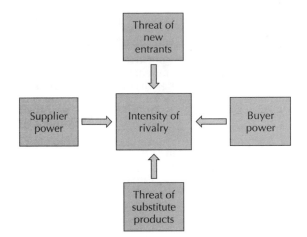

Figure 6-1. Porter's five forces model. (From Porter [7].)

Porter's five forces model is visually depicted in Fig. 6-1. At the center of the diagram is the intensity of rivalry among incumbents. This force is considered central, because the other four forces affect it. The other four forces also help to broaden the competitive analysis to include a value-chain perspective: what is the relative ability of players along the value chain (e.g., buyers, suppliers) to capture the value created in the industry?

Intensity of Rivalry

Rivals (incumbents) in an industry or market compete for market share. This competition is typically based on a combination of price and nonprice (e.g., quality) attributes of the products or services rendered. Three factors that promote this internal rivalry flow directly from market structure (Table 6-1). The simplest of these is the number of competitor firms. The greater the number, the more difficult it is for firms to coordinate their behavior and the more likely it is that any one firm will behave individualistically (e.g., lower price to grab more market share) and hope that others will not notice. Another factor, the heterogeneity of firms in the market, exerts a similar effect, making it difficult to coordinate firm behavior and increasing the uncertainty about what one's competitors might do. A third factor, the size distribution of firms in a market, can be measured in any number of ways. The two most popular methods are:

Table 6-1. Porter's "five forces" analysis: intensity of rivalry.

1. Number of competitors in market
2. Heterogeneity of competitors
3. Equal size distribution of competitors in market
4. Asset specificity
5. High fixed costs
6. Excess industry capacity
7. Variable demand
8. Product homogeneity
9. Low switching costs
10. Potential big savings in switching
11. Large infrequent sales orders
12. Invisible terms of sales transactions by others

1. the four-firm concentration ratio (total share accounted for by top four firms)
2. the Hirschman–Herfindahl Index or HHI (sum of the squared market shares of all firms in the market).

Internal rivalry increases as the market becomes less concentrated, i.e., as the top four firms account for a smaller percentage of total market share, or as firms in the market have more equal shares. The greater the equality of market share, the greater the likelihood of antagonism and direct rivalry among competitors. In such cases there is no dominant firm that leads and guides the behavior of others in the market.

Factors other than market structure can promote internal rivalry. A second set of factors stems from the industry's physical assets and capacity. One such factor is asset specificity, i.e., assets that are specific to that industry and cannot be used in other businesses. When the firm has such assets, it is rational to continue to deploy them in markets with relatively low returns, because they have few other uses. The assets thus have low opportunity costs; they also pose barriers to exit from the industry. For such reasons, specific assets promote greater internal rivalry. A related set of factors is the presence of high fixed costs and excess industry capacity. Under such conditions, there is an enormous emphasis on maximizing the use of one's physical capacity to gain short-term economies of scale. However, given the excess capacity there is a "volume-grubbing contest" to gain as much share as possible to fill your capacity. All of

these factors are accentuated to the degree that demand fluctuates and causes greater excess capacity in the face of high fixed costs.

A third set of factors that increase internal rivalry concerns product differentiation and the role of the consumer. Rivalry increases to the extent that consumers view the products as homogeneous. When products are homogenous, firms are left to compete only over price. Rivalry also increases when the consumer's cost of switching to competitors is low. Switching costs are low when products are nonspecialized, commodity items that require little effort to learn to use.

A final set of factors that can promote internal rivalry concerns the nature of the sales process itself. If sales are based on large, infrequent orders, then firms will compete more vigorously for contracts. Firms will also compete more vigorously if they cannot easily observe the terms of sales transactions by their competitors. This increases uncertainty and makes coordinated behavior more difficult.

Threat of Substitute Products/Services

Substitute products are defined as competition from related markets. This competition can come from products that serve the same function for the same set of customers. The extent of this competitive threat is measured by the cross-elasticity of demand, i.e., the change in the quantity demanded for one product based on a change in the price for a substitute product. The factors that increase the threat of substitution include the existence of close substitutes for the firm's product or service, the performance characteristics of these substitutes, the propensity of buyers to substitute, and the switching costs they face in doing so (Table 6-2).

Product substitution has several effects. First, it means that some firms gain market share whereas others lose it. Second, as a result, it intensifies internal rivalry over existing shares. Third, it influences the firm's ability to raise its prices or change its products. The threat of substitutes is especially keen in markets where there are few rivals, where demand is rising rapidly, and where it is difficult to increase industry supply (capacity) in the short term.

Table 6-2. Porter's "five forces" analysis: substitute products.

1. Existence of close substitutes for the product/service
2. Equivalent price-performance characteristics of substitutes
3. Propensity of buyers to substitute (their responsiveness to changes in relative prices)
4. Low switching costs faced by buyers

Buyer Power

Buyer power is defined as the ability of customers to (1) negotiate purchase prices that extract profits from the sellers or (2) influence the level of product quality. This ability hinges on two sets of conditions: the buyer's price sensitivity, and the buyer's bargaining power relative to the seller (Table 6-3).

The buyer's sensitivity to the seller's price motivates greater search behavior, tougher negotiating behavior, and greater switching behavior. Price sensitivity is associated with the proportion of the buyer's total cost accounted for by the seller's product, the profitability of the buyer's firm, and the intensity of competition among firms in the buyer's market. Price sensitivity will also be associated with low differentiation among the seller's products, low brand identity among these products, and a lower importance of the supplier's product to the quality of the buyer's product or service.

As with internal rivalry, the buyer's bargaining power depends partly on market structure. To the extent that buyers are concentrated, i.e., limited in number, they enjoy some bargaining power because they can threaten to shift their business to other sellers. Similarly, if the buyers have large size relative to sellers, buyers are relatively more powerful.

Another set of factors concerns product differentiation and the role of the consumer. If the products are standardized (undifferentiated), buyers face lower switching costs and thus enjoy relative power. If the transactions and transaction prices between sellers and buyers are open and visible, the buyer faces lower search costs, has more information, and enjoys more power. Moreover, the willingness of the buyer to shop

Table 6-3. Porter's "five forces" analysis: buyer power.

Buyers' *price sensitivity* is associated with:
1. Product cost is a big percentage of customer's total costs
2. Customer suffering from poor profitability
3. Intensity of competition among buyers
4. Low product differentiation
5. Lower importance of supplier's product to the quality of the buyer's product or service

Buyers' *relative bargaining power* is associated with:
1. Small number of buyers, each making large purchase
2. Buyers have large size relative to sellers
3. Products are standardized
4. Openness of transactions
5. Customers know their suppliers' costs
6. Degree of internal rivalry in seller industry
7. Customers have learned that supplier badly needs the business to soak up excess capacity
8. Sellers invest in relationships with buyers that locks in sellers
9. Buyers can integrate backwards

around for the best price increases the degree of internal rivalry among sellers. In addition, if the buyers know the sellers' costs and/or know that sellers badly need the business to soak up excess capacity, then buyers enjoy greater power.

A third set of factors that increases buyer bargaining power concerns vertical exchange relationships with sellers. If sellers invest in relationships with buyers that lock in the sellers ("relationship-specific assets"), buyers enjoy an advantage. If buyers have the potential to integrate backwards into the sellers' business and obviate any contracting with sellers, the buyers enjoy bargaining power.

Supplier Power

Supplier power is essentially the opposite of buyer power. It is defined as the ability of input suppliers to negotiate prices that extract profits from their customers. The relative bargaining power of suppliers rests partially on the suppliers' market structure (Table 6-4). Suppliers enjoy power to the degree that there are a few large suppliers that account for most of the supplier market (concentrated supplier market), and whose size exceeds that of their customers.

Table 6-4. Porter's "five forces" analysis: supplier power.

Suppliers' *relative bargaining power* is associated with:
1. Small number of suppliers, each making large sales
2. Suppliers have large size relative to buyers
3. Low standardization of products
4. Low amount of open information
5. Buyers are locked into relationship-specific investments
6. No credible threat of backward integration by buyers
7. Some credible threat of suppliers to integrate forwards

Table 6-5. Porter's "five forces" analysis: threat of new entrants.

1. Few economies of scale
2. Low capital requirements of getting established in industry
3. Small learning curve effects
4. Product homogeneity
5. Few pioneering brand advantages
6. Few marketing advantages of incumbents
7. Unrestricted access to channels of supply/distribution
8. Low governmental barriers
9. Low legal barriers
10. Low costs of exit that encourage entry
11. Little threat of retaliation by incumbents

Supplier power also depends on low product standardization (high product differentiation), low amounts of open information and visible transactions, and thus higher switching costs for customers. Finally, supplier power over customers increases to the extent that customers make relationship-specific investments in contracting with certain suppliers, and to the extent that suppliers can credibly integrate forward into the customers' market.

Threat of New Entrants

New entrants erode the profits earned by firms in an industry in two ways: first, by stealing business and dividing up market share among a greater number of firms; second, by decreasing market concentration, intensifying internal rivalry, and reducing profit margins.

A number of conditions may foster the threat of new entry (Table 6-5). The first is the absence of economies of scale, or the ability to achieve them with a small organization. Low economies of scale mean that a new entrant can quickly gain the minimum scale or market share needed to be an efficient producer. Low economies of scale are typically found in more labor-intensive industries that have a high variable cost component. As volume or output rises, there are minimal economies to be reaped. A second, related factor is low capital requirements for getting established in an industry. Labor-intensive industries typically have divisible (rather than indivisible) capital requirements, such that a new entrant

can make the technological investments needed to efficiently produce even at a small scale of production. A third, related factor is the absence of strong learning-curve benefits accruing to firms that accumulate experience with the product/service as the volume grows. The slope of the learning curve, which reflects decreasing production costs as aggregate output volume rises, is typically flatter in more labor-intensive industries.

Another set of factors that can increase the threat of new entrants deals with product characteristics and branding. If there is little product differentiation, new entrants face fewer obstacles in overcoming the customer loyalty enjoyed by incumbent firms. If incumbents have pioneered few branding advantages, there is likely to be less customer investment in existing products, less customer risk avoidance toward new firms in the industry, fewer potential costs to the customer of purchasing from a new entrant, and lower overall customer uncertainty which might favor familiar incumbents over unfamiliar new entrants. Finally, if incumbents enjoy fewer marketing advantages (e.g., umbrella branding of their products), new entrants face lower advertising costs and overall costs of new product introduction.

The threat of new entry is also likely to be greater when incumbents have not developed preferential and/or long-term contracts with suppliers and customers that limit or crowd channel access. New entry is also more likely when governmental barriers to entry are low (e.g., low licensing costs, low regulatory compliance costs), when legal barriers are weak (e.g., patents), where exit costs are low (e.g., low asset specificity, low failure rates), and where incumbents are not known to retaliate aggressively toward new entrants.

Overall Impact of Five Forces

The joint effect of the five forces is hard to estimate. All five forces may not point in the same direction at the same time (e.g., buyer power may be strong but supplier power may be weak). Moreover, those forces that do point in a consistent direction may exert multiplicative rather than additive effects (e.g., buyer power in the presence of strong internal rivalry). In addition, the relative importance of the specific factors associated with each force is unknown and will vary from one industry to another.

Collectively, however, the five forces account for a substantial share of the variability in industry profitability. In a recent analysis, McGahan and Porter decomposed the variation in profits for 12,296 business segments in 628 different industries over a 14-year period (1981–94) [9]. They found that industry-level effects (such as those embodied in the five forces) explained 19% of the variation. By contrast, business-specific (firm-level) effects explained a much larger 32% of the variation. Other researchers have reported similar findings about the relative importance of firm-level and industry-level effects, although the differential may be even wider [10]. Nevertheless, McGahan and Porter report that the effects of industry are stronger in the service sector (such as health care). In a subsequent article, they also find that industry-level effects on profitability attenuate more slowly over time than firm-level effects [11]. Thus, industry factors explain a considerable portion of the variability in a firm's profits and exert a more enduring influence on these profits.

Competitive Positioning

Given the overall assessment of these five forces, the firm is in a position to identify its strengths and weaknesses relative to the industry, i.e., relative to the causes underlying the five competit-

ive forces, e.g., how strong is the firm compared to substitutes or potential new entrants? As the answers to such questions will differ for each firm in each industry, there is no discussion here of this assessment. What is important to note is that the firm gauges its strengths and weaknesses relative to the five forces, and does not mindlessly engage in an assessment of "what we are good at and not so good at doing".

Once this assessment has been completed, Porter suggests three avenues that might be undertaken. First, the firm can engage in a defensive strategy to position itself against the five forces. Here, industry and market conditions are taken as given and immutable, and the firm seeks either to find a position it can exploit in the industry where the forces are weakest or to build its defenses against forces considered the strongest. Second, the firm can undertake a more offensive-minded strategy to alter some of the factors underlying the five forces in the firm's favor, e.g., firms can undertake mergers and acquisitions that reduce the number of competitors in the market and potentially increase power over both buyers and suppliers. Third, the firm can seek to anticipate shifts in these underlying factors and exploit the changes occurring in the industry or market.

These three avenues are not easy. As competitive pressures intensify across industries, finding and then exploiting weaknesses become more difficult. In addition, changes in technology and consumer demand (e.g., web-based technology, use of the Internet) break down traditional industry divisions and create the potential for new entry by firms that can take advantage of these changes. The firms that may be best situated to take advantage are those that have not invested in traditional technologies, because such investments may be a barrier to adaptation. Finally, forecasting changes in the environment is subject to enormous error [2].

Porter described some "generic strategies" that the firm could pursue to position and defend itself against these five forces and outperform other firms over the long term. These generic strategies include low-cost leadership, product/service differentiation, and focus on occupying a particular market niche. The low-cost leader approach can rest on a number of factors, including economies of scale, heavy capital investment, large market share, learning curve advantages, and tight cost control. The product differentiation strategy rests on a number of dimensions, including branding, design advantages, customer service advantages, technological sophistication, product features, and channel advantages. Finally, the focused approach rests on serving a particular niche of the market well, and much better than a generalized producer can. In this manner, the focused firm achieves either a low-cost or product differentiation advantage in dealing with one small segment of the market.

To be sure, there are multiple requirements to pursuing these generic strategies. Porter states that their implementation requires different resources and skills, but his work is not as thorough in describing what these resources and skills are. This discussion is critical, because it really informs an analysis of what the firm's real strengths and weaknesses are in dealing with the external opportunities and threats posed (and identified) by analysis of the five forces.

Fortunately, several new streams of thinking in competitive strategy have emerged which focus on the internal requirements needed to confront the five forces. The key stream of thinking, and the one considered here, is the "resource-based view" of the firm. According to this school of thought, the principal basis of strategy is the firm's bundle of unique resources and capabilities that can achieve competitive advantage. These resources and capabilities underlie Porter's generic strategies, and they may even serve as the foundation behind some of the five forces (e.g., source of entry barriers).

There are thus two sources of competitive advantage. On the one hand, the analysis of the five forces, the identification of opportunities and weaknesses in the industry structure, and the subsequent development of generic strategies to deal with them define an external source of competitive advantage for firms that can exploit them. On the other hand, the firm's resources and capabilities serve as an internal source of competitive advantage to the degree that competitors do not share them. Thus, while Porter emphasizes similar (generic) strategies that firms undertake to deal with common industry conditions, the resource-based view emphasizes the differences

among firms in their resources and capabilities that can be exploited.

Assessment of the Firm's Resources and Capabilities

What are resources and capabilities? Drawing on Grant, resources consist of tangible, intangible, and human resource stocks which the firm has accumulated and developed over time [12]. Capabilities are bundles of skills and knowledge, embodied in and exercised through organizational routines and processes, which tie these resources together and deploy them in productive ways.

Organizational Resources

Tangible resources include both financial resources (e.g., balance sheet strength, financial ratios, internal revenue generation, credit rating) and physical resources (scale of plant, age of equipment, technological sophistication, flexibility in the use of plant and equipment for alternate purposes, reserves of raw materials). In gauging the strategic value of these resources, managers should consider what opportunities there are for more efficient use of these assets and/or for employing them in more productive venues.

Intangible resources encompass stocks of proprietary technology and intellectual capital (e.g., patents), infrastructure to support innovation (e.g., research facilities, technical and scientific expertise, research and development [R&D] staff), organizational culture, and the firm's reputation or brand image. *Human* resources encompass the motivation and commitment of employees, their training and skill levels, their interpersonal and team process skills, and their ability to adapt.

Resources do not automatically confer competitive advantage. Some resources are less easily duplicated or acquired by competitors than other resources, e.g., the firm's culture or employee loyalty develops over time in ways that are not easily understood by outside firms. They are not to be appropriated by competitors simply by hiring away employees from the firm. In addition, resources need to be coordinated internally

—either overtly by management or through organizational processes—in order to be productive. That is how firms develop capabilities.

Organizational Capabilities

Capabilities refer to the firm's capacity for undertaking some productive activity [12]. This requires the integration of resources, skills, and knowledge. The key managerial challenge involves the integration of skills and knowledge within and across employees. The former is accomplished through specialization and the division of labor, the latter through rules and routines. Rules and routines tie human resources together in productive ways. Rules—guidelines, protocols, directives—transfer and integrate explicit specialized knowledge across the firm. Routines involve teams of individuals undertaking a sequence of closely coordinated activity [13]. They are based on the firm's tacit knowledge, which is invisibly embedded in teamwork and interpersonal processes in the organization, and they are resistant to formalization. Capabilities thus tend to focus on the firm's ability (1) to coordinate and manage activities and (2) to learn.

There are several approaches for defining and classifying a firm's capabilities. Most researchers define capabilities in comparison to other firms. Thus, the presence of capabilities denotes strategic differences from one's competitors in terms of what each knows how to do well. As with individuals, firms cannot excel at everything they do; they have a limited stock of productive knowledge. Management researchers refer to this condition as *bounded rationality*. Resources and capabilities are thus to the firm what skills and human capital are to the employee. Hamel and Pralahad further distinguished "core capabilities" as those that make a disproportionate contribution to customer value or to the efficiency with which that value is achieved [14]; core capabilities provide a basis for entering new markets.

Another approach is to examine the functional areas of the firm and identify the capabilities that may be critical for performance and competitive position. In the firm's marketing area, these capabilities may consist of brand promotion and management, listening to customers, customer service, and gauging demographic trends and tastes. In the firm's manufacturing division, these capabilities may consist of efficient production, ability to mass customize, and continuous quality improvement skills. In the firm's research and development division, these capabilities may include the ability to innovate, the ability to exploit new technology, the speed of product development, and the ability to partner with other firms in new product development.

This last point introduces a newly identified set of capabilities dealing with the firm's ability to learn from other firms in its environment. This capability derives from the costs and uncertainties of developing capabilities. As McEvily and Zaheer have recently argued, acquiring capabilities involves uncertainty about the value of the capability and the benefits it bestows on the firm [15]. Firms are advantaged by having networks of knowledgeable contacts that can provide reliable information about the options for enhancing competitive capabilities, information on the costs and benefits they entail, and even access to some of the capabilities themselves through strategic alliances. To the degree that competitors do not participate, this networking behavior and the alliances they spawn constitute a "relational capability." This can also be viewed as a capability to collaborate, i.e., to create and transfer useful knowledge through interorganizational networks. The richness and uniqueness of the firm's external network ties become another source of firm heterogeneity and thus competitive advantage.

Assessing Resources and Capabilities

Once the resources and capabilities of the firm are identified, the manager must evaluate their potential for earning above-average profits in the industry (what strategy theorists call "rents"). These rents are a function of three factors. The first factor is the extent of the competitive advantage that they bestow. As with organizational power, the extent of competitive advantage is based on two attributes of the resources and capabilities: they are in scarce supply in the industry and they are important desired characteristics of success [16].

The second factor is the sustainability of the competitive advantage. Sustainability is based on the durability, immobility, and nonreplicability of the resources and capabilities. Durability reflects the productive lifespan of the assets and thus the length of time that profits can accrue. Immobility reflects the difficulty that competitors face in buying or otherwise transferring these assets. Such difficulties may exist because the assets are firm specific (e.g., brand reputation), decline in value after transfer (e.g., hiring away of executive talent), or are subject to incomplete information. Non-replicability reflects the difficulty that competitors face in trying to build or develop the assets on their own. These difficulties reside in the complex organizational systems, cultures, interpersonal networks, and processes that are needed to make the assets productive, but are not visible and understandable to outside firms. Researchers refer to these capabilities as "sticky" in nature, because they are not easily exchanged or transferred.

The third factor is the appropriability of the competitive advantage. This appropriability is itself a function of: the property rights associated with the assets (i.e., is there clear intellectual property?), the embeddedness of the resources in organizational routines not easily understood by outsiders, and the firm's ownership claim to these assets over the individual employee (such that employees cannot take the assets with them when they leave the firm).

Creating Strategies to Exploit Resources and Capabilities

Although the Porter five forces analysis suggests where the firm should compete, the resource-based view of the firm suggests how it should compete. Porter's model indicates what industries or market segments might be attractive to enter by virtue of offering defensible cost positions, differentiation positions, or niche positions. The source of these defensible positions (the source of Porter's generic strategies) is, however, the set of resources and capabilities possessed by the firm. Strategy is thus concerned with matching the firm's resources and capabilities to the opportunities presented by the external environment (industry, market). This argument

has most recently been made by Shoemaker and Amit [17]. To the degree that the environment is changing, resources and capabilities provide a more solid foundation for the firm's long-term strategy [12].

Strategy is thus bounded by the structure of competition within the firm's industry and markets, which suggests some positions to occupy. But, within these bounds, strategy and strategic decision-making consist of a "war of movement" between firms engaged in developing resources and capabilities that confer competitive advantage. The building blocks of competitive strategy, then, are not the firm's products or services but rather the firm's business processes and infrastructure. For Porter, these processes and infrastructure enable the firm to pursue one of three generic strategies: be the low-cost producer; develop differentiated (new) products and services; or identify and serve niche markets. For others, these processes and infrastructure enable firms to develop three "value disciplines" (similar to strategies) that maximize different types of customer value: operational excellence (e.g., low price and dependability), customer responsiveness (e.g., customized product, personalized service), and performance superiority (high technical performance, innovation) [18]. Each type of strategy rests on a distinctive stock of resources and capabilities that firms need to develop leverage.

Competitive advantage rests partly on the stocks of resources and capabilities with which a firm is endowed. Such endowments reflect either favorable conditions at the firm's founding or the firm's historical development ("path-dependent" capabilities), and are thus not amenable to imitation and appropriation. In addition to being historically endowed, firms must give their resources and capabilities leverage to gain competitive advantage. According to Hamel and Pralahad [14], resources can be given leverage by *concentrating* them on specific goals, *linking* them with complementary resources and capabilities for synergistic effects, *conserving* them by recycling them for other uses (similar to economies of scope) or co-opting them from other firms via trading alliances, or *recovering* them to achieve quicker returns on investment by reducing cycle times [12].

A growing number of strategy researchers now focus on the firm as a bundle of processes. Ghoshal and Bartlett argue that these processes include managerial entrepreneurship, sharing knowledge and skills across the firm's dispersed operations, and continuous renewal of the firm and its operations [5]. In a related vein, Szulanski emphasizes the capability of transferring knowledge and best practices within the firm [19,20].

Dynamic View of Resources and Capabilities

Finally, it is important to view the firm's resources and capabilities in dynamic rather than static terms. As mentioned earlier, the presence of superior economic returns attracts new entrants to an industry or segment, which will increase internal rivalry and may drive down profits. The firm's competitive advantage is continually subject to erosion by rivals and new entrants by virtue of the fact that they respond to the firm's strategy. They might seek to imitate or appropriate the firm's capabilities, or they might innovate and develop new resources and capabilities of their own that establish a new source of competitive advantage.

Given this fact of life, the firm can either try to erect barriers to imitation, which impede competitors from appropriating its competitive advantage, or decide to continually invest in developing new resources and capabilities. Barriers to imitation include intellectual property and patents, retention of key personnel, and embedded resources in internal teams or external network ties. The process of resource renewal includes investment in research and development, upgrading existing abilities with continuous quality improvement techniques, acquiring/investing/partnering with other firms, and developing the firm's infrastructure.

Conclusion

In sum, competitive strategy involves both deliberate and nondeliberate elements. The former is typically referred to as strategic planning; the latter is called organizational learning. This chapter

has focused on the former, but has discussed learning in so far as it develops into an organizational capability, i.e., team-based interpersonal activities that promote the sharing of information and knowledge.

Strategic planning requires both an external, environmental analysis of industry conditions and an internal assessment of the firm's resources and capabilities. The former highlights the "where" of competitive advantage by suggesting weaknesses and opportunities in industry structure that the firm might exploit. The latter highlights the "how" of competitive advantage by identifying the unique routines and processes (capabilities) within the firm that coordinate its resources to exploit industry weaknesses and opportunities. This matching process is not a simple comparison of (1) the firm's strengths and weaknesses with (2) the environment's opportunities and threats, as SWOT analysis proposes. Rather, it is based on a rigorous analysis of industry conditions using Porter's five forces analysis and an assessment of the firm's capabilities relative to both these forces and its competitors' capabilities.

References

1. Mintzberg H. Strategy formation. Schools of thought. In: Frederickson JW, ed. *Perspectives on Strategic Management*. New York: Harper Business, 1990: 105–235.
2. Mintzberg H. *The Rise and Fall of Strategic Planning*. New York: Free Press, 1994.
3. Brews PJ, Hunt MR. Learning to plan and planning to learn: Resolving the planning school/learning school debate. *Strategic Manage J* 1999; **20**: 889–913.
4. Collins JC, Porras JI. *Built to Last*. New York: Harper Business, 1994.
5. Ghoshal S, Bartlett CA. Changing the role of top management: Beyond structure to process. *Harvard Business Rev* 1995; **73**(1): 86–96.
6. Burns LR. Polarity management. The key challenge for integrated health systems. *J Healthcare Manage* 1999; **44**(1): 14–31.
7. Porter ME. *Competitive Strategy*. New York: Free Press, 1980.
8. Porter ME. *Competitive Advantage*. New York: Free Press, 1985.
9. McGahan AM, Porter ME. How much does industry matter really? *Strategic Manage J* 1997; **18**. 15–30.

10. Brush TH, Bromiley P, Hendrickx M. The relative influence of industry and corporation on business segment performance: An alternative estimate. *Strategic Manage J* 1999; **20**: 519–47.
11. McGahan AM, Porter ME. The persistence of shocks to profitability. *Rev Economics Statistics* 1999; **81**(1): 143–53.
12. Grant RM. *Contemporary Strategy Analysis*, 3rd edn. Malden, MA: Blackwell Publishers, 1998.
13. Nelson R, Winter S. *An Evolutionary Theory of Economic Change*. Cambridge, MA: Belknap Press, Harvard University Press, 1982.
14. Hamel G, Pralahad CK. *Competing for the Future*. Boston, MA: Harvard Business School Press, 1994.
15. McEvily B, Zaheer A. Bridging ties. A source of firm heterogeneity in competitive Capabilities, *Strategic Manage J* 1999; 20: 1133–56.
16. Thompson JD. *Organizations in Action*. New York: McGraw-Hill, 1967.
17. Shoemaker PJH, Amit R. The competitive dynamics of capabilities: Developing strategic assets for multiple futures. In: Day GS, Reibstein DJ, eds. *Wharton on Dynamic Competitive Strategy*. New York: Wiley, 1997: 368–94.
18. Day GS. Maintaining the competitive edge. Creating and sustaining advantages in dynamic competitive markets. In: Day GS, Reibstein DJ, eds. *Wharton on Dynamic Competitive Strategy*. New York: Wiley 1997: 48–75.
19. Szulanski G. *Intra-firm Transfer of Best Practices Project*. Fontainebleau: INSEAD, 1994.
20. Szulanski G. Exploring internal stickiness. Impediments to the transfer of best practice within the firm. *Strategic Manage J* 1996; **17**(Winter Special Issue): 27–43.

7

Personal Behavior in Medical Management

Charles C. Lobeck

Unacceptable behavior by physician executives will, at the very least, reduce their effectiveness, and it often leads to dismissal or reassignment. As disciplinary actions can be disguised as changes for "personal" reasons, such as the desire to "return to clinical work," their numbers are hard to track. The author's own long experience in academic medical management suggests that this type of "career change" is more common than we might assume.

This chapter presents some of the most common elements of personal behavior and their effects on the organization. It is important for the medical executive to know what constitutes unacceptable behavior and why it is unacceptable. The science of business administration emphasizes how we manage an organization, and exhibit the values, political sense, and vision to be an effective leader. It does not dwell on the importance of the personal behaviors of the executive that can enhance his or her effectiveness or indeed destroy it.

Further, the fact that the executive is a physician complicates the picture. Medical training and custom set boundaries between professional and nonprofessional conduct. A physician in the clinic knows the limits that will be tolerated in the presence of patients and usually behaves accordingly. When the patient is not present, or is not conscious, behavior may change dramatically. Physicians who become managers and leaders may not understand the need to maintain a constant professional demeanor in their new role.

Determination of Personal Behavior

There is no need to emphasize to health professionals the importance of genetics and early life influences on behavior. Parents, peers, and community acting on our genetic templates are the major determinants of our personalities. In adulthood, our professional education teaches us many new behaviors associated with our profession.

Medical and health professional students are a highly selected group. All are very bright and have a reputation of integrity and a desire to help and care for people. In the US, they are assumed by the public to have great power because of their special knowledge and skills. They increasingly represent both sexes and many cultural minorities. As they mature they develop a personal style that becomes an important attribute of their personality. They bring this to their executive position.

Style

Personal style can be defined as the way a person does his or her work. Style itself should echo the important characteristics that the manager wishes to instill in the organization. Our styles are closely observed and sometimes emulated by employees. To some extent, personal style is immutable and a fundamental part of the personality, but it can be modulated at the margins. Some important issues deserve emphasis.

Dress and Grooming

> Toughness doesn't have to come in pinstripe suits.
> Dianne Feinstein

Dress and grooming are often overemphasized as an indicator of professionalism, but they are still important determinants of the tone of an office. Employees often assume that the dress and appearance of the physician executive set the limits for their own dress and grooming. Informal dress by an executive may make a personal statement about wanting to be approachable, but it also reduces the appearance of professionalism and promotes informal attitudes in the organization. There are no hard-and-fast rules on dress, but its importance to the atmosphere of an office should be recognized as a controllable element.

Language

> Proper words in proper places, make the true definition of a style.
> Jonathan Swift

The choice of words and the way they are used by the physician executive is another important component of style. The use of titles when addressing colleagues or employees creates a barrier of formality that is not now in vogue, but it serves to keep a distance between employees and executives. Although titles promote formality, they are often pleasing to the person being addressed. Allowing your own title to be used is often a way of demonstrating respect for the position, not just yourself.

The way in which members of the organization address one another has an important effect on personal relationships. The use of nicknames for people below the level of the executive can be perceived as a power play. They should be used carefully. Crude language should be avoided if one wants to maintain respect and credibility. Even though unrefined language may be used by many employees, executives should realize that their own use of language is more likely to be emulated by others.

Humor: The Most Important Element of Style

> If you lose the power to laugh, you lose the power to think.
> Clarence Darrow

Perhaps the most important element of personal style is the proper use of humor. Humor is an action tending to cause laughter. It should not be used solely to attract attention. At its best, it makes the listeners and observers feel good. If the humor does not have an ulterior motive, such as exposing another's weaknesses, it will demonstrate an informality and a desire to increase laughter and reduce tension.

The executive is often the butt of humor in the office, especially when he or she is not present. This should be taken as one of the prices of leadership. Knowing which personal qualities are considered humorous may lead to examination of correctable personal attributes.

Sometimes it is assumed that humor about ethnicity, sex, race, or handicap is permissible when no one with the referred to characteristics is present. This is not true; such humor reveals the speaker's prejudices, and it will not be forgotten by listeners when they are in other situations. This principle holds true even when the executive makes humorous remarks about his or her own ethnicity, race, or sex.

Style: Not Synonymous with Integrity

> Do not speaketh one thing and privily meaneth another.
> Castiglione

Some people still believe that style and integrity are synonymous. This is regularly proven wrong. Style is how the work of the executive gets done; it is not the sole indication of underlying character. Everyday behavior is far more important than appearance in promoting an image of integrity. Style cannot substitute for integrity.

These remarks about personal style are not exhaustive. The elements of style interact in complex ways that a good physician executive learns to adjust over time. They should always reflect underlying integrity.

Personal Actions and Environmental Factors That Can Determine Success in the Organization

There are some conditions in the workplace which, coupled with personal actions, can make or break the career of the physician executive. Many of these are not discussed in the literature because they are considered self-evident and, in some cases, immutable, but their importance is undeniable and they should be mentioned.

Everyone is Watching. Nowhere to Hide

> There is only one thing in the world worse than being talked about, and that is not being talked about.
> Oscar Wilde

The power of an executive position makes constant observation by employees axiomatic. In the clinic, there are so many health professionals that personal idiosyncrasies are often overlooked, but in the office of a health care organization the style of the physician executive stands out. As with parents who try without success to hide their natural behavior from their children, executives find it impossible to hide their own characteristics from peers and employees. A health professional who engages in abusive, dishonest, or intemperate behavior will be evaluated harshly.

The Gatekeeper or Confidant(e)

> You see but do not observe.
> Sir Arthur Conan Doyle

It is important to have a gatekeeper or confidant, a person in the workplace who will alert the executive to how he or she is being perceived in the office. Information received in this way can often reveal areas in which executives should modify their behavior. It is also important to have some information about office morale and the personal problems of others, and a confidant(e) can help keep the executive informed. Paradoxically, it is not a bad idea to be the last to know about office love affairs and the behavioral abnormalities of co-workers. There is a very fine line between prying into the affairs of others and useful observation.

Confidentiality and Secrets

> If you do not want another to tell your secrets, you must not tell them yourself.
> Seneca

Confidences cannot be kept when physician executives are unable to keep their own secrets. It is funny to see how fast information spreads through an organization after it has been told in confidence to a single colleague. This is not to say that no one keeps confidences; close assistants of the executive are usually very responsible. It is the executive who is most likely to leak the information.

The rules of confidentiality learned in the clinic usually allowed information about patients to be shared with a professional colleague in order to get another opinion. In the office of the health care organization this cannot be done, mainly because information there concerns personnel or business operations.

Sex Issues

> The principle which regulates the existing social relations between the two sexes—the legal subordination of one sex to the other—is wrong in itself, and now one of the chief hindrances to human improvement; and . . . it ought to be replaced by a principle of perfect equality, admitting no power or privilege on the one side, nor disability on the other.
> John Stuart Mill in 1869

No area of personal behavior is more important or dangerous than that related to sex. Personal attraction between people who work together daily happens in every organization and should be accepted as a norm. If the attraction results in a sexual liaison, however, the power relationships in the workplace are always changed.

If executives understand that sexual attractions in the office are unavoidable, they should also recognize how explosive for morale their consummation can be. Sexual relationships cannot be kept secret for long. The example of the actions in the White House by President Clinton is a good one. Though his actions did not lead to dismissal or career change, they undermined his effectiveness.

A common set of sex issues are those related to touching, e.g., in some offices hugging as a form of greeting is common and seemingly innocuous, but even this can be interpreted as power play. The most cautious path is to avoid intimate physical contact with employees so that there can be no ambiguity about relationships. This is difficult to do when the executive wishes to be responsive and warm, but the danger is always there. Of course, overt sexual behavior is one of the quickest routes to trouble. Every office sexual affair that I have observed has had serious consequences.

The use of proper terminology for the sexes is increasingly important. Avoiding "girl" and "boy" and sensitivity to Ms, Mrs, and Dr titles are important. Again, having a confidant(e) will help the executive to know when he or she is using an incorrect title.

Sexual harassment is beyond the scope of this discussion, except that seemingly innocuous sex references and behaviors can be the beginning of a formal complaint.

Omnipotence

> It is difficult to esteem a man as high as he wishes to be esteemed.
> Vauvenargues

Many executives develop a very high opinion of themselves. This "ego trip" almost always accompanies high executive office. It provides a measure of the confidence and security needed to make decisions affecting an entire organization. It also has its dangers.

A feeling of self-importance can lead to a perception that the rewards of the position are insufficient. This can lead to misuse of funds, embezzlement, or other major violations of organizational rules. Stealing from the organization and misusing privileges have led to the dismissal of many executives.

Alcohol and Drug Intoxication

> An effective and widely available solvent of the super-ego is alcohol.
> Anonymous

As every physician knows, intoxication with alcohol or other drugs presents a complex problem. The alcoholic is expert at hiding his or her condition, and some of the more difficult personnel decisions are those that arise from the suspicion of alcoholism or drug dependence.

Chronic alcoholism is beyond the scope of this discussion, but there are other ways in which intoxication can become a problem for physician executives. Office parties present a common danger. The opportunity to relieve tension and to lower barriers of formality with colleagues and employees can be welcome, but intoxication can lead to disaster. The spur-of-the-moment statement or evanescent sexual attraction will be closely observed, and in the worst cases it will damage the executive's career.

Guarding against impulsive behavior caused by intoxication in the workplace is difficult. In the workplace, drinking and drug use are usually apparent to all. It is necessary to control one's personal behavior in order to have the credibility to take action with those who have a pathological drug or alcohol problem. Of course, the same is true, in the modern world, for smoking tobacco. One cannot enforce "no smoking" rules if they surreptitiously smoke themselves. As a result of the residual odors on clothing and other evidence, this is never a secret.

Ageism and Other Distinctions

> Youth is a blunder; manhood a struggle; old age a regret.
> Disraeli

Subtle distinctions made between people of differing ages, handicaps, races, and religions are common in the workplace. Age is the least well known of these discriminations. The physician executive is often tempted to consider age when dealing with colleagues and employees. It takes considerable introspection to recognize this bias. This kind of discrimination is much less publicized than sex, race, or religious prejudice, but it can cause loss of credibility for the executive.

Conclusion

The preceding review could be filled with anecdotes from my 35 years of experience. I can attest to having observed all of these behaviors during my career as dean of a medical school and departmental chair. Often they left me puzzled as to how those involved could have done such things. Disasters in the careers of otherwise superb managers could have been avoided by observing the cautions presented in this chapter. Many of these people are still active in academic medicine or medical management, but they have had major career setbacks.

Executives must be sensitive to the workplace environment and must avoid secretive behaviors, however, innocuous. That "no one will ever know" is never the case. I have often been amazed at the surprise shown by physician executives when they are reprimanded for a serious behavioral lapse. This is probably the result of the fact that much of their behavior is intuitive and comes from their clinical experience. Perhaps being a physician desensitizes executives to the need for professional behavior.

It strikes me as important to discuss these problems thoroughly with physicians during their education for management careers. They should not be viewed as abnormal behaviors, but as aberrations of normal behavior. The style of the medical manager, coupled with how his or her integrity holds up in personal dealings, will, I believe, become a major determinant of success.

Nothing in this discussion is meant to detract from the importance of analyzing how organizations are structured, how they are led, and how they get work done. The issues discussed in this chapter complement the leadership studies of most authors [1,2], are clearly important to the organizational environment [3], and play a major role in the recruitment and retention of personnel. The point is that even the most skilled and motivated managers and leaders can lose their positions because of errors in behavior, a tragedy that should not happen.

References

1. Badaracco JL, Ellsworth RR. *Leadership and the Quest for Integrity*. Boston, MA: Harvard Business School Press, 1989.
2. Kotter JP. *A Force for Change: How leadership differs from management*. New York: The Free Press, 1990.
3. Pierce JL, Dunham RB. *Managing*. Glenview, IL: Scott Foresman/Little Brown Higher Education, 1990.

8

Health Care Accounting and Finance

Mark A. Covaleski

Introduction to Financial Accounting

Financial accounting information is the result of a process of identifying, measuring, recording, and communicating the economic events of an organization (business or nonbusiness) to interested users of the information. This information is summarized and presented in three important financial statements: the balance sheet, the income statement, and the statement of cash flows. As these statements communicate financial information about an enterprise, accounting is often called "the language of business." An understanding of financial statements provides the users of this information important insights about the economic status of the health care organization.

Users of Financial Accounting Information

Most users of financial accounting information have a direct financial interest in evaluating the economic status of the health care organization, such as investors and creditors. Other parties, such as taxing authorities, regulatory agencies, labor unions, customers, and economic planners, may have an indirect financial interest in the health care organization and would also use financial accounting information. However, our major concern is to understand financial accounting from the eyes of investors and lenders.

Investors typically have a predominant financial interest in a health care organization. One of the unique features of the health care industry is that the term "investor" reflects a variety of

different roles, depending on the organization's mission. Some investors are owners of stock in for-profit health care organizations. The daily market price of such shares, which are exchanged publicly, are indicated in such financial publications as the *Wall Street Journal*. The term "investors" can also describe a nonprofit group of physicians who exchange stock for cash or other assets. This stock is not sold publicly.

More typical than either of the preceding examples are situations in which there is no stock exchange to identify the investor/owner group. These types of investors include the classic nonprofit organizations, such as religious organizations or community hospitals, or the large nonprofit private systems. These traditional nonprofit health care organizations have no explicit investor group (as reflected by shares of stock), but they can stand for the community at large, whether defined in terms of religion, geography, or common interests, who have donated and generated wealth over the years, thus implicitly representing the investor group. And although this implicit investor group does not receive financial remuneration such as dividend payments, it expects these nonprofit organizations to reciprocate through such paybacks as charity care and education.

All of these different types of health care investor groups have a *board of directors*. Whether the health care organization is for-profit or nonprofit, or does or does not issue stock, the board of directors has a critical responsibility for fiscal stewardship, i.e., the board of directors, as an elected subset of the investor/owner group, is responsible for assuring the economic viability of the health care organization to the investors who own it. Earlier we said that investors are predominant users of financial accounting information because of their direct financial interest in the organization. This relationship of investor to organization becomes crystallized or operationalized in the relationship between the board of directors and the management of the health care organization.

Lenders constitute the second broadly defined group with a direct financial interest in the economic status of the health care organization. Again, there are different types of lending groups, such as commercial lenders, banks, etc. Furthermore, these lending sources are generally the same for both for-profit and nonprofit organizations. As one of the two dominant sources of financial capital, they, too, expect remuneration. Such remuneration is not in the form of a cash dividend, but instead is in the form of interest payments received by the lenders from the health care organization. Just as the investors' interests are represented by the board of directors and the power of governance that comes with investor ownership, the lenders (as nonowners) represent their interests through the contract of the debt instrument, which often specify financial parameters that must be achieved by management, with clear consequences for failure to achieve them.

In summary, creditors are the predominant users of financial accounting information because of their direct financial interest. They do not simply read the financial statements, however; they also actively pressure management to achieve desired parameters within these financial statements. This critical pressure point between top management (the CEO or president of the organization) and the financial capital market (investing community and lenders) eventually makes its way down to lower levels of management in the form of budgets, pricing strategies, cost-cutting strategies, etc.

The Significance of Regulation

As a consequence of the Great Depression of the 1930s and the resultant widespread collapse of businesses and the securities market, the federal government began regulating financial statements and accounting standards. A direct result of this collapse in the financial markets was the creation of the Securities and Exchange Commission (SEC) as an independent regulatory agency of the US government. The SEC has the legal power to enforce the form and content of financial statements for companies that wish to sell securities to the public. To do this the SEC developed a set of standards for financial reporting that is generally accepted and universally practiced. These common standards are called generally accepted accounting principles (GAAPs). These standards indicate how to measure and report economic events. If a company does not follow GAAPs, the SEC will not allow it to issue securities. The SEC believes that financial statements prepared according to GAAPs provide investors, creditors, and other interested parties with useful information to make informed decisions.

For the most part, the SEC has delegated the responsibility for establishing GAAPs to a rule-making body called the Financial Accounting Standards Board (FASB). The FASB is a private organization, the mission of which is to establish and improve standards of financial accounting and reporting. The FASB has been granted the power from the SEC to establish GAAPs because it has the financial resources and expertise to tackle many different financial reporting issues. More specifically, GAAPs can be defined as a set of objectives, conventions, and principles that have evolved through the years to govern the preparation and presentation of financial statements. These principles apply to the area of financial accounting, as distinct from other areas of accounting such as managerial accounting and tax accounting.

FASB has the authority from the SEC and the private resources to rule on financial reporting issues, but this does not guarantee that accountants will work in the manner FASB prescribes. This leads to a third group: the American Institute of Certified Public Accountants (AICPA), the professional association of accountants that has substantial influence with its membership, much like the relationship that the American Medical Association (AMA) has with physicians. The AICPA creates the rules and documents (e.g., there is an Audit Guide for the Health Care Industry) that public accounting firms and individual certified public accountants (CPAs) follow when auditing an organization's financial statements. The auditor's report is a letter from the outside auditor, giving an opinion on whether or not the firm's financial statements are a fair presentation of the results of operations, cash flows, and financial position in accordance with GAAPs. Essentially, these AICPA rulings and audit guides govern the accounting profession, and they align the work of professional accountants with GAAPs as espoused by FASB.

In summary, the AICPA, in its political wisdom, has wisely acquiesced to the FASB by ruling that the pronouncements of the latter carry the weight of competent authority. If public accounting firms or individual CPAs choose not to follow AICPA rulings and documents, the professional is subject to strong sanctions by the AICPA. In turn, if the AICPA rulings and documents—as the authority of the profession—choose to stray too far from the guidance of GAAPs as prescribed by the FASB, the profession runs the risk of facing the wrath of the SEC. It should be no surprise that the field of financial accounting is classified as a social science rather than a physical science, given the evolutionary and political nature of the discipline.

The Financial Statements

The three primary types of financial statements are the balance sheet, the income statement, and the statement of "cash flow." Each of these statements has strengths and weaknesses for determining the financial condition of the organization. A thorough and continuing analysis of the financial statements can highlight potential problem areas and aid in determining corrective action.

The Balance Sheet
The balance sheet may be thought of as a snapshot of the financial condition of the firm at a given point in time. The assets (A) side of the balance sheet lists the total resources owned by the health care organization in dollar terms. Equities are rights or claims against these resources. Equities may be further subdivided into two categories: claims of creditors (liabilities) and claims

of owners (owners' equity). This equation ($A = L + OE$) is often referred to as the *basic accounting equation*. Assets must equal the sum of liabilities and owners' equity. As creditor claims are paid before ownership claims if a health care organization is liquidated, liabilities are shown before owners' equity in the basic accounting equation.

The balance sheet can present the financial position of the organization at any point in time. This can be the end of the year, the end of the month, or any other time desired by the administrator. Its reliability is determined by the accuracy of the accounting information and the appropriateness of generally accepted accounting principles and regulations for the decision being made. The FASB and other professional accounting organizations issue guidance through pronouncements and opinions on appropriate accounting practices for presenting fair financial statements, e.g., the physical assets of the organization are typically carried at their initial acquisition costs, and the amounts carried in inventory and accounts receivable are a function of the accuracy of the record-keeping system and the time selected for the report. Some organizations will use the calendar year as their reporting period. Others may use another fiscal period that is more appropriate in terms of patient services and census, e.g., a December 31 cutoff date for the balance sheet may have been selected more as a matter of tradition than because it is a proper time to analyze the financial position.

Assets. The common characteristic possessed by all assets is *service potential* or *future economic benefit*, i.e., the capacity to provide future services or benefits to the entities that use them. The balance sheet is broken down into a logical organizational structure. There are four major categories of assets: current assets; long-term investments; property, plant, and equipment; and other assets.

The components of the balance sheet are typically classified into definite groupings, e.g., the current assets section includes cash and other assets that are normally converted into cash within a year or within an operating cycle, whichever is longer. The current assets are primarily on hand to reflect the liquidity the organization has to pay the current liabilities. This relationship between current assets and current liabilities is referred to as *working capital*. Within current assets, there is cash, which is money in the checking account or savings account, and short-term marketable securities, which represent short-term investments of cash in highly liquid, low-risk securities such as US Treasury bills or prime commercial paper. The marketable securities investment is normally carried on the balance sheet at cost, with the market value of the securities listed in the notes to the financial statements. It is not necessarily desirable to optimize the dollar amount in cash and short-term marketable securities, as these are relatively low-income-generating assets. The combination of cash and short-term marketable securities is kept on hand to pay the short-term bills or in preparation for moving it to a longer-term asset, such as a long-term investment or the purchase of property, plant, and equipment.

Patient accounts receivable represent amounts due to the health care provider for services that have been rendered but not yet paid. The patient accounts receivable amount is listed on the balance sheet, minus an allowance for discounts, charity care, and bad debt write-offs. Health care providers' billing systems usually start with a "gross" accounts receivable amount and then subtract the various adjustments to reflect the "net" billing to be collected. These adjustments from the gross billings are tracked in the clinic's internal information—its managerial accounting system—but are no longer part of the external financial reporting. Before the 1991 *AICPA Audit Guide for Health Care Organizations* (New York: American Institute of Certified Public Accountants), financial statements used to start with the gross accounts receivable amount and then reflect the subtractions from that amount, including the discounts, charity care, and bad debt expenses. Now this detailed information is not reported in the body of the audited financial statement. The bad debt allowance is typically shown in the footnotes, and only some narrative about discount and charity care policy will be reflected in the footnotes.

Another current asset—inventories and supplies—primarily reflects the health care provider's investment in inventory. Again, consistent with the other current assets, it is not necessarily desirable to maximize this number. A

certain buffer amount is necessary, but more and more organizations are trying to drive inventory investment toward zero through aggressive inventory management.

To summarize the current assets section of the balance sheet, the primary purpose served by these current assets is liquidity. These are not very lucrative income-generating assets. Money in the checking or savings accounts earn little or no interest. Short-term marketable securities provide a somewhat better return, but not as much as securities locked into longer time periods. Accounts receivable, of course, provide no return as essentially this amount represents promises to pay. It would be desirable to drive receivables to zero through collections to convert this asset to cash. Finally, inventories and supplies also represent investment in items that provide no return because they sit on the shelf. Organizations try to streamline these current assets while providing a reasonable amount of liquidity buffer, a process known as working capital management.

The second major asset category is *long-term investments*. This is the money that the health care provider has set aside in the form of various income-producing investments such as stocks, bonds, and other higher-yielding investments. A footnote to this balance sheet item will usually reveal the details about the types of investments held by the organization. When we discussed current assets, we suggested that organizations try to have only some reasonable amount to pay the current liabilities. The benefit of such prudent management of working capital would be that more money could be moved into long-term investments, where the returns are higher. The various management efforts to streamline working capital should enhance interest revenue in the income statement.

The third major asset category would be *property*, *plant*, and *equipment*. These assets, compared with current assets, are highly illiquid and are used over long periods of time by the provider. They are listed at historical cost less accumulated depreciation as of the date of the balance sheet. Accumulated depreciation represents the cumulative total dollars of depreciation that have been charged off (the annual charge-off is seen on the income statement as a depreciation expense) against the historical cost of the organization's fixed asset base. Depreciation expense is neither a measure of the using up of an asset nor an indication of its loss of market value. Accounting depreciation is only an expense item that allocates the historical cost of an asset to the years of its useful life. This allocation is typically done by straight-line depreciation, i.e., dividing the historical cost of an asset over its useful life. The quotient is the asset's annual depreciation expense, which is the annual charge reflected in the income statement.

The fourth major asset category is *other assets*. This is really a catch-all category of miscellaneous items that may or may not be very significant. An example of a significant other asset is goodwill. Goodwill is an intangible asset, in contrast to the three other major asset categories, which have physical form and substance. Intangible assets such as good credit standing, skilled employees, and original services and products do not have any physical form and, as such, are not typically recorded on the financial statements because of the difficulty in precisely measuring the vale of intangible assets.

However, the one type of intangible asset that is allowed to be recorded—goodwill—is particularly relevant to the health care industry because it is born out of the merger and acquisition of organizations, e.g., if a health care organization was to purchase a physician practice, the price paid for that practice establishes a reasonable minimum value on the asset. Then a market value of the specific tangible assets of the acquired physician practice is established. The difference between the price paid for that practice and the market value of the specific tangible assets is presumed to be the intangible asset called goodwill. Accountants are essentially willing to allow the intangible asset called goodwill to be shown on the financial statement for the excess amount (excess over market value of the specific tangible assets) that the acquiring organization paid for the practice. The logic is that the only reason one would pay more than the value of the group practice's tangible assets is because the practice has valuable intangible assets. Otherwise the purchaser would simply have duplicated all of the tangible assets instead of buying the practice.

Liabilities.   Offsetting the asset accounts are the liabilities and equity accounts of the organization. Liabilities consist of both short-term (current liabilities) and long-term (payable over more than 1 year) debt. Liabilities are creditors' claims on total assets. Most claims of creditors attach to total enterprise assets rather than to the specific assets provided by the creditor. In the event of nonpayment, creditors may legally force the liquidation of a business. In that case, the law requires that creditor claims be paid before ownership claims. The liabilities section of the balance sheet also follows a logical organizational format. *Current liabilities*—those debts that will fall due within 1 year or operating cycle—are listed first. *Long-term debt* (more formal debt instruments that fall due beyond 1 year) are listed second.

Current liabilities include such items as the currently due portion of any long-term debt, accounts payable to the organization's suppliers, and various categories of accrued expenses. Accounts payable and accrued expenses represent expenses that have been incurred as of the balance sheet date but have not yet been paid in cash. Accounts payable generally pertain to amounts due to vendors for supplies. Items such as salaries and wages due to employees, interest due on loans, accrued utilities expenses, and similar items would be included as accrued expenses. As mentioned in the discussion of current assets, one extremely important balance-sheet relationship is that of current assets to current liabilities. The difference between these two balance-sheet categories is referred to as working capital. The working capital number gives the reader some sense of the short-term liquidity of the provider. As mentioned in the discussion of current assets, the idea is not necessarily to maximize this working capital (which ties too much up in nonincome-producing assets), but to generate a comfortable buffer.

An important current liability in a capitated environment is an item referred to as *incurred but not reported* (IBNR). The uniqueness of the capitated environment is that we know that for any given period a health care organization will have captured all of its premium revenue. This is the amount that is billed out on the first of the month. Whether the cash has been received or the billed amount is still in premiums receivable, we have still recognized the amount in the income statement as revenue for the period. However, at the end of the period there may still be a number of expenses related to services for our enrollees that have not yet been recognized. Many of the expenses will naturally be recognized and matched to the appropriate period, i.e., those in the beginning or middle of the month. But those costs of services near the end of the month may still be in the pipeline, e.g., if the organization subcontracts out for those services, they may not have been billed yet for these services incurred during the month. Alternatively, even if the services are provided in house, the episode of care related to monthly premium dollars might straddle into the next time period, thus resulting in a need to estimate the cost of those services. Thus, one of the last accounting entries typically done in a capitated environment is to record one more current liability—IBNR—the offsetting entry for which goes to the income statement as an expense of business. The expense of treating the enrollee is now properly matched to the month receiving the premium revenue. Again, these expenses are typically end-of-the-period treatment costs that have not yet surfaced in our information systems, as a result of either slowness in billing or the natural straddling of services into the next period. They must be brought back (through the current liability IBNR) and matched to the earlier period that recognized the revenue.

The long-term debt represents the more formal and legal forms of borrowing. This section lists any long-term debt owed to banks and other creditors and any obligations under capital leases. Usually, detailed information about the specific characteristics of the long-term debt is disclosed in the footnotes to the financial statements.

Two basic policy initiatives by the federal government fueled the 1972–85 trend toward greater bond indebtedness in the health care industry. One initiative was that Medicare and Medicaid reimbursement reduced the risk involved with debt finance by reimbursing 100% of interest and allowing full recovery of the physical capital costs (depreciation on the asset). A second initiative, off-budget financing, appeared during the Nixon administration and encouraged investment banking firms and local governments to create tax-exempt financing authorities to issue tax-exempt hospital bonds. These financing authorities organized by state governments have greatly aided hospitals in issuing tax-free debt by reducing the riskiness of the securities. These securities typically offer high yields and have proven to be very attractive to large buyers (banks, mutual funds). Essentially, then, the impact of these two developments on debt financing was that the increased demand for debt financing (as a result of Medicare and Medicaid reimbursement policies) were matched by an enlarged infrastructure (off-budget financing) for the issuing of that debt.

Another important event took place around this time from within health care organizations. The 1969 American Hospital Association (AHA) *Statement on the Financial Requirements of Health Providers* (Chicago: American Hospital Publishing) demanded that various payers pay for capital costs (both financial in terms of interest and physical in terms of full cost of the asset through depreciation). This AHA statement became the effective precursor of the Medicare and Medicaid reimbursement policy in the early 1970s, but it was also making the demand of commercial payers. This really gave hospitals the financial independence they needed. This AHA statement, combined with the generous Medicare/Medicaid reimbursement, opened up access to debt/equity markets, turning hospitals into quasi-commercial enterprises. Critics of such generous reimbursement of capital assets and related debt financing have argued that these hospitals, in demanding payments for depreciation and interest, implicitly assumed that communities would benefit by their perpetual recapitalization regardless of future changes in technology, population, disease, and performance. It has been argued that the AHA statement essentially ended any sense of strong planned capital payments. This implicit "perpetual recapitalization" was indeed reflective of the 1970s and most of the 1980s, but the move toward a fixed-revenue environment, combined with the increasing power of the purchasers of health care, have dramatically changed the nature and inherent risks and incentives in capital financing.

Owners' Equity. The ownership claim on total assets is known as owners' equity. Equity accounts are composed of the initial capital investment of the owners and the earnings retained in the organization from providing services. Equity accounts for not-for-profit organizations are sometimes called fund balances. The amounts reflect what has been retained in the organization after the amounts due to external creditors have been subtracted from the total assets (total assets minus total debt equals equity/net worth/fund balances). Balance sheet accounts are usually considered to be permanent accounts, i.e., they do not close at the end of each accounting period. As discussed earlier regarding the amorphous nature of the ownership of health care organizations, this ownership claim is also referred to in a number of ways: stockholders' equity, fund balance, net worth, and net assets. We will use the term "owners' equity," but the various terms all mean the same thing: it is the amount equal to total assets minus total liabilities.

The logic goes as follows: to determine what belongs to the investors (whether explicitly recognized, as in for-profit organizations, or implicit, as in not-for-profit ones), we subtract creditors' claims (the liabilities) from assets. The remainder (owners' equity) is the investors' claim on the assets of the health care organization. The owners' equity section of the balance sheet consists of two parts: contributed capital and accumulated earnings. Contributed capital is the term used to describe the total amount paid in by stockholders (investors). The accumulated earnings section of the balance sheet is the accumulation of earnings from the income statement (minus any dividends paid out in the case of a for-profit organization) over time that have essentially been reinvested in the organization.

The asset and liability sections of the balance sheet are pretty much the same across all health care organizations. However, the owners' equity sections tend to differ (in presentation, but not economic substance) because of the different forms of ownership in health care delivery that we discussed earlier. Perhaps, more importantly, the sophistication of the capital markets to which a for-profit health organization has access creates real differences in the magnitude of dollars raised.

One unique feature of many nonprofit health care organizations is that they might have additional balance sheets to reflect the economic status of the organization. These additional balance sheets represent the fact that, if the organization receives restricted donations, they are required to have at least two funds or accounting entities: general funds and donor-restricted funds. The AICPA defines a fund as "a self-contained accounting entity set up to account for a specific activity or project." This organizational unit (accounting entity) has assets, claims against those assets, and a fund balance. General funds represent all resources not restricted to identified purposes by donors and grantors. The general fund therefore would have the characteristics of assets, liabilities, and owners' equity as we have discussed. Donor-restricted funds, such as special funds, plant funds, or endowment funds, account for resources restricted by law or contractual agreement to use for a specific purpose. These restricted funds may represent resources legally designated to finance fixed assets. Endowment funds are permanently or temporarily restricted by their donors to investments that generate income. The assets of these funds cannot be consumed; they must remain intact. Restricted contributions and gifts impose legal and fiduciary responsibilities on the health care organization's trustees to carry out the written specifications of donors.

These donor-restricted funds have their separate balance sheets where the assets, by definition, must equal the liabilities plus the net fund balance. However, the composition of these assets, liabilities, and fund balance differ significantly from the balance sheet in the general fund. The restricted funds follow the same broad framework and definitions as presented previously, but there is little complexity in these restricted balance sheets, e.g., restricted fund assets are primarily made up of long-term and perhaps some short-term investments. The idea is to have this money set aside in a separate restricted fund where it can generate income revenue to support other activities of the health care organization. Thus, the assets are primarily investments. You would not see much of the various other types of assets that are part of the general fund. Likewise there would be minimal complexity on the right-hand side of the balance sheet. There probably would be few or no liabilities of any sort, current or long term. This is because the health care organization is not conducting business from these restricted funds; it essentially has money set aside to earn more money. Thus, the right-hand side of the balance sheet would primarily consist of the fund balance. In summary, most of the assets of a restricted fund would be reflected in long- and short-term investments, and most of the liabilities and fund balance would be reflected in fund balance. There are journal entries that are involved in transferring money between funds, but the detail of this is beyond the scope of this book.

The Income Statement

If the balance sheet may be visualized as a snapshot type of financial statement, the income statement may be thought of as a flow type of financial statement. The income statement presents the flow of revenues and expenses through the health care system in a given year. Basically, the income statement feeds into the balance sheet. The net income for the year is closed into the owners' equity section of the balance sheet, thus enhancing the wealth, by the net income amount. The core components of the income statement are the following: revenues minus expenses equals net income (or loss). Revenues are the gross increase in owners' equity primarily resulting from clinical activities entered into for the purpose of earning income. Generally, revenues result from the performance of services, resulting in an increase in assets. Expenses are the cost of assets consumed or services used in the process of earning revenue. Expenses are the decreases in owners' equity that result from operating the business. Expenses represent actual or expected cash outflows (payments). When revenues exceed expenses, net income results. When expenses exceed revenues, a net loss results. When a health care organization is economically successful it generates net income.

The income statement basically measures the results of providing services over a period of time. It, too, is prepared in accordance with generally accepted accounting principles. One of the important measurement concepts in accordance with GAAPs is the accrual concept, which has three aspects: the measurement of revenue, the measurement of expenses, and the matching of revenues and expenses to produce income. The first aspect of the accrual concept states that revenue earned does not necessarily correspond to the receipt of cash. Earned revenue is recognized when there has been a critical event that indicates that a service has been provided, creating a corresponding economic obligation by the purchaser. The asset received in exchange for the services may be cash but more often is accounts receivable. The same logic applies on the expense side, where the accrual basis of accounting recognizes that the critical event is the economic obligation related to the services provided.

The accrual method (matching of revenues and expenses), the depreciation method (straight-line, accelerated), and the inventory valuation method can each have a decided impact on reported income. Under the accrual method of accounting, and where noncash expenses such as depreciation are included, the income reported on the income statement is not the same as cash; in fact, using this method, it is possible to report high income and still experience a serious cash shortage. The rationale behind the use of the accrual method ties back to our discussion of the objectives of financial statements, i.e., to portray the economic status of the organization. It can be argued that the cash basis of accounting fails to do this as well as the accrual method.

Generally, revenues result from the performance of services, resulting in an increase in assets. In a fee-for-service environment, this means the sale of traditional health care services, such as per day, per test, and per ancillary services. In a capitated environment, the sales represent the insurance contract, i.e., the dollar amount contracted for to guarantee the health care for a given population. Therefore, the primary source of revenue is expressed as some sort of premium. The revenue accounts should be segregated by payer categories. The amounts shown as revenues do not include contractual allowances, discounts, and charity care. Only amounts that have been billed to payers will be included. Bad debts or amounts expected not to be collected are included as an expense account instead of a deduction from revenue. Charity care is shown only as a footnote to the summary statements and is no longer shown as a deduction from revenues. Nonpatient service revenues are shown as operating gains and losses after the determination of net income from providing services to patients. Interest earned from investments would not typically be shown as patient care revenues and should be shown after net patient care income has been determined, in order to correctly identify the revenues earned from providing services to patients. In health maintenance organizations (HMOs), interest earned can be shown as an operating revenue.

Donations would also be part of this interest revenue category. Some nonprofit organizations with large, well-endowed foundations rely on this type of revenue. An issue to consider, however, is not to become overly reliant on this investment and interest revenue. It could disguise some operational inefficiencies such that, if the investments do not succeed as a result of downturns in the market, the health care provider could be at some risk.

Finally, the third revenue category is other revenue. With the increasing pressures on the pricing of health care services, these organizations are looking to increase their revenues in other ways. Other revenues can come from certain donations, as well as parking lot fees, consulting services, renting of space, or income from shared services. A nonprofit health care organization needs to be careful not to generate excessive revenue from other sources tangential to the health care mission, at the risk of having its nonprofit status revoked by the Internal Revenue Service. The organization would do better to spin off the money-making business into a for-profit corporation and pay its taxes.

Expenses are the cost of assets consumed or services used in the process of earning revenue. Expenses are the decreases in owners' equity that result from operating the health care organization. Details about the cost behavior of these line items are not really part of the financial accounting information. Such details appear in the managerial accounting information. Expenses represent actual or expected cash outflows (payments). They are typically presented on a functional basis and reflect the amounts expended to provide the services responsible for the revenues shown in the income statement.

In summary, income statement accounts are considered to be temporary accounts, because they are zeroed out at the end of each accounting period to prepare them for the next accounting period. Net income represents an increase in net assets, which are primarily available (exclusively available in the case of a nonprofit organization) to reinvest in the organization. With for-profit health care providers, all or part of the net income is then available to distribute to stockholders as a reward for their invested capital. Cash or other assets distributed to stockholders are called dividends. Dividends reduce retained earnings, but they are not considered an expense. The organization first determines its revenues and expenses, and then computes net income or loss. At this point, it may decide to distribute a dividend.

The Statement of "Cash Flow"

The third financial statement that is required by GAAPs is the statement of "cash flow." This statement uses data from the balance sheet and income statement to provide information about changes in the cash balances that result from the provision of services, investments, and financing decisions for the period covered by the financial statements. The statement of cash flow can be an important indicator of financial solvency. This statement separates the effects of normal operating activities from financing and investing activities. The effects of three major strategies and determinants of fiscal success are separated and shown in terms of their cash flow impact.

The statement of cash flows is a relatively new financial statement that has been added to the annual report in response to demands for better information about firms' cash inflows and outflows. Although the balance sheet provides a snapshot balance of cash for the final day of the period, it does not give the details of how that balance occurred. In the statement of cash flows, the unit of analysis is the difference between the ending cash balance and the beginning cash balance. The statement of cash flows details where cash resources come from and how they are used so that the reader understands why and how the cash position changed. This change is not evident in the balance sheet. Indeed the income statement tells only part of the story. Net income is a major, but not exclusive, source of cash. From a cash flow perspective, several adjustments must be made to this net income figure before we can make any conclusions about the amount of cash contributed by operations.

Furthermore, cash may be raised by methods that do not appear on the income statement, e.g., the health care provider may have raised cash by floating some debt or selling off some assets. These issues are considered in the statement of cash flows. Finally, even though cash increased from operations (with adjustments) and other sources, cash also went out. Again, we do not see this on the income statement, but cash might have been spent to purchase more assets or pay off some debt. These are essentially transactions within the balance sheet that affect the cash position. These sorts of items would also be in the statement of cash flows.

In short, the statement of cash flows provides more valuable information about liquidity than can be obtained from the balance sheet and income statement. The statement of cash flows shows where the health care organization got its cash and how it used it over the entire period covered by the financial statement. In this respect it resembles the income statement, which shows revenues and expenses for the entire accounting period. However, the statement of cash flows is more inclusive than the income statement in that it also considers nonincome statement impacts on cash flow (intra-balance sheet transactions) such as purchasing assets or retiring debt.

Therefore, the statement of cash flows is divided into three major sections: (1) cash from operations; (2) cash from/to financing activities; and (3) cash to investing activities. The operating activities are those related to the revenue- and expense-producing activities reflected in the income statement. These activities are adjusted by noncash amounts such as depreciation expense, as well as several other more complicated adjustments. The working capital portion of the balance sheet is also considered among the ordinary activities of the firm, so the changes in these amounts are also factored into cash from operations. The financing activities of the organization involve borrowing money and repaying

it, issuing stock, and paying dividends. All of these financing activities are potential nonincome statement sources of cash (or drains on cash in terms of repaying debt or paying out dividends). Finally, the investing activities of the health care organization are also potential nonincome statement uses of cash related to the purchase and sale of fixed assets and securities.

Introduction to Managerial Accounting

As important as the statements produced by financial accounting systems are, other analyses of the accounting system information are even more important for management. Managerial accounting deals with formulating budgets, analyzing fiscal performance in comparison to what was budgeted, projecting the effects of management decisions on future financial accounting statements, identifying actual costs of producing services, calculating "full" costs of services using cost allocation formulas, and dealing with other related issues of cost and payment (e.g., internal transfer pricing, income distribution mechanisms, and maximizing third-party payments related to cost).

Users of Managerial Accounting Information

Although financial accounting information is critically important to outside investors and creditors, managerial accounting information is critically important to health care managers. One of the main distinctions between managerial and financial accounting is unit of analysis. The economics of sublevel units of analysis such as by program, by department, by capitated contract, etc., are important managerial concerns. This is the level at which managerial responsibilities are often defined and therefore the level with which managerial accounting is mainly concerned.

These managerial accounting data can be compiled to address normal operations such as routine budgeting processes, income distribution, or pricing decisions, all dealing with internal divisions of the organization. They can also be compiled for special projects such as assessing alternative modes of delivery, projecting the profitability of a particular capitated contract or Diagnostic Related Groupings (DRG) classification, or establishing or revising income distribution systems. Again, these special projects all address sublevel units of analysis that the managerial accounting system stands ready to address.

This leads to a second important distinction between financial and managerial accounting information: the needs of the users. The focus of managerial accounting is primarily on the needs of managers within the organization, rather than interested parties outside the organization. The purpose of managerial accounting information is to serve management decisions better. The third critical dimension on which to compare managerial and financial accounting information pertains to the audit process. In contrast to financial accounting, managerial accounting basically has no audit process and related GAAP rules to follow. Managerial accounting information primarily stays inside the health care organization; thus there is no need for an audit process to assure the external capital markets as to the quality of the information. Organizations typically have more confidence in the accuracy and cleanliness of their financial statements than in their managerial accounting information systems for two reasons: (1) the units of analysis make financial accounting easier; and (2) there is audit process to ensure the accuracy of the managerial accounting information. This anarchy in managerial accounting information is often revealed after two organizations merge, whereupon they have tremendous difficulty getting the two managerial accounting systems to be compatible.

This leads to the fourth important distinction between financial and managerial accounting information: timing. Although financial accounting has the comfort of retrospectively recording and reporting events, managerial accounting information is for the most part very forward looking. This predominantly forward-looking aspect of managerial accounting is filled with all sorts of cost projections, price-setting commitments, and special decisions that take place before the start of the year. One of the consequences of these timing differences is the certainty of information. Again, although it may not seem so, financial accounting contains a relatively cleaner and more

defined information set. Managerial accounting, on the other hand, has to deal with the uncertain future. As we embark on budgeting and price setting we are always dealing with assumptions. Combining this with the fact that we have no generally agreed-upon rules in managerial accounting makes for a wide latitude for interpretation. Remember, financial accounting simply measures past events and categorizes according to a rule-making body. Managerial accounting primarily projects future events and compiles information to serve the managerial decisions at hand, with little or no concern for rules.

The increasing competition in the health care industry is forcing managers to produce high-quality services at the lowest possible cost. This means that there is increasing pressure on the revenue structure of health care organizations. This pressure gets responded to in one of the two remaining parts of the income statement: decreasing the health care organization's underlying cost structure and/or decreasing profits. These requirements are placing ever-greater demands on the information provided by managerial accounting systems.

Cost Behavior

A critical part of managerial accounting is the measurement of costs. The relevant definition of health care costs depends on the context and the environment. A fundamental concept of cost accounting is that there are different costs for different decision-making purposes. Understanding these purposes enables the managerial accountant to provide appropriate cost data to the managers who need it. In general, the term "cost" describes a measurement of expenditure directly associated with providing a given health care service. The cost per service for pricing purposes is different from the cost per service for management control purposes. The cost per service for long-range planning purposes may differ from the cost per service for short-term pricing purposes. Different costs may be determined for the various objectives or purposes for which the health care manager desires to measure activity.

A working framework for defining cost uses two dimensions: space and time. Regarding space, we return to the principle that managerial accounting focuses on costs at a subunit level of analysis: by department, by service, by capitated contract, etc. As mentioned previously, the relevant cost definition depends on the managerial responsibility or managerial decision at hand. The ability of most managerial accounting systems to measure and report costs at these subunit levels is, however, mixed.

Many costs (perhaps 50% of a health care organization's cost structure) can typically be identified with certainty at a subunit level. These are what are referred to as *direct costs*, e.g., regarding the costs of a clinical department, we will find that many costs are unique to that clinical department—this person works only in that department, or this equipment and these supplies are used only in that department. These are the direct costs of that clinical department. They can be measured with certainty but they constitute only a subset of the department's entire cost structure. The remaining resources used by this department are shared resources, e.g., this clinical department shares the physical space of the organization as well as the related infrastructure. These support costs are known as overheads, or *indirect costs*. These indirect costs, in contrast to direct costs, are much more difficult to measure for the precise reason that they are shared resources.

Breaking the expenses of the income statement out by their direct and indirect nature is often referred to as the *functional format* of measurement and presentation. This functional format brings with it the difficult issue of measuring indirect costs. This is discussed later in the chapter. For now, we can simply state that both types of costs—direct and indirect—need to be captured to enhance management decision-making.

The second dimension within our working framework from which to define costs pertains to the issue of time, i.e., how costs behave over time. As stated earlier, much of managerial accounting pertains to issues in the future. In dealing with the future, there is always the unknown volume, such as the number of patient days, visits, or enrollees. Therefore, our definition must include some sense of the volume sensitivity of costs within a certain time period. Some costs are more or less locked into over a time period and therefore are insensitive to volume. These are the health care organization's *fixed costs*, e.g., salaried workers, such as base-level staffing and supervisors, as well as many of the capital expenditures, such as equipment, facilities, and information systems, are considered fixed costs. Once the organization has purchased these items, they are locked into them, regardless of volume. On the other hand, other resources are acquired as volume dictates. These are *variable costs*. Examples might include some of the clinical staffing, as is often seen in the use of agency nurses. Buying the use of capital equipment through some sort of renting arrangement, such as on a per-procedure basis, would be a variable cost. Subcontracting for resources on an "as-needed" basis is a variable cost.

Breaking the expenses of the income statement out by their fixed and variable nature is often referred to as the *contribution format* of measurement and presentation. The next section identifies critical issues involved in distinguishing between fixed costs and variable costs.

Fixed and Variable Costs

The income statement is set up in a contribution format (i.e., it delineates between variable and fixed costs) to address the expected changes in costs resulting from changes in activity. Activity refers to a measure of the organization's output of services and can include such measures as the number of days in the hospital, number of visits, number of procedures, or number of enrollees in an HMO plan.

Health care managers want to know how costs will be affected by changes in the organization's activity. The relationship between cost and activity, called cost behavior (or the underlying cost structure), is relevant to the management functions of planning, control, and decision-making. The critical issue in trying to define an organization's underlying cost structure is the ability to forecast costs at a particular level of activity. Managers must be able to anticipate whether programs, services, or contracts are profitable or not. As both total costs and average cost per unit differ depending on the level of activity, the revenue per unit of activity may be greater or less than the cost per unit, so profitability is uncertain.

Variable costs change in direct proportion to a change in the level of activity. If activity increases by 20%, total variable costs increase by approximately 20% as well. Although total variable costs increase or decrease proportionately with the activity change, unit variable cost remains the same.

In contrast to variable costs, total fixed costs remain unchanged as the level of activity varies. Whether activity increases or decreases, total fixed costs remain the same. Examples of fixed cost include depreciation of equipment and facilities, salaried administrators, managers, and staff. The important point of this declining fixed cost per unit is that the fixed cost structure is where health care organizations can benefit from economies of scale.

The inverse of this is also true, i.e., the fixed cost structure risks the consequences of diseconomies of scale. If volume decreases, the fixed cost per unit increases, because there is less volume in which to spread the fixed costs. This increase in fixed cost per unit, in turn, translates into higher average costs per unit. The variable cost structure is not exposed to these risks of diseconomies of scale. If volume were to decrease, the total variable costs would decrease proportionately, and thus the cost per unit would remain the same.

One other point should be noted about fixed-cost behavior, i.e., fixed costs do not remain constant forever. At some increased volume, additional fixed costs must be incurred in the form of new equipment, more base staffing, etc. Likewise, we might expect that if volume shrinks enough we would be shedding some of our fixed cost base. Nevertheless, our predominant assumption is that, within "relevant ranges" of volume, the fixed cost structure will remain constant. For the most part, we will be working with cases and illustrations that stay within these relevant ranges.

Cost–volume–profit (CVP) analysis is an analytical technique that articulates the contribution format to address various managerial planning and control decisions involving the uncertainties of the future. This technique summarizes the effects of changes in a health care organization's volume of activity on its costs, revenues, and profit. In short, CVP analysis is a four-variable model (volume, revenue, costs, and profits) that provides management with a comprehensive overview of the effects that changes on three of the variables have on the fourth as managers consider alternatives in short-term decisions. This four-variable CVP analysis allows management to project income statements at various anticipated volume levels.

Previously, we examined the distinction between direct and indirect costs. We identified the functional format as that form of measurement and reporting that delineates direct and indirect cost areas, so that costs per unit in each department can be calculated. The goal of cost allocation is congruent with the broader objectives of a good managerial accounting system, which is to trace as many costs as possible directly to the activities that cause them to be incurred. Health care organizations would like to track costs patient by patient, doctor by doctor, and disease by disease. They employ computerized databases to help them organize and maintain the data that they need to make cost-effective decisions in treating patients. This process of comprehensive cost definition is vital to important management objectives such as pricing strategies and cost control.

The competitive health care environment has made it imperative for health care organizations to eliminate nonvalue-added costs in the delivery of their services. Nonvalue-added costs are the costs of activities that can be eliminated without harming service quality, performance, or perceived value. It is important that overhead costs, not just direct costs, be traced as meaningfully as possible so that they can be evaluated in terms of the value they add to the delivery of services. As always, the benefits of more accurate assignment of costs must be weighed against the cost of data collection.

The health care industry certainly needs to improve on its legacy of very poor cost allocation systems. Before the inception of Medicare and Medicaid programs in the mid-1960s, accurate definition of the full costs of providing services to patients was not the basis for pricing and therefore did not exist. Pricing was based on informal and intuitive cross-subsidization, with shortages being made up each year by donations, some local grants, and unrestricted price increases to patients. Since the introduction of Medicare and Medicaid, the health care industry's costing practices have revolved around the Medicare cost report. To some extent this contributed to cost definitions becoming worse, not better. Medicare and Medicaid regulations were written to ensure that the government paid for most of the costs of providing services to their patients. The result of this contractual arrangement between the government and health care providers was that many providers developed their managerial accounting systems to load up on allocating costs to government-sponsored patients. In short, managerial accounting systems and their underlying cost allocation systems became oriented to revenue maximization, not cost finding.

So the health care industry regressed from essentially no accurate cost finding in pre-Medicare and Medicaid days to knowingly wrong cost definitions (but it did maximize revenue!). The introduction of fixed-rate payments in the 1980s in the form of DRGs for the government and capitation for commercial payers (and now Medicare and Medicaid) was a rude awakening. Health care providers did not have much of an idea of what it really cost to treat different types of patients. Interestingly, now that much revenue comes from various forms of fixed-rate payments with no explicit tie to costs, accurate cost definitions are more important for providers than ever before. Many excellent health care organizations are rising to the challenge.

A critical part of cost determination is the allocation of overhead costs. Cost allocation is an internal pricing process in which one department in a health care organization allocates costs to another department. This pricing process is metaphorical, not real, because there is no exchange of dollars to objectively establish a price for overhead services. Thus, the issue for cost allocation is how to establish such an internal price for the service provided by one department for another.

Much of the pressure for more accurate cost allocation systems is coming from the "customers" or recipients of overhead services. As the managers come under increasing pressure to optimize economic performance, their attention to the fairness or appropriateness of the allocated costs has heightened. These managers are being held accountable to control both direct and indirect costs. The consequences of economic performance now affect everything from year-end bonuses to decisions on expanding or dropping services. These incentives that did not exist in the health care industry 20 years ago.

An important first step in understanding the cost behavior in any organization is identifying the cost drivers on which various types of costs depend. A cost driver is a characteristic of an event or activity that causes costs to be incurred by that event or activity. In most organizations different types of costs respond to widely differing cost drivers. It is an oversimplification to lump all clinical overhead costs together and say that they are driven by the quantity of patient days, visits, or revenue dollars generated. In state-of-the-art cost management systems, accountants are careful to separate various types of costs into different cost pools and identify the most appropriate cost driver for each pool.

In identifying a cost driver, the health care organization should consider the extent to which a cost or pool of costs varies in accordance with the cost driver. The higher the correlation between the cost and the cost driver, the more accurate will be the resulting understanding of cost behavior. Modern management cost systems use an activity-based costing (ABC) approach, which proposes that often there is some specific activity that causes overhead costs to be incurred. Investigation will identify the crucial causal activity and will enable us to select a volume measure that can be used to assign the costs of that activity to different product lines. The main difference between ABC and traditional costing is the avoidance of allocation based on simple statistical data (such as allocating on revenue dollars or labor hours) in lieu of more meaningful cost drivers that reflect the usage of the overhead item. Not only does this improve cost allocation, but it also provides information to help control costs. Once the true costs are clearly identified, managers can eliminate nonvalue-added processes.

In short, the central concept of a rigorous costing system such as ABC is to assign the costs of each activity to the services provided on the basis of how each service area consumes the cost driver identified for that activity. The idea is to infer how each service area consumes the activity by observing how each product line consumes the cost driver. The cost information generated will be more accurate, with the result that better decisions can be made. Furthermore, employees will be more cost conscious because the overhead amounts that they are being assigned are based on cause-and-effect activity, not presumed correlations to overhead cost behavior.

To assign costs from one area to another, there must be a cost pool (a numerator) and a cost driver (a denominator). A cost pool is any grouping of costs to be allocated. A cost driver is the criterion on which the allocation is to be made, e.g., we could choose to allocate costs based on patient days. In that case, the number of patient days would be the cost driver. Alternatively, cost could be allocated based on hours. It is common to allocate housekeeping costs based on hours of service provided. The total number of housekeeping service hours becomes the cost driver. When the cost driver is divided into the total costs for providing housekeeping services, the result is an overhead allocation rate—in this case, a cost per hour of housekeeping service. Each time a patient day is incurred, one would apply the overhead allocation rate to that patient. So now, in addition to the direct costs of treating a patient such as labor and supplies, the patient would also be assigned the allocation rate for housekeeping services. The development of meaningful overhead application rates serves to provide management with information needed for price negotiations, evaluation of the profitability of specific types of patients, and other important decisions.

Budgeting

Budgeting is an important part of planning a health care organization's economic activity. The budget is probably the most fundamental financial document in an organization and most likely the first encounter that a health care manager has with accounting information. The organizational budget is the basic tool for tying together the planning and control functions of management. More specifically, budgeting involves detailed plans, expressed in quantitative terms, that spec-

ify how resources will be acquired and used during a specified period of time. The bulk of this quantified plan is expressed in economic parameters. Furthermore, many of these economic parameters pertain to costs and revenues; thus budgeting applies much of our knowledge of cost accounting as defined earlier.

This quantified economic planning is not a detached analysis done by the accountants. The derivation and use of this plan should infiltrate the entire health care organization. Thus, the budgeting process also serves to facilitate communication and coordination throughout the organization. Each manager must be aware of the plans made by other managers for the organization to be effective as a whole; essentially this process integrates the plans of each manager in an organization. Finally, the budgeting process and the resulting budget serve to allocate limited organizational resources among competing uses. These three major uses of the organizational budget—to quantify economic planning, facilitate communication and coordination, and allocate organizational resources— form the front end of budgeting processes and are the focus of this section.

The richness and particular relevance of budgeting, however, go beyond the planning, communicating, and allocating processes. There is also a back end to the budgeting process in which budgets are used in a feedback mode. Budgeting serves to help control operations and related profits. Plans are subject to change, and the budget serves as a useful benchmark with which actual results can be compared with planned activity. Comparing actual results with budgeted results helps managers to evaluate the performance of individuals, departments, product lines, and capitated contracts. As budgets are used to evaluate performance, they can also be used to provide incentives for people to perform well. Furthermore, the information about what actually happened versus what was planned is incorporated into future plans to improve the accuracy of the planning process. In this way, the budget process forms a continuous loop of information—planning, implementing, controlling, feedback.

Budgeting is an important application or subset of managerial accounting, and it is where we particularly appreciate the dimensions that separate financial from managerial accounting. The budget process very much involves the various subunits of a health care organization, e.g. the operating budget helps us to plan and control costs and revenues by various departments, product lines, individuals, or special projects. The *user* of budgeting, as stated previously, should be the entire management team, not just the accountants and probably not the external capital markets.

Forecasting volume and services becomes the starting point for revenue and expense projections. A slightly inaccurate volume forecast, coming at the very beginning of the budgeting process, will throw off all of the revenue and expense projections. Once a patient-volume forecast exists, it is possible for managers to determine revenues, appropriate staffing, and the need for clinical and other supplies. Essentially, the operating budget provides the plan for the revenue and expenses for the coming year. Some departments have responsibilities for both, and budget accordingly. They are referred to as profit centers or revenue centers. Other departments are held accountable for only expenses. These are referred to as cost centers. Assumptions about inflation for the coming year also need to be made.

An important trend in the budgeting process is the increasing focus on the continuum of health care when planning the efficient delivery of health services. In developing their models for improving the health of the population, health care organizations are refocusing the system from the delivery of discrete health care services to managed health. Such planning is done by using models that include risk assessment and prevention, continuous care management across the health care delivery spectrum, and disease management. A relatively small number of diagnoses account for most of an organization's costs of delivery. By providing a focus on prevention and then channeling patients into a specialized continuum of care, the organization will deliver the best outcomes at the least cost.

One major health care provider already classes its services in eight product lines: cancer, cardiology, diabetes, behavioral health, workers' compensation, women's services, senior care,

and emergency services. They believe that this disease management approach to planning and budgeting will give the company a competitive advantage with managed care in marketing these lines of health care services. Such an approach incorporates into the budgeting philosophy the idea that long-term profitability will be developed by demonstrating value to patients, employers, and the community through decreased health care costs combined with improvement in the health of the population served. One hospital has also saved money by mapping out treatment schemes in such detail and having this underpin their budgeting process. Finally, a major clinic is spending $80 million on a disease-management center in which to structure their plans and control of health care costs and outcomes.

Behavioral Aspects of Budgeting

There is no other area of accounting where the behavioral implications are more important than in the budgeting area. A budget affects virtually everyone in the organization. The human reactions to the budgeting process can have considerable influence on an organization's overall effectiveness. One important area is negotiation. Budgets are often prepared by the managers of the departments. This ensures that the budgets are based on realistic information and expectations. These proposed budgets are then submitted to the finance department of the organization, which compiles the master budget. This budget must be approved before it can be implemented. Often, however, the departmental budgets do not combine into a feasible overall budget. Critical questions are asked about the managers' requests. Even if a department's budget is reasonable, there may still be limitations on what the organization can, or will, approve. Thus there is an interplay between the various budget actors before it all comes together. The changes are often made through a process of negotiation, as top managers try to find the areas where budget cuts would do the least damage.

A more authoritarian or top-down approach to the budget involves little negotiation from most of the staff. This orientation has the advantages of being relatively expeditious and reflecting top management perspective. On the other hand, it has the disadvantages of lacking the involvement, communication, and commitment that can result from a more participatory budget process. The participatory approach to budgeting perceives the budgeting process from the standpoint of responsibility management. Most people will perform better and make greater attempts to achieve a goal if they have helped to set the goal. The idea of participative budgeting is to involve employees throughout the organization in the budgetary process.

Another behavioral aspect of budgeting involves work standards and task analysis, both sensitive issues to the staff doing the work. Any control system has three basic parts: a predetermined or standard performance level, a measure of actual performance, and a comparison between standard and actual performance. On the first issue, a predetermined or standard cost is set. One indicator of future standards and costs is historical data. In a mature and predictable health care delivery process, historical standards and costs can provide a good basis for predicting future costs. These predictions will often need to be adjusted to reflect movements in price levels or technological changes in the production process. However, even a minor change in the way a service is provided can make historical data almost totally irrelevant. As we have stated previously, many health care organizations are making major changes to the way in which they plan and control costs.

Finally, the behavioral dimension of budgeting is particularly acute when it is used in the process of performance evaluation. Budgeting lays down a set of expectations. Managers must review the budget as approved and begin to carry out whatever activities are necessary to comply with the budget. After the budget is in place and the new year begins, managers will start to receive feedback as actual results are known. The actual results are then compared with these expectations to evaluate performance. This feedback will require investigation to understand the causes of any differences between the plan and the actual results.

Budgeting as a Planning and Control Tool

The budgeting process and the resulting output, the approved operating budget, are probably among the most valuable short-term tools available to the manager. The organizational budget is the basic tool for tying together the planning and control functions of management. More specifically, budgeting involves detailed plans, expressed in quantitative terms, that specify how resources will be acquired and used during a specified period of time.

Budget preparation and implementation yield the following benefits to the organization:

- Communication is improved throughout the organization. If the budget reflects the goals and objectives of the organization, the preparers and readers of the document will know these objectives. Through its allocation of resources, the budget communicates what is important.
- Coordination is improved, because the completed master budget ensures that all preparers are working with the same data on anticipated patient loads and expenses. Estimated demand and services to be supplied are made explicit.
- Control is improved, because the budget authorizes certain levels of expenses and clarifies what revenues are to be anticipated. Comparison with actual results enables management to become aware of deviations from the budget as they occur.
- Motivation is improved, because people who have participated in the budget feel a greater loyalty to the organization. They know what is anticipated and what is expected of them.
- Finally, comparison of the plan with actual results facilitates performance management. Variances can be computed to focus management interest on results not in accordance with the budget.

To achieve these benefits, certain things must be done:

- Top management must be involved with and committed to the budgeting process. The completed plan must be used for decision-making.
- There should be a formal system with well-defined goals and objectives, formalized reports, and responsibility accounting. Training sessions for supervisors and department heads are usually needed to provide the proper guidance and motivation.

- Sufficient time should be allowed for preparation, negotiation, and review by interested parties. Typically, a minimum of 90 days should be scheduled for the budget process.
- Supervisors with responsibility for cost control and/or revenue generation should be actively involved in the preparation of the budget. This joint effort ensures that the budget is a participating budget, not just a management budget.
- Finally, there should be accurate data for expense and revenue projections and a statistical base in terms of work and dollars involved, e.g., reimbursement levels from third-party payers must be anticipated and used in the budget plan. Formal recognition of these constraints will make the budget more realistic and useful for planning purposes. The inflation rate must be estimated and included in the planned expenses for the next period. Inflation rates should be determined for each major cost element in order to obtain the best possible expense budget.

Budgets cannot control costs; only people can control costs. The budget, by itself, is only a tool to help managers and supervisors make decisions. An effective process will involve all levels of management and supervision in the preparation of the budget. However, because of the dynamic nature of providing health care services, performance information must also be provided periodically to those same managers and supervisors if corrective action is to be taken. Timely budget reporting provides this information.

An effective budget reporting system provides information using a responsibility center concept, e.g., the budget report received by a manager or supervisor would identify those costs that are controllable by that person. For revenue centers, the report would focus on the contribution margin or the difference between revenues and expenses. The purpose is to encourage the provision of services in ways that will enhance the total dollar amount of the contribution margin.

In summary, reports must be designed to meet the needs of the user. What is appropriate for one organization may not be effective for another. The level of detail, the type of information, and the timeliness of the report depend on the management training and the style of the manager.

Pricing Strategies

An important part of managerial decision-making pertains to decisions about establishing or accepting a price for health care services, e.g., in a fee-for-service environment, health care organizations need to determine whether they should offer discounts for large volume to valued payer groups such as large HMOs or business coalitions. In a capitated environment, the organization needs to determine the premium amount within which it is willing to risk responsibility for the provision of health care services. In the case of payers such as Medicare and Medicaid, where the health care organization is basically a price taker, the organization still needs to understand the impact of this *de facto* decision to sell services to the government. Understanding how to analyze product costs, such as costs by service, by DRG classification, or by enrollment population, is important for making such pricing decisions. Even when prices are set by overall market supply and demand forces (or by government power) and the health care organization has little or no influence on prices for services, the organization still has to make decisions about the extent and mix of services offered. In short, an important function of management accounting is to supply the cost information that helps support pricing decisions.

Pricing strategies ultimately tie back to a concern for the financial statements. As most providers get the bulk of their revenue from providing services, it is essential that health care managers establish prices that will generate revenues sufficient to meet the organization's total financial requirements, which include the full cost of doing business. It is also important that the revenue function be able to provide for the replenishment of existing assets, the costs of assets to expand into new services, and, in the case of for-profit organizations, the dividend rewards to the investors.

One of the critical underpinnings of the past pricing strategies of health care organizations was cross-subsidization, which meant the overcharging for many routine services, such as radiology and ancillary services, while under-charging for others and supporting teaching and services for the poor. Such cross-subsidization helped many hospitals to function as full-service institutions.

Major purchasers are no longer interested in having cross-subsidies built into their prices. Health care organizations that continue to cross-subsidize will contribute to two adverse selections. One of these will be that the healthier population will move away from the organizations that cross-subsidize toward the providers with prices that reflect the real value to the purchasers. A second adverse selection will be the movement of the less healthy population or certain types of services to the organizations that continue to offer these services below value. This will challenge the latter providers' ability to function as full-service institutions.

Managed care covers a range of pricing philosophies, from fee for service, where the challenge is in setting discounts, to semi-flat rate such as DRGs and commercial product line pricing, where some risk is assumed by the provider, to fully capitated arrangements that expose the provider to significant risk if utilization goes unmanaged.

Fee-for-service pricing puts the provider at little or no risk, other than the discounts at which services are offered. There is a positive incentive for the health care organization to use more tests and more procedures, to keep the patient in the hospital longer, and to admit more patients to the hospital. The only way the provider can hurt on this payment arrangement is if the discount on the fee-for-service price is so great that the revenue does not exceed the full cost (in the long run) or marginal cost (in the short run).

DRG payment, or the related commercial product line payment, such as fixed-price contracts for kidney transplantations, now provides negative incentives for the hospital to increase either utilization resource-by-resource or the length of hospital stays. However, under this payment philosophy, it is still in the hospital's interest to maximize the number of admissions pertaining to this DRG or commercial product line into the hospital.

Finally, the capitated payment philosophy provides negative incentives for the health care provider to maximize utilization at any level, whether resource by resource, length of stay, or number of admissions. The whole focus of managed-care systems as they move from fee-for-service toward capitation is to change the view of a hospital from that of a revenue center to that of a cost center. The focus becomes moved to a target-costing approach to pricing strategies, in which providers compete on premium prices established in the marketplace and work backward to get their cost structures in line with these market-defined prices. Part of this effort involves cascading health care services down to the lowest-cost mode of delivery (i.e., moving away from the hospital as our major cost center) while maintaining quality. One CFO from a multi-system stated that "we don't consider ourselves as being in the hospital business.... we view our hospital as a cost center, not as a revenue center as in the past." Essentially, the premium dollar has moved outside the hospital toward more outpatient, nursing home, and home health care services. As a health care organization moves from fee-for-service to prepaid practice, the primary emphasis moves from revenue production to cost control.

9

Ending the Blame Game: Economic Forces Behind our Health Care Problems

Timothy D. McBride

Introduction

In the last century, the US has considered major health care reform six times, and only once (in 1965) was it passed. This suggests that US citizens have often believed that we face a "health care crisis". Indeed, in 1991, 91% of Americans apparently believed that the US faced a "health care crisis" [1]. This perception led to the introduction of major health care reform proposals in 1993–94, including the much-publicized proposal introduced by President Clinton in October 1994.

Despite widespread agreement over the existence of a health care crisis and the nature of the problem, the public appears to be unaware or has been misled about the *causes* of the current health care morass that we face.

Most Americans have a good idea of whom to blame for our health care problems. When asked to identify the causes of the health care crisis, politicians, business owners, and health care providers commonly blame each other. Patients like to blame insurance companies for the uninsured problem and the American Medical Association (AMA) for escalating costs. Insurance companies blame doctors for escalating costs and the government for excess regulation and gaps in insurance coverage. Doctors and other providers blame government, the judicial system, and insurance companies for our health

care problems. Conveniently, few major players like to blame themselves for our health care problems and few people point the finger of blame at the recipients of the care, the patients.

In a 1993 survey of voters, Blendon found evidence to support this "blame game" behavior [2]. When Americans were asked which two groups were "most responsible for the high costs of health care," the responses were: insurers (48%), physicians (47%), hospitals (33%), and lawyers (33%). However, only 5% of voters (patients) listed patients as the group most responsible for the high costs of health care.

This "blame game" is not constructive. It solves very few of our problems to lay blame at the doorstep of any single group in the health care system. A careful study will reveal that no one group should be "blamed" for our current health care morass. Instead, the problems that we now observe are the inevitable outcome of natural forces within a health care "system" that has been poorly conceived, if it can be argued that the system was "conceived" at all. In this chapter, the author argues that economic forces have played an extremely important role in shaping our current health care system and its associated problems.

Why is it so important to understand these forces? Only if we develop an understanding of these causes of the health care crisis can we begin to develop intelligent solutions to it.

The Problems in the US Health Care System

Most people would identify the two major problems with the US health care system as: (1) the problem of escalating health care costs, and (2) the problem of access to health care for the uninsured and underinsured.*

Although there is common agreement on the problems, few understand the complexities of the issues and the causes of these problems. How did we get to this point of crisis? What is wrong with our health care market, and do we need the government to get involved to solve the problem?

If health care markets worked perfectly, nearly every economist and most other people would argue that there would be no reason for the government to become involved in health care. Most people understand the superiority of well-functioning free markets.

Unfortunately, it is not obvious that health care markets work very well. In fact, the root causes for the access and cost problems lie in the functioning of the markets. In most cases, these markets developed naturally, whereas, in other cases, government interventions exacerbated natural forces and, in still others, social and political forces unrelated to economics led to the outcomes we see today.

When markets fail for whatever reason, it is also intuitively clear to many Americans, but perhaps fewer economists, that there is a role for government. Most Americans understand that government is the only entity that can provide for national defense and that natural monopolies such as utility companies would exploit their market power if not regulated by the government. There is broader disagreement over the proper government role in education or protecting the economically disadvantaged. Yet almost everyone agrees that the markets for many goods and services, such as electronic products, automobiles, and personal services, operate very well with little government intervention.

* In addition, the author likes to identify a third problem: the problems associated with delivering *long-term care* to elderly and disabled people. However, there has been little discussion of this issue in recent health care reform debates.

This helps to explain the perpetual debates over health care reform. Most people seem to agree that the government should intervene in the health care market. The disagreement is over how much intervention is appropriate. To make such decisions, policymakers and average voters both need to understand how our health care crisis came about.

The Problem of Escalating Costs

The first major problem is escalating health care costs. Americans spend more money on health care than they do on food and housing combined. In 1997, health expenditures totaled almost $1.1 trillion, a figure that represents 13.5% of the gross domestic product (GDP) and about $3925 for each person in the country [3].

Although the health care sector is now enormous, it is the growth in health care spending that has caused consternation. Until recently, the rate of growth in spending has been staggering. Health care spending in 1997 was almost 100 times higher than it was in 1950 ($12.7 billion), when it equaled only 4.4% of the GDP (Table 9-1). On average, health care spending increased by over 10% per year from 1960 through 1997, and it is projected to increase at similar rates in the future.

Why Do We Care about Escalating Costs?

The mere existence of a huge growth rate in health care spending does not prove that there is a problem. An economist is likely to say: "So what if health care spending is rising? It must mean that people are willing to pay that much for health care". Indeed, health care's huge share of the GDP and its fast growth rate may simply be evidence of Americans' strong desire for health care and the incredible success of health care providers at selling their services. To put it another way, consider what the reaction would be if Table 9-1 had portrayed car sales as a percentage of GDP. A great deal of attention is paid to the health of the auto industry, and huge increases in auto sales would certainly be applauded by executives at Ford and GM.

Table 9-1. National Health Expenditures: Calendar Years 1960–1997 and Projections, 1998–2007. (Source: Health Care Financing Administration, Office of the Actuary, National Health Statistics Group (1999); and author's calculations).

Year	TOTAL ($ million)	Percentage of gross domestic product	Per capita amounts (2001 $)	(1998 $)
1960	26,850	5.1	141	766
1961	28,768	5.3	149	799
1962	31,268	5.3	159	847
1963	34,067	5.5	171	898
1964	37,647	5.7	187	967
1965	41,145	5.7	202	1028
1966	45,263	5.7	219	1087
1967	50,969	6.1	245	1175
1968	57,684	6.3	274	1264
1969	64,792	6.6	305	1333
1970	73,243	7.1	341	1411
1971	81,018	7.2	373	1480
1972	90,943	7.4	415	1594
1973	100,838	7.3	456	1650
1974	114,265	7.6	513	1670
1975	130,727	8.0	582	1737
1976	149,856	8.2	662	3949
1977	170,375	8.4	746	1975
1978	190,601	8.3	827	2035
1979	215,201	8.4	924	2044
1980	247,273	8.9	1052	2049
1981	286,908	9.2	1208	2133
1982	322,978	10.0	1346	2238
1983	355,291	10.1	1466	2362
1984	390,076	10.0	1594	2462
1985	428,720	10.3	1735	2588
1986	461,228	10.4	1848	2706
1987	500,502	10.7	1985	2805
1988	560,379	11.1	2201	2986
1989	623,536	11.5	2423	3137
1990	699,361	12.2	2690	3303
1991	766,783	13.0	2919	3440
1992	836,537	13.4	3151	3604
1993	898,496	13.7	3350	3721
1994	947,717	13.6	3500	3790
1995	993,725	13.7	3636	3829
1996	1,042,522	13.6	3780	3867
1997	1,092,385	13.5	3925	3925
Average Annual Growth rates (%)				
1960–97	10.5	2.7	9.4	4.5
1960–70	10.6	3.3	9.2	6.3
1970–80	12.9	2.3	11.9	3.8
1980–90	11.0	3.2	9.8	4.9
1990–97	6.6	1.5	5.5	2.5

Remember the adage, "what's good for GM is good for America." Whether this is true or not, we should remember that health care is a business like many others, so that may make us wonder whether rising health care costs is really a problem at all.

The Money's Worth Question

One reason rising health care costs are perceived to be a problem is that people are asking the inevitable question: if we are spending more than any other country on health care, are our health and health care so much better? Most people feel that the health care we receive is the best in the world. International comparisons show that US health care expenditures are the highest in the world, by far [4]. Despite this, there is little evidence that these vast expenditures have significantly improved our health. Our higher-than-average mortality and infant mortality rates suggest that spending has not eliminated all problems [5]. Most epidemiological studies suggest that the major advances in public health occurred long before the explosion in health care costs [6]. Improvements in public sanitation, the environment, immunizations, and education did far more to improve our health than any of the machines in hospitals. In addition to problems with health measures, skeptics note that 16% of US citizens lack health insurance and perhaps lack access to health care.

Although the money's worth argument is a compelling complaint about the US system, it may go too far. This is because international health care cost comparisons are flawed. Not only are these comparisons subject to exchange rate variations and purchasing power parity problems, but slower increases in health care costs as a percentage of the GDP could occur simply because the GDP grew faster in one country than it did in another [7].

Perhaps more important is the problem of finding an objective criterion for comparing health care systems across countries. Indicators such as mortality rates are the best that are available, but it is easy to see that the health care system is only one factor that affects mortality rates. Other factors—such as higher murder rates, drug abuse, higher use of cars, many guns, more income inequality, and other social problems—contribute more to the difference in mortality rates across countries.

The Burden of Health Care Costs

If Americans are spending more of their money on health care, then they must be spending less in percentage terms on everything else. And few people, except perhaps hypochondriacs, are happy to subject themselves to medical interventions. Businesses are paying higher health insurance premiums, government budgets are being squeezed by health care costs, and individual consumers are facing higher and higher out-of-pocket costs.

The evidence shows that health care is a bigger burden on everyone's budgets. But, although most of the increases in health care costs in the 1950s and 1960s were borne by businesses and government, in the 1970s and 1980s a concerted effort was made to shift much of the burden of health care costs to households [8]. It can be argued that this trend explains much of the increasing crescendo for health care reform.

Is the Market Working?

Although the "burden" of health care costs may be a valid political explanation for the demand for health care reform, it is not a compelling reason from an economist's point of view unless it can be shown that the market is not operating efficiently. This is because consumers in a perfect market who choose to increase the burden of health care expenditures on their budgets could simply be making a rational choice to do so.

An economist would argue that the increase in health care spending would not be a problem if we were getting the best health care for the money spent (an economist would ask: is the provision of health care efficient?) and if the consumers wanted the high level of health care expenditures. If these conditions were met, then it could be argued that there is no problem—the market is working properly. If, however, there is evidence that there are problems in the health care market, a high level of health care spending might be a public policy problem. Unfortunately, there is evidence of problems in the health care market and evidence that these problems have contributed to the cost escalation problem.

Table 9-2. Breakdown of Average Annual Growth in National Health Spending: 1960–2007. (Source: Author's calculations based on Table 9-1.)

| Years | Percentage increase in total | Average annual growth in: | | Total | Average annual growth in Real per capita spending: | |
| | | Population | General inflation | | Total attributable to: | |
					Prices	Utilization
1960–97	10.5	1.1	4.9	4.5	1.9	2.7
By decade:						
1960–70	10.6	1.3	2.9	6.3	1.6	4.7
1970–80	12.9	1.0	8.1	3.8	0.4	3.4
1980–90	11.0	1.1	5.0	4.9	3.3	1.6
1990–97	6.6	1.0	3.1	2.5	2.3	0.2
In 1990s:						
1993–97	8.7	1.1	3.5	4.1	3.8	0.2
1993–97	5.0	1.0	2.7	1.3	1.2	0.1
Projection:						
1997–2007	6.9	0.8	2.7	3.4	1.2	2.1

What Factors Account for the Increases in Health Care Costs?

When the public was asked by pollster Robert Blendon in 1994 to identify the factors contributing "a great deal" to high health care costs, the responses were: malpractice lawsuits (59%), waste and fraud (58%), fraudulent claims (50%), doctors practicing defensive medicine (44%), AIDS (44%), new and expensive drugs (43%), new technology (39%), urban problems such as crime and drugs (34%), the aging population (29%), and the expectations of the public for "best" treatment under any condition (25%). Moreover, 83% of the public agreed with the statement: "Cutting waste, greed, and profits is the most practical way to finance national health care." Despite these opinions, what does the evidence show? Table 9-2 displays the annual growth rates in health care spending and breaks down these increases into various factors that account for that growth. Overall, health care costs increased by an average of 10.5% per year from 1960 to 1997. However, this is the growth in *overall* health care spending. This spending will increase for a couple of reasons that are unrelated to what is going on in the health care sector. In particular, spending will increase because of increases in

(1) general price inflation and (2) population. Table 9-2 shows that the average increase in general inflation between 1960 and 1997 was 4.9%, whereas the population increased by an average of 1.1% annually.

Removing these effects isolates the increases in real per capita health care spending, which is shown to have increased by 4.5% annually from 1950 to 1997 (Table 9-2). Analysts have attributed these increases to various factors, although a great deal of attention has been paid to health care price inflation (in excess of general inflation). Table 9-2 shows that medical care inflation has increased by 1.9% per year faster than general inflation. This leaves 2.7% annual growth that is entirely the result of "volume intensity," i.e., increases in either the volume of services used per person or the intensity of service use per person.

Many analysts have pointed out that the health care component of the consumer price index (CPI), as measured by the Department of Labor, is not a good measure of health care inflation because it does not adequately account for changes in the *quality* or even *quantity* of health care services that might result in health care price inflation [9,10]. Thus, the distinction drawn in Table 9-2 may not be so meaningful. Obviously, health care prices may have increased faster than the rate of general inflation over the last few decades, but the health care component of the CPI overstates increases in health care prices because it does not account for these quality and quantity changes. Thus, we need to turn to other explanations for rising health care costs.

Economic Forces Behind Escalating Costs

It is difficult to understand any of the forces shaping our health care system without understanding the important role uncertainty plays in the system. Although it is true that few events in our lives occur with certainty, it is obvious that few, if any, health-related events occur with certainty. Instead, uncertainty is pervasive throughout the health care sector, with profound consequences on the behavior of everyone involved.

The most important consequence of uncertainty is that it has led to the development of the entire health insurance industry. Uncertainty leads to the demand for health insurance, because we believe that most patients have a well-founded and rational desire to minimize the amount of financial risk that they face [11]. Thus, they will forgo a sum of money (an insurance premium) on a regular and predictable basis, rather than face irregular and potentially catastrophic health bills, even if the total of their lifetime health insurance premiums exceeds their lifetime medical costs. Not only have economic theorists shown that consumers will behave in this way, but simple observation of the widespread demand for health insurance has demonstrated its utility.

Uncertainty plays other important roles in the health care system and contributes to other big problems with the system, e.g., doctors and other providers are often uncertain about the efficacy of the care they provide. It can be argued that this may lead them to purchase insurance to protect them against malpractice lawsuits, and perhaps to provide excessive services, including excessive tests and unnecessary operations, when the decision to avoid these services could lead to negative outcomes and, most important, malpractice lawsuits. This "defensive medicine" has been cited as a major cause of the increase

in health care costs, although academic studies suggest that the size of this problem has been vastly overstated [12].

Insurance Market Problems

It is obvious that usually health insurance is a valuable benefit that makes the recipients of insurance better off, if mostly from the peace of mind that it offers. In addition, insurance provides the essential funds to purchase expensive health care that would otherwise be inaccessible to almost everyone.

Despite the obvious benefits of insurance, problems in the insurance market are the root cause of most the problems facing the US health care system today. Although it is widely believed that these insurance market problems are the result of devious and money-hungry profiteers in the health insurance industry, it is more accurate to describe the structure of our insurance system, with its myriad problems, as the natural outcome of competition between insurance companies, shaped by historical, social, and political forces.

In the US, health insurance is mostly provided through employers. This is the case because employer group insurance filled the natural void that was left when federal and state government policymakers decided in the 1920s and 1930s, and again in the 1950s, not to set up a system of national health insurance. Many factors contributed to this decision, including the power of interest groups (particularly the AMA), the influence of anticommunism and anti-Germanism, and the natural proclivity of Americans to distrust the government [6].

When political and social forces led to the decision not to provide national health insurance, it was almost inevitable that employers would form the groups that would purchase insurance for their workers. This is because insurance requires that risk be shared by all members of a group, and employers were natural groups for this risk sharing. It might have been possible for individuals to use other social groups to purchase insurance, such as trade unions or social clubs. However, the development of employer group insurance was encouraged in the 1940s when wage and price controls during the Second World War coincided with the development of health insurance and provided a strong incentive for employers to provide compensation to workers through means other than direct wage payments [13]. Employer-provided insurance was further encouraged by the union movement [6].

Once the US had decided to provide health insurance mostly through employers, the natural economic forces driving the insurance market toward the problems we face today were set in motion. Not only has the simple presence of health insurance contributed to the problem of escalating costs, but insurance market problems today have contributed to the access problem. It can be argued that insurance markets initially worked well in providing the financial means to pay for health care. However, competition among insurers and the slow but steady increase in health care costs eventually led insurers to develop practices that have exacerbated the access problem.

What are the insurance market practices and problems that have contributed directly to the health care crisis? Experts list many culprits.

Insurance and Induced Demand

The commonsense proposition that consumers will purchase more of goods or services if the price drops has long been one of the central tenets of economic analysis. It should come as no surprise therefore that economists would predict that insurance should lead consumers to purchase more health care goods and services. This is because health insurance acts as a mechanism that drops the price of health care *at the point of purchase.** Sometimes, the price is

equal to the deductible (typically a few hundred dollars), plus some percentage of the costs above that amount (equal to the co-payment, typically between 10% and 20%). Sometimes, consumers receive health care services at zero price, with no deductibles or co-payments (typical for people covered by health maintenance organizations or HMOs). In any case, it should come as no surprise that individuals would use more health care services when the purchase price is zero or nearly so.

There is no doubt among economists that health insurance increases the consumption of health care goods and services [9]. However, there is some disagreement about the magnitude of the effect. Some seem to argue that nearly all of the increases in health care costs are attributable to this factor [13]. On the other hand, others have concluded that the research suggests that the effect is smaller than one might otherwise believe [14,15]. Primarily this is because of the uniqueness of health care services. It is obvious that many, if not most, expensive health care services are perceived by patients to be essential and life-saving when provided. Therefore, patients choose the amount of health services to consume without regard for the price of these services, especially when the disease is life threatening. Patients facing life-threatening health problems will not behave like rational consumers (as economists require) and will not worry about how they will pay for services that may be charged against their estates. Thus it has been found that health care price elasticities are relatively small for health care services in general, ranging from -0.17 to -0.22 for all medical expenditures [9]. Elasticities are smallest for services such as hospital services, although they are higher when purchasing less acute services such as doctor's well visits, outpatient care, or dental care. Thus, the effect of insurance on the quantity and price of health services is less pronounced than would be expected, especially because it is difficult to separate this effect from physician-induced demand. Owing to the low estimates of price elasticities, Aaron [14] and Newhouse [15] have concluded that increased insurance coverage has accounted for between 5% and 10% of the increase in health care spending since 1950.

---

* Although consumers will have to pay for the cost of health care consumed eventually through increases in health care premiums, it also clear that many consumers are likely to act as though the purchase price of a health care service is reduced by the amount paid by insurance. This is because every dollar of increased health care costs, if it is eventually reflected in the insurance premium at all, will only increase an individual's premium by ($1/n$) $\times f$, where n is the size of the insurance group and f is equal to the loading fee. The larger the size of the group, the smaller is this amount, through its direct effects on $1/n$ and through indirect effects on the size of the loading fee, e.g., the loading fee for a group with 5000 people is estimated to be only 5%, so an additional dollar of health care expenditures should increase a person's premium by less than 2/100ths of a cent ($1.05 \times 1/5000$). In contrast, the loading fee for a small group of five people is typically 40%. Thus, a $1 expenditure for a person in this group should lead to a 28-cent increase in premiums.

Moral Hazard

Insurers have been long been fearful about the effects of insurance on the use of health care. Pauly [16] coined the term "moral hazard" to describe any behavioral changes that lead to increased health care costs. Clearly this could include the effect described previously as insurance-induced demand. However, economists have identified another possible response that increases health care use. Insurance may induce some people who are covered by insurance to engage in risky activities when insurers insulate them from the costs of these activities, e.g., people who smoke might consider the potential costs of treating cancer if they had to pay for the costs of that treatment out of their own pockets. On the other hand, if health insurance paid for the costs of this treatment, insurers fear that consumers would simply increase their cigarette consumption. Although it might seem incredible that individuals would consider only the costs of health care and not other costs when deciding to smoke, it is nevertheless indisputable that insurance lowers the costs of negative behaviors such as smoking, drinking, or unsafe sex, and contributes to the "moral hazard" that people will engage in these risky behaviors.

Insurers have a few tools available to control the increased costs brought on by the problems of moral hazard, including induced demand. They may use underwriting to deny coverage to people who engage in risky behaviors, if they can be identified. This is possible only because most private health insurance in the US is optionally renewable [13]. Alternatively, insurers may enact preexisting condition exclusions to exclude from coverage procedures that treat problems associated with negative behaviors (e.g., cancer, liver, and AIDS treatments). Finally, they have developed experience rating to match the health care cost experience of an individual or group as closely as possible to the premium they are charged (more on this later). Thus, the creation of methods for controlling health care claims are the natural response of insurance companies to an insurance market problem. But this response creates its own problems—the insurance practices have led to increased complaints about access problems and have increased the number of uninsured people.

Insurance and Technology

Many economists who have looked at the reasons for rising health care costs have concluded that *rapidly increasing technology* is the major reason costs have risen [14,15].

Almost everyone has been exposed to the miracles of modern medicine. In our lifetimes we have seen the development of computed tomography (CT) and magnetic resonance imaging (MRI), the introduction of procedures such as organ transplantations and sophisticated surgical procedures for curing heart problems, the development of drugs that cure a host of important problems, and the rapid advances in medical education leading to well-trained nurses and physicians. Experts conclude that more than half the increases in real per-capita health care costs have been caused by the increased use of these sophisticated technologies.

What has not been discussed in great detail is the role that health insurance plays in the development of these technological innovations. Many of these machines and procedures are very expensive, but improve health and survival rates only slightly. In these cases, it is doubtful that the economic value of these procedures is higher than their costs. If patients were paying the full costs of these procedures, they might not purchase them, just as we decide not to purchase consumer goods that we feel are not worth the price. However, when insurance lowers the price of medical care to a small fraction of its total costs, it is much more likely that people will choose to use expensive new technology and that providers will choose to adopt it. It is this insulation from the costs of new technology— provided by insurance—that has fueled the rapid growth in technological innovation. Goddeeris [17] developed a model that demonstrates how health insurance induces innovators to switch from cost-reducing innovations to cost-increasing innovations.

Tax Policy and Insurance Coverage

In the US, income tax policy encourages people to purchase more expensive insurance [18]. This occurs because the tax code essentially subsidizes the purchase of insurance, as health insurance premiums are not taxable to employees who receive them. The amount of this subsidy is equal to the tax the person pays on wages.[†] It is important to note that the amount of this subsidy could be quite large—ranging from a low of roughly 15% for a low-wage worker to a high of over 50% for a worker with a higher income living in a state with an income tax.

The policy problem created by this tax policy is that the amount of the subsidy increases as the size of the tax-deferred premium increases. A person who chooses an expensive (so-called "Cadillac") health insurance plan receives a larger subsidy than a person who chooses a lower-priced plan. Thus, the tax policy encourages people to choose policies with more generous benefits that lead to higher health care costs, e.g., suppose that an employee is choosing between two plans—one generous plan with a premium of $4000 and another with a premium of $3000. Without the tax break, the difference in costs between these plans is $1000. But with the tax break, the after-tax cost of these plans for a person facing a marginal tax rate of 40% are $2400 and $1800, respectively. Thus, the tax code lowers the price difference between the plans to $600 from $1000, and may encourage this employee to enroll in the more generous plan.

Information Asymmetry and Physician-induced Demand

When consumers and producers have access to the same information, the market should function well. Consumers will understand what they are buying and know how much it is worth to them, how much they can afford, and what the "going price" is. On the other hand, sellers will realize that consumers have access to information, so they will not be able to sell consumers more than they want or charge them a price that is higher than the market price. Unfortunately, when either the consumer or seller has more

---

[†] The purchase of health insurance is subsidized through the tax code by the following mechanism. Employers are allowed to deduct, as a cost of doing business, the full compensation paid to employees, including the amount they pay for premiums. On the other hand, employees do not pay tax on the health insurance premiums paid by their employer (and in some cases on the amount paid out of pocket if they can set up a tax-free flexible spending account). Thus, if premiums were taxable, then employees would have paid a tax on these premiums, equal to the tax rate times the premium.

information than the other party, then this well-functioning market breaks down [19].

It is commonly believed that doctors and other health care providers have more information than their patients. There are many reasons why this information asymmetry may exist. First, health care providers usually have much more experience and training in the health field. Second, health care technology changes so rapidly that even diligent consumers cannot keep up with their doctors. Third, there is a historical tradition to respect doctors: nearly every poll reveals that the average person trusts their doctor more than anyone else. Fourth, consumers may not be rational when they receive their medical care. In other words, if they are so worried about their condition, especially if it is life threatening, then they will not question the recommendation of their doctor. For these reasons, many people argue that doctors can induce their patients to consume more health care services than their patients would otherwise agree to use.

The process might go something like in this hypothetical example:

> Hype O. Chondriac is a patient covered by fee-for-service insurance with no deductibles or copayments. Recently he has been feeling ill, so he made an appointment with his doctor, Dr Mal O. Practice, to discuss the problem. At the appointment, Hype explained to Dr Practice: "Doctor, my arm is really hurting these days. I don't know what the problem is. This medical care is so confusing, I don't know what I need. Do you have any idea about what to do?" Dr Practice, thinking for a moment, glanced at the insurance form in front of him, which reminded him of Hype's health insurance coverage. "Well Hype, I am not sure. I think I need to order an MRI and a few other tests before I can draw a conclusion." Hype wondered for a moment about how expensive these tests would be, then quickly dismissed the thought because he knew he would not pay for them. "Whatever you say, Doc," he concluded. With that, Dr Practice ordered the tests and Hype left, satisfied that the American health care system had served him well again.

If a well-informed consumer would not have agreed to these tests, it can be argued that the doctor induced the consumer to use more medical care services.

Unfortunately, there are incentives for doctors and other providers to induce their patients to use more medical care. First, many health care providers can increase their income by ordering more tests and procedures. The financial stake that many doctors have in their businesses only increases these incentives. Second, health care providers are trained according to the Hippocratic Oath, which says that "the health of my patient will be my first consideration" [20]. Thus, costs should not be the first consideration and, what is more, the Oath underscores that patients shall not be discriminated against on the basis of social standing or ability to pay. Finally, health care providers might be severely penalized through malpractice suits if they order too few tests or procedures. Unfortunately it is impossible to tell whether a doctor made the decision in order to avoid malpractice or to increase his or her income. The AMA and many doctors like to argue that all excess tests and procedures are the result of fears of malpractice—so-called "defensive medicine." Certainly defensive medicine is part of the problem, but evidence suggests that this accounts for only about 5% of total health care spending [12]. Thus, the other two explanations are more likely.

What is important about this example is the way that insurance-induced demand and physician-induced demand interact with each other. Together they are a formula for disaster. The problem is that consumers have no incentive to close the information gap because they pay little or none of the costs. When purchasing a car, we often will buy *Consumer Reports* and attempt to close the information gap. But, if a person belongs to an HMO and pays nothing out of pocket for health care costs, why question the doctor's advice?

To make an absurd analogy, suppose that you recently purchased food insurance to cover all of your grocery bills, and you know nothing about food. At the grocery store, you tell the manager, "I'm hungry and I have food insurance. Could you pick out some food for me?" The elated manager will return with a cart of groceries filled with lobster, caviar, steaks, and duplicates of many other unnecessary items.

To be sure, this absurd analogy is not an accurate depiction of the health care market. There are a few mechanisms to help control this sort of behavior. First, some patients have become diligent, learning about the appropriate procedures and tests for many health problems. Second, health care providers are taught ethics and presumably behave in the best interests of their patients, not only in their own financial interests. Unfortunately, these important checks on the behavior of health care providers may not be enough in all cases to overwhelm either the behavior of the patients or the strong incentives for providers to "order the extra test." Thus, many people feel that physician-induced demand is a reality.

The Insurer's Response: Managed Care and Administrative Costs

The problem we have described occurs because there are *three* players involved every time a health care decision is made, but only *two* participate in the decision. Health care decisions are made by the patient and the provider. But a third party, the insurance company, is paying the bill and passing it back to employers. The problem is that these third parties were not in the room when the decisions were made. They cannot say, "Hey, that costs too much. Isn't there a cheaper choice?" Of course, insurance companies have not been passive about increasing health care costs. First, they have tried to pass most of the cost increases through as increases in premiums. Sometimes they can do this. But as the insurance market has become very competitive, it has become more difficult for them to pass these costs along. Thus, insurers have turned to other methods. As insurance companies feel left out of the decision-making process, they have recently injected themselves into it. Insurance companies have set up elaborate mechanisms to "manage care" where unknowledgeable patients are replaced with knowledgeable managers of care, often nurses, who work for the insurance company.

Managed care in health insurance plans started with the introduction of HMOs and preferred provider organizations (PPOs) in the 1970s. The number of people insured by HMOs and PPOs has grown considerably. The share of the insurance market controlled by HMOs and PPOs grew from only 4% in 1977 to 86% by 1998 [21]. This is only part of the revolution in health insurance. Besides HMOs and PPOs, most other insurers in "conventional" plans have turned to managed care to help them control health care costs.

The shift to managed care was designed to help control costs. The recent slowdown in the growth of health care expenditures (Table 9-1) has been credited by some to the managed care revolution. However, all of the increased management of health care adds to the already high administrative costs of running the US system, estimated to total 20–30% of US health care costs [22]. These costs include other administrative costs, but the extra burden is the cost of operating 1500 or more insurance companies. There are no studies to show how quickly these costs are rising. However, these costs are much higher than they are in countries with national health insurance systems, or at least many fewer insurance plans, e.g., only about 10% of health care costs go for administrative costs in Canada [23].

Do These Factors Account for Rising Health Care Costs?

In Table 9-2, an attempt was made to account for the factors that cause health care costs to increase. Available data allow for the removal of general inflation and population growth. However, we were unable to easily explain the 4.5% average annual increase in real per-capita health care costs from 1950 to 1997.

Do the market factors we have just discussed explain any portion of this 4.5% annual increase? In my opinion, the health economics literature has identified the following as important factors in real per-capita health care cost increases.

Increases in Health Care Inflation (Above General Price Inflation)

Table 9-2 shows that this has been computed by the Department of Labor to be 1.9% per year. However, for the reasons previously cited, most people conclude that part of this increase measures changes in the quality and quantity of services provided. Although the flaws in the medical care CPI make it difficult to attach exact

numbers to various effects, it is still possible that health care price inflation has exceeded general inflation. In fact, the problems of insurance-induced demand and asymmetric information contribute to this by effectively removing the consumer from health care decision-making. Although a 1.9% annual increase is too high, many analysts have concluded that health care price inflation accounts for roughly 1.0% of the increase in real per-capita costs [14,15].

Insurance-induced Demand

If insurance induces increased demand for health care services by dropping the price of health care at the point of purchase, increases in health insurance coverage since 1960 should account for some increase in health care costs. However, this effect is dampened by low price elasticities of demand. Thus, insurance-induced demand accounts for only about 10% of the increases in health care spending, i.e., about 0.5% of the average annual increase.

Aging of the Population

Although much discussed, this factor has accounted for only about 0.5% of the increase in real per-capita health care costs [14,23].

Increases in National Personal Income

Most people believe that health care is a luxury good, i.e., its use increases when income increases. International studies of the relationship of health care spending to national income have confirmed this. These studies have computed the income elasticity for health care spending [24], and this in turn can be used to measure the impact of increases in national personal income on health care spending. From these international studies, we can conclude that approximately 1.0–1.3% of the 4.5% increase has resulted from increases in national income.

Other Factors

Many authors have identified other factors that account for the increase in health care costs, including increased malpractice costs and defensive medicine and increased administrative costs. Although the costs of defensive medicine account for about 5% of health care spending and administrative costs account for 10–20%, there have been few studies of the increase in these costs in recent years.

The factors described so far account collectively for about 3.0–3.3% of the 4.5% average annual increase in real per-capita health care costs since 1950. What accounts for the rest of the increase?

Insurance and Technology

From this analysis, increases in health care technology account for roughly 1.2–1.5% of the average annual increase in real per-capita health care costs. From this breakdown, we can see that three factors—health care price inflation, income growth, and technological change—account for most of the increases in real per-capita health care spending in the last 40–45 years.

The Problem of Access for the Uninsured

Although we spend more money than any country in the world on health care, skeptics point out that we are the only industrialized country in the world (other than South Africa) to leave a significant portion of our citizens without health insurance coverage [25]. One out of seven people do not have health insurance coverage. In addition, many who have health insurance have inadequate coverage. This creates a host of other problems. Either these people go without health care, or they face huge expenditures on health care, or hospitals and other providers must pick up the tab for the care they receive. In fact, the evidence suggests that all three of these outcomes occur.

As indicated by Table 9-3, 84% of nonelderly people are covered by health insurance in the US.* The vast majority (70%) are covered by "private" insurance, including employment-based insurance or other privately purchased insurance. About 24% are covered by public insurance (primarily Medicare, the federal government program that covers the aged, blind, and disabled, or Medicaid, the program designed to

cover the poor). This means that 16% of people are "uninsured," i.e., they are not covered by any health insurance policy.

The latest estimate of the number of uninsured at any given point in time is 44.3 million, based on a 1998 estimate from Current Population Survey (CPS) (US Bureau of the Census 1999). Part of the reason for the concern about the uninsured is that the number is increasing (Table 9-3).[†] Most of this increase has resulted from increases in the US population, but there is a slight increase in the percentage of the population that is uninsured.[‡]

The issue of the number of uninsured has become a source of controversy [26]. Some commentators have argued that the number of uninsured people is overstated because many are short-term uninsured [27,28]. However, this argument is flawed, because it stems from a misinterpretation of recent research findings [26]. The data show that 28 million people are "chronically" uninsured for over 1 year, and over 20 million are chronically uninsured for more than 2 years. Moreover, approximately 58 million people in the US will lose health insurance for at least 1 month over a 1-year period [29]. Many of these people lose their insurance when they change jobs, but this shows that, over a 1-year period, almost 25% of us will face the problem of being uninsured. This may not be a problem for many people, but going without health insurance for only 1 month may be catastrophic for someone who just happens to face an illness in that month, especially if the illness creates a preexisting condition that then makes them ineligible for health insurance.

[†] As a result of the change in the CPS questions in 1988 (adding the cover sheet questions for children), this percentage change is not directly computable. However, the number of uninsured people increased by 30% from 1979 to 1990 (from 30.4 to 39.6 million) and by 8% from 1990 to 1992 (from 34.7 to 37.3 million), using consistent definitions. Putting these growth rates together gives an estimated increase in the uninsured population of roughly 40% from 1979 to 1992.
[‡] It is difficult to derive an exact time series of the number of uninsured people, mostly because of changes in the survey questionnaires used to measure them. Reconstructions of the estimates using the old methods do show an increase in the percentage of people who are uninsured from 13.7% to 15.9% from 1979 to 1990 (excluding the cover sheet children) and from 13.9% to 14.7% from 1990 to 1992 (including the cover sheet children).

---

* The discussion is restricted here to nonelderly people, because the vast majority (99%) of elderly people aged over 65 are covered by Medicare.

Table 9-3. Sources of Health Insurance Coverage, 1987–98.

| | | | | Percentage of people with insurance | | | | | |
| | | | | Private | | Public* | | | |
Year	Total population (millions)	Total (%)	Total (%)*	Employer (%)	Total (%)	Medicare (%)	Medicaid (%)	Percentage uninsured	Number of uninsured
1987	241.2	87.1	75.5	62.1	23.3	12.6	8.4	12.9	31,026
1988	243.7	86.6	74.7	61.9	23.3	12.7	8.5	13.4	32,680
1989	246.2	86.4	74.5	61.6	23.3	12.8	8.6	13.6	33,385
1990	248.9	86.1	73.2	60.4	24.5	13.0	9.7	13.9	34,719
1991	251.4	85.9	72.1	59.7	25.4	13.1	10.7	14.1	35,447
1992	257.3	85.0	71.1	57.9	25.8	12.9	11.5	15.0	38,641
1993	259.5	84.7	70.2	57.1	26.4	12.7	12.2	15.3	39,713
1994	261.2	84.8	70.3	60.9	26.8	12.9	12.1	15.2	39,718
1995	264.3	84.6	70.3	61.1	26.4	13.1	12.1	15.4	40,582
1996	266.8	84.4	70.2	61.2	25.9	13.2	11.8	15.6	41,716
1997	269.1	83.9	70.1	61.4	24.8	13.2	10.8	16.1	43,448
1998	271.7	83.7	70.2	62.0	24.3	13.2	10.3	16.3	44,281

* Some persons have both private and public coverage or multiple sources of public coverage. (Source: US Census Bureau World Wide Web table H1–1, retrieved November 1999.)

Who are Uninsured People?

One reason for the concern about uninsured people is that any of us could become uninsured. Popular stereotypes depict uninsured people as poor, young, and unemployed, but the facts show that they are a very diverse group. Although it is true that people under age 25 are more likely to be uninsured, it is also true that more than half of uninsured people are over the age of 25. Similarly, the poor are more likely to be uninsured. But over 70% of uninsured people live in families with incomes above the poverty level, and 21% have incomes that exceed three times the poverty level.

Probably the most erroneous stereotype about uninsured people is that they are likely to be unemployed. As most insurance is provided through employers, many of us believe that almost every working person has insurance. In fact, it turns out that 84% of uninsured people come from a family where someone is working, and 68% come from a family where someone is working full-time (US Bureau of the Census 1999). Thus, only 16% of uninsured people fit the stereotype.

These facts are shocking to many people. How could it be possible that some people in the US could be working full-time and still not have health insurance? There is no simple answer to this question, but this has occurred largely because our system of employer-provided health insurance is falling apart.

Why are People Uninsured?

As noted, 16% of the US population at a given time is without health insurance. Employers are the most important source of health insurance (62% of nonelderly people obtain insurance through an employer). However, 86% of the uninsured are members of a family in which someone is working. The remainder live in families without a worker. In this case, they have not obtained either private, nongroup insurance or public insurance. Why would they not be covered by these sources of insurance? And why would workers? There are two main reasons for this: (1) insurance premiums are not affordable, or (2) insurance is not available.

Economic Forces Contributing to the Uninsured Problem: Affordability

To the extent that it is possible, insurance companies who face escalating health care costs will pass these on to employers through higher premiums. When faced with these escalating premium costs, employers face several choices. Usually they will pass these increases on to their employees through lower wages (or at least wages that do not increase as fast as they would otherwise) or through higher premiums charged directly to employees. In this case, some employees may decide to forgo coverage because of high premiums. Long and Marquis found that 10% of employees were offered health insurance by their firms, but turned down the coverage [30].* Some of these decisions may result from a misperception of their health risks, but some people (especially people in the 18–24 age group) may find that no insurance is worth the price charged (because they are healthy and unlikely to use insurance).

If employers cannot or do not want to pass premium cost increases through to employees, they may decide to eliminate insurance coverage when premium costs increase.† This has also contributed to the uninsured problem. Only 77% of employees worked for firms that offered insurance in 1989 [31]. Moreover, in a recent survey of small business owners, 13% of them indicated that they had dropped insurance coverage in the last 3 years [32].

Economic Forces Behind the Uninsured Problem: Availability and Insurance Market Problems

Although escalating costs have contributed directly to the problem of the uninsured, there are other reasons why insurance has become very difficult to obtain. In particular, insurance companies have developed elaborate ways to rid themselves of insurees with high health care costs. These methods have led to substantial criticism from policymakers and others who contend

---

* In an employer survey conducted by the Health Insurance Association of America, 86% of employers who did not provide insurance cited "expense" as an important reason for not offering insurance. Other reasons cited as important were: low or unstable profits (76%), future cost (70%), and low employee interest (52%) [31].
† It is important to note that 8% of employees who turned down the coverage had other insurance coverage. Only 2% turned down coverage and remained uninsured. However, another 6% of employees were ineligible for insurance coverage (probably because of preexisting conditions), and 18% of employees worked for firms that did not offer them insurance coverage.

that the insurers are ruthless, uncompassionate, greedy, or all of the above.

The Problem of Adverse Selection

Though it is easy to blame the insurance companies, a closer examination of the insurance market suggests that many of their behaviors are the inevitable result of market forces, in particular, adverse selection.

What is adverse selection? People who are high risks for large medical costs will obviously have the strongest demand for health insurance. Moreover, when faced with a choice of health insurance plans with different premiums but similar services, consumers will be likely to choose the plan with the lowest premium in relation to their expected health care costs. Thus, the natural behavior of individuals should lead them to *self-select* into health insurance plans with premiums below their expected health care costs. This entire process of self-selection is described as adverse selection. Left unchecked, it will bankrupt insurance companies, because, without controls, such plans will be filled with "bad risks." If the premium exceeds their expected costs, people will either choose another plan or choose to remain uninsured. It is easy to see how this process could be very unstable if not controlled. As good risks choose other insurance plans or choose to remain uninsured, the first plan's premiums will rise, driving more insurees out of the plan, and so on.

The Response to Adverse Selection

Insurance companies are well aware of the natural process of adverse selection and have developed many ways to control its effects, e.g., if insurance companies have information about the presence of high-cost conditions among certain people, they may impose a "preexisting condition" exclusion on these people, under which the insurance will not cover procedures to treat illnesses present on enrollment. Sometimes they may simply deny coverage for people with preexisting conditions. If insurance companies have less information about prospective insurees, they can "redline" entire industries, denying coverage to firms that are likely to have workers with high insurance costs [33]. This leads to an obvious policy problem: controls like these may be rational responses to adverse selection, but they exacerbate the problem of the uninsured. It is not surprising therefore that most health care reform proposals call for the elimination of many of these insurance practices.

Although insurance companies respond to the existence of induced demand, moral hazard, and adverse selection through the techniques previously described, it is important to understand that another possible response is to charge premiums that closely match expected health care costs. Thus, insurance companies can observe the response of their insurees to the provision of insurance. Any increase in health care costs can be matched with subsequent increases in premiums to cover the costs. This insurance practice is known as "experience rating," the matching of insurance premiums to the health care cost "experience" of the group. Experience rating is literally that: insurers adjust premiums from year to year to account for the cost experience of the group.

Note that the natural forces of the market would lead to a preference for experience rating. Why? If firm A charges all of its customers the same premium (a procedure called "community rating," by which every person in a community is charged roughly the same premium equal to the community's average health care costs, not adjusted for actual experience, plus administrative costs), then firm B can use experience rating to offer a lower premium to firms with favorable health care cost experience. In this case, all "good risks" will flock to firm B, and firm A will be left insuring all the "bad risks" and will eventually lose money.

This occurred in the US in the 1950s and led to the situation today where experience rating procedures dominate the insurance market. When Blue Cross/Blue Shield (BC/BS) dominated the insurance market in the 1950s, it used community rating exclusively. BC/BS could afford to charge these premiums as long as it was the dominant insurer in the market. It was inevitable, however, that other private insurers, such as Aetna and Prudential, would eventually come into the market and offer lower premiums to some firms, thereby "skimming off" the good risks. This competition eventually forced BC/BS and nearly every other insurer to adopt experi-

ence rating, because they would otherwise be left only with bad risks. Thus it has been the natural forces of competition and innovation in the insurance market that have led to the development of practices that have encouraged many firms to drop insurance coverage.

Although experience rating is a natural response of insurers to their marketplace, it has driven some consumers out of the insurance market when the premiums become unaffordable. Even if people can obtain insurance, their premiums may be so high as to make them essentially uninsurable.

Insurance and Small Business

The problems in the insurance markets are particularly acute for small businesses. In the US, over two-thirds of the uninsured workers work for firms with fewer than 100 employees, and over one-half of the uninsured work for firms with fewer than 25 employees (US Bureau of the Census 1999).

Small firms face big problems in insurance markets, because insurance companies that use experience rating (as almost all do) usually charge small employers larger premiums, if they offer to cover them at all. This is because the costs of loading fees charged by insurance companies are higher in age terms for smaller employers, e.g., small firms with fewer than five workers will be charged 40–60% (of expected health care costs) for administrative costs, whereas large firms will be charged only about 5–6% for administrative costs [31]. Insurance companies charge lower loading fees to large firms for three major reasons:

1. the ability to spread fixed costs (such as sales commissions and other administrative costs) across more employees in a large firm
2. economies of scale in the processing of claims for large firms
3. the higher risk associated with insuring a small firm.*

---

* Mathematically, the coefficient of variation for expected health care expenditures will be lower for large firms because of the large number of employees covered. Insurance companies use this measure of risk to build in a portion of the loading fee to cover "risk and profit" [31].

Even if a small employer wants to cover his or her workers, many small businesses cannot obtain insurance. This is usually because insurance companies feel that the firm is too high a risk, even if they are willing to pay a higher premium. This is most likely to occur to small firms with one or two workers with cancer, AIDS, or another expensive disease. Sometimes, the insurance company will offer the firm a Hobson's choice: either drop coverage for the ill worker or we will not offer insurance to your firm. Although this may be a heartless choice by the insurance company, it is really a rational decision by a profit-making firm.

Insurance and Changes in the Workforce

Recent changes in the workforce have contributed to the problem of the uninsured. In the 1970s and 1980s, workers' real wages grew only slightly, if at all. (In part this occurred because most of the increases in compensation were applied to rising health insurance premiums.) In addition, workers had more difficulty obtaining insurance because of "industrial restructuring" [34], including a big shift in employment from manufacturing jobs to service-sector jobs and from unionized to nonunionized jobs. Although some service workers receive high wages, the employment shifts have contributed to the problem of the uninsured because, on average, service sector and nonunion employees are much less likely to receive insurance coverage through their employers [35].

Gaps in Government Insurance Coverage

People not insured through an employer may be able to obtain insurance directly from an insurance company. This is an option chosen by many, especially self-employed people. For some people, however, privately purchased insurance is either not available or very expensive, primarily because the loading fees are typically 60% of expected benefits and, in some cases, may exceed 100% of expected benefits [10].

If insurance is not available or affordable from a private insurance company, why is public insurance not filling the gap? In the US, about 10% of the population receives insurance through public programs, primarily Medicaid or Medi-

care. But neither of these programs can reach all remaining uninsured people.

Medicare is designed to cover elderly people aged over 65 and disabled people aged under 65. Medicare covers nearly everyone aged over 65, but gaps remain in the coverage for elderly retired people. First, Medicare does not cover the millions who retire before age 65. Some of these people are covered by retiree health insurance coverage offered by their previous employers or private coverage purchased elsewhere. The second problem is the large out-of-pocket costs that many aged Medicare recipients must pay. Medicare does not cover prescription drugs, has very little coverage for long-term care, has a large deductible (over $600) for each hospital stay, requires 20% co-payments for physician costs, and does not cover hospital costs if a person stays longer than 90 days.

Medicaid is the program designed to cover poor people. Over 50% of Medicaid's budget pays for the long-term care costs of older people who have become poor by exhausting their resources. The remaining portion of the budget is supposed to cover nonelderly poor people. Unfortunately, only 47% of nonaged poor people are covered by Medicaid [36], mostly because in most states Medicaid coverage is provided only when the person is also receiving benefits under the Aid to Families with Dependent Children (AFDC) program. In many states the eligibility requirements for this program are very stringent, allowing many poor families to slip through the safety net. In some states, Medicaid is available on a short-term basis to cover people who are literally bankrupted by their health care expenditures. This option is not, however, available in all states.

In almost all cases, "working poor" and near-poor families cannot obtain insurance either through their employers or through Medicaid. It is through this gap in our safety net that many uninsured people fall.[†] Sociologist Paul Starr has described the predicament that these people face as "the Medicaid-private insurance corridor, the purgatory of categorical social welfare systems" [6].

[†] Twenty-nine percent of the population in poverty and 27% of the population with incomes between 100 and 133% of poverty were uninsured in 1991 [31].

Why Do We Care? What Are the Consequences of Being Uninsured?

The existence of the uninsured population does not, on the face of it, suggest that there is a public policy problem that needs to be solved. Instead, we have to ask why we care, i.e., what are the *consequences* of having a large population of people without health insurance? The problems fall into two categories: equity problems and efficiency problems.

Equity Problems

When discussing the goal of equity it is important to distinguish between equality of access and equality of result. Several studies have found that the uninsured use less health care than the insured [37,38], e.g. Lefkowitz and Monheit [39] found that the expenditures of insured people are 44% higher than the expenditures of uninsured people. For some, this result is *prima facie* evidence of an equity problem. However, does the simple existence of a difference suggest that there is a public policy problem? Not necessarily. To answer this question, we need to consider why uninsured people use less health care than the insured population. It is obvious that one reason for this is the induced demand effect, i.e., the price of health care is cheaper at the point of purchase for insured people. However, studies of health care use have identified two other explanations for the difference.

First, the difference in health care use is partially explained by adverse selection—those with higher health care costs are more likely to purchase health insurance. If some uninsured people use less health care simply because they are healthier than the insured, the difference in health care use may simply reflect this difference [38]. In fact, many studies show that uninsured people as a whole are more healthy, especially uninsured people aged under 25 [38].

Does adverse selection explain all of the difference in health care use? No. Lefkowitz and Monheit [39] found that insured people in excellent or good health had 64% higher health care expenditures than uninsured people with the same health status, whereas insured people in fair or poor health had 110% higher health care expenditures than uninsured people in fair or

poor health. Freeman *et al.* [37] found that almost 20% of uninsured people said that they needed health care but did not receive it, 17% said they chose to forgo health care for economic reasons, and 71% said that they had serious symptoms but did not see a physician. In perhaps the most persuasive study, Hadley *et al.* [40] found that insured patients, admitted for the same reason as uninsured patients, were more likely than the uninsured patients to stay longer in the hospital and receive more services while there, and they were more likely to be discharged alive. Hadley *et al.* concluded that much of the difference resulted from implicit or explicit provider choices, because many costs would not be borne by the patients. Thus, providers are choosing to "ration" fewer services to those who are less likely to pay their bills.

Thus, there are three explanations for the difference in health care use between insured and uninsured persons: (1) self-selection, (2) induced demand, and (3) provider rationing. Clearly, the first of these explanations poses no public policy problem. However, the last two are tied to the ability of the patient to pay. Many if not most people believe that this is a public policy problem, because they believe that people should not be denied medical care simply because they are unable to pay for it. In other words, many Americans now believe that everyone has a right to health care.

Although it may be charitable to believe this, the existence of a right to health care is very difficult and expensive to implement in practice [41]. How is this right defined? Does every person have a right to treatment, or does it depend on the illness? For example, do alcoholics with liver disease have a right to a liver transplantation? Does a smoker have a right to a heart transplantation, or should these precious hearts be preserved for people who have not smoked? If some of these decisions are to be made, who will make them? These difficult ethical decisions about the rationing of health care will need to be raised if we legislate a right to health care.

Efficiency Problems

Besides an equity problem, the existence of uninsured people raises an efficiency problem as well. As uninsured people are not likely to have a regular source of care, they may be more likely to seek care from an emergency room when the need arises [37]. Alternatively, if uninsured people are not obtaining care when they should, but choose to seek care in a later stage of their disease, this delay could increase the total cost of treating the problem when care is eventually received. Typically, uninsured people will not seek care for routine problems from physicians in their offices as many insured people do. Instead, they may wait until a simple problem, such as a cold, escalates into pneumonia or another infection and then seek care from an emergency room. In either case, uninsured people are more likely to use the emergency room, e.g., 18% of uninsured people use the emergency room as their usual source of ambulatory care, and 44% used the emergency room in a recent year, compared with only 36% of insured people [37]. The problem is that care provided through the emergency room is usually more expensive than treatment provided on an outpatient basis or through a doctor's office. Thus, health care could be provided more efficiently if uninsured people had a regular source of primary care.

If uninsured people choose to seek the health care that they need despite the fact that they cannot pay for it, there are two possible outcomes. One, they will be forced to pay the full costs of their health care, perhaps over a long period of time. This could represent a significant economic burden. For serious problems, it would not be uncommon for health care costs to exceed a person's income and assets by 10 or 15 times, thus requiring payback over many years. The other possible outcome is that uninsured people may never pay for any, or at least some, of their health care services. Overall the evidence suggests that "uncompensated care"—care provided for which the hospital or provider is never paid—represented 6.1% of hospital revenues in 1989 (up from 5.3% in 1981). The evidence shows that the burden was heavier on public hospitals, teaching hospitals, and rural hospitals [36].

If uninsured people do not pay for the costs of their health care, who pays? There are four possible sources of payment: (1) government subsidies, (2) outside donations (charity), (3) hospitals or other providers (pro bono), or (4) cost shifting. To the extent that this is possible, hospitals or other providers might seek to cover the costs of uncompensated care by raising the rates charged to others who have a source of payment. This *cost shifting*, as it has come to be called, is very controversial, especially to insurance companies who have to pay the bills. There is no doubt that some cost shifting has occurred. The problem has been exacerbated by the perceived shifting of costs from Medicaid and Medicare patients to insured patients, because the reimbursement rates for Medicare and Medicaid patients have been cut in recent years [36]. However, hospitals and other providers have found that the proliferation of managed-care plans has made it much more difficult to shift costs. One potential solution for hospitals who cannot shift costs and either cannot, or seek not to, pay for uncompensated care out of profits or reserves is to close emergency rooms or simply refuse to treat uninsured patients. In some cases, hospitals faced with substantial uncompensated care bills may close down entirely, especially in inner cities and rural areas [40].

Some people have argued that uncompensated care is not a serious problem because the costs will eventually be paid by someone. This might be a valid argument if uncompensated care costs were distributed fairly to all in society. Instead, some hospitals and providers bear little of the uncompensated care burden, whereas others are forced to close emergency rooms or close entirely. In any case, people who could have purchased health insurance but chose not to because they knew that their costs would be passed on to others could be considered "free riders". Government may have a role in forcing such people to prepay for their health care costs through health insurance.

Ending the Blame Game

In the perpetual debates over the topic of health care reform, the blame game always starts. But, as we have seen, no single interest group is to blame for the problems we now face. Instead, we should realize that the current situation is the natural result of economic, social, and political forces that created the health care "system" we have today.

And there are rational explanations for everyone's behavior in this market. Thus, it is the system itself that is to blame.

On observing this phenomenon, health policy analyst Robert Blendon has pointed out that a famous philosopher, the sagacious cartoon character Pogo, had some words of wisdom on this subject:

We have met the enemy, and it is us.

References

1. Blendon RJ, Donelan K. The public and the future of U.S. health care system reform. In: Blendon RJ, Edwards JN, eds. *System in Crisis: The case for health care reform.* Washington, DC: Faulkner and Gray's, 1991: 173–94.

2. Blendon RJ, Hyams TS, Benson JM. Bridging the gap between expert and public views on health care reform. *JAMA* 1993; **269**: 2573–8.

3. Levit K, Cown C, Lazenby H *et al.* Health spending in 1998. *Signals Change Health Affairs* 2000; **19**(1): 124–32.

4. Schieber GJ, Pouiller J-P, Greenwald LM. U.S. health expenditure performance. An international comparison and data update. *Health Care Financing Rev* 1992; **13**(4): 1–23.

5. Donham CS, Maple BT, Levit KR. Health care indicators for the United States. *Health Care Financing Rev* 1992; **13**(4): 173–99.

6. Starr P. *The Social Transformation of American Medicine.* New York: Basic Books, 1982.

7. Evans RG, Lomas J, Barer ML *et al.* Controlling health expenditures—the Canadian reality. *N Engl J Med* 1989; **320**: 571–7.

8. Levit K, Cowan CA. Business, households, and governments: Health care costs, 1990. *Health Care Financing Rev* 1991; **13**(2): 83–93.

9. Newhouse JP. *Free for All? Lessons from the RAND health insurance experiments.* Cambridge, MA: Harvard University Press, 1993.

10. Phelps CE. *Health Economics.* New York: Harper Collins, 1992.

11. Arrow KJ. Uncertainty and the welfare economics of medical care. *Am Economic Rev* 1963; **53**: 941–73.

12. Danzon P. *Medical Malpractice. Theory, evidence, and public policy.* Cambridge, MA: Harvard University Press, 1985.

13. Haislmaier EF. *What's Wrong with America's Health Insurance Market? A policymaker's guide to the health care crisis,* part III. Washington, DC: The Heritage Foundation, 1992.

14. Aaron HJ. *Serious and Unstable Condition: Financing America's Health Care.* Washington, DC: Brookings Institution, 1991.

15. Newhouse JP. An iconclastic view of health care cost containment. *Health Affairs Supplement* 1993; **12**(1): 152–71.

16. Pauly M. The economics of moral hazard. *Am Economic Rev* 1968; **49**: 531–7.

17. Goddeeris JH. Insurance and incentives for innovation in medical care. *Southern Economic J* 1984; **51**: 530–9.

18. Pauly MV. Taxation, health insurance, and market failure in the medical economy. *J Economic Literature* 1986; **24**: 629–75.

19. Akerlof GA. The market for "lemons". Qualitative uncertainty and the market mechanism. *Q J Economics* 1970; **84**: 488–500.

20. Kaplan RM. The Hippocratic predicament. Affordability, access and accountability. In: *American Medicine.* San Diego: Academic Press, 1993.

21. Employer Health Benefits. *Annual Survey.* Menlo Park, CA: Kaiser Family Foundation, 1999.

22. Himmelstein DV, Woolhandler S. Cost without benefit: Administrative waste in U.S. health care. *N Engl J Med* 1989; **314**: 441–5.

23. Congressional Budget Office. Projections of national health expenditures. *Update.* CBO Memorandum, 1993.

24. Jonsson B. What can Americans learn from Europeans? *Health Care Financing Review* 1989 Annual Supplement.

25. Leader S, Moon M. *Changing America's Health Care System: Proposals for legislative action.* Washington, DC: American Association of Retired Persons, 1989.

26. McBride TD. Whither the health care crisis? Misinterpretations of chronically uninsured estimates. Unpublished manuscript. University of Missouri, St Louis, 1994.

27. McBride TD, Swartz K. *Spells Without Health Insurance. What Affects Spell Durations and Who Are the Chronically Uninsured?.* Urban Institute Working Paper. Washington DC: The Urban Institute, August, 1991.

28. Swartz K, Marcotte J, McBride TD. Spells without health insurance. The distribution of durations when left censored spells are included. *Inquiry* 1993; **30**(1): 77–83.

29. Swartz K. Dynamics of people without health insurance: Don't let the numbers fool you. *JAMA* 1994; **271**(1): 64–6.

30. Long SH, Marquis MS. Gaps in employer coverage. Lack of supply or demand? *Health Affairs Supplement* 1993; 282–93.

31. Congressional Budget Office. *Rising Health Care Costs. Causes, implications, and strategies*. Washington, DC: Congressional Budget Office, 1991.

32. Zellers WK, McLaughlin CG, Frick K. Small business health insurance: Only the healthy need apply. *Health Affairs* 1992; **11**(1): 174–80.

33. Edwards JN, Blendon RJ, Leitman R, Morrison E, Taylor H. Small business and the national health care reform debate. *Health Affairs* 1992; **11**(1): 164–73.

34. Swartz K. *The Medically Uninsured. Special Focus on Workers*. Urban Institute Working Paper, Washington, DC: The Urban Institute, 1989.

35. Short P, Monheit A, Beauregard K. A profile of uninsured Americans. DHHS, National Center for Health Services Research and Health Care Technology Assessment. *National Medical Expenditure Survey Research Findings 1, Publication #89-3443*. Rockville, MD: Public Health Service, 1989.

36. US Congress, House of Representatives, Ways and Means Committee. *Green Book: Overview of entitlement programs*. Washington, DC: Government Printing Office, 1993.

37. Freeman HE, Aiken LH, Blendon RJ, Corey CR. Uninsured working-age adults. *Characteristics Consequences Health Services Res* 1990; **24**: 813–23.

38. Marquis MS, Reinisch EJ. *Health Status and Health Care Use of Uninsured Workers*. Los Angeles: Rand Corporation, 1990.

39. Lefkowitz DC, Monheit AC. *Health Insurance, Use of Health Services, and Health Care Expenditures. DHSS, Public Health Service National Medical Expenditure Survey Research Findings*. Rockville, MD: National Center for Health Services Research and Health Care Technology Assessment, 1991.

40. Hadley J, Steinberg EP, Feder J. Comparison of uninsured and privately insured patients. *JAMA* 1991; **265**: 374–9.

41. Rhodes RP. *Health Care Politics, Policy, and Distributive Justice*. Albany, NY: State University of New York Press, 1992.

10

Capital Finance

Louis Gapenski

Whereas accounting provides a rational way to measure a business's financial performance and assess operations, *capital finance* provides the concepts and tools needed to help managers make better decisions about the acquisition and use of capital. Of course, the boundary between accounting and capital finance is blurred; certain aspects of accounting involve decision-making, and much of the application of capital finance requires accounting-derived data.

This chapter introduces the essential components of capital finance: business financing, the cost of capital, and capital investment decisions. It is impossible to cover all relevant information about capital finance in just one chapter (for more information on accounting and capital finance, see Gapenski [1]; for a more in-depth treatment of capital finance, see Gapenski [2]). Still, our goal is to acquaint you with the key concepts so you will better understand why good capital finance practices are vital to the financial well-being of all businesses.

Debt Financing

If a business is to operate, it must have assets. To acquire assets, it must raise *capital*. Capital comes in two basic forms: debt and equity. Historically, capital furnished by the owners of investor-owned businesses was called *equity* capital, whereas capital obtained by not-for-profit businesses from grants, contributions, and retained earnings was called *fund* capital. Both types of capital serve the same purpose in financing businesses—providing a permanent financing base without a contractually fixed cost or maturity—

so today the term "equity" is often used to represent nonliability capital regardless of ownership type.

In addition to equity financing, most health care businesses use a considerable amount of *debt* financing. In fact, *Value Line* reports that, on average, health care providers finance their assets with 5% short-term debt, 30% long-term debt, and 65% equity. Thus, over one-third of providers' financing comes from creditors.

The Cost of Money

Money (capital) in a free economy is allocated through the price system. The *interest rate* is the price paid to obtain debt capital, whereas in the case of equity capital in for-profit firms, investors' returns come in the form of *dividends* and, hopefully, *capital gains*. The four fundamental factors that affect the supply of and demand for investment capital, and hence the cost of money, are investment opportunities, time preferences for consumption, risk, and inflation.

To see how these factors operate, visualize the situation facing Mark Vogel, a physician–entrepreneur who is planning to open a new medical practice. Mark does not have enough personal funds to start the business, so he must go to the debt markets for additional capital. If Mark estimates that the business will be highly profitable, he will be able to pay creditors a higher interest rate than if it is barely profitable. Thus, his ability to pay for borrowed capital depends on the business's *investment opportunities*. The higher the profitability of the business, the higher the interest rate that Mark can afford to pay lenders for the use of their savings.

The interest rate that lenders will charge depends in large part on their *time preferences for consumption*, e.g., some potential lenders may be saving for retirement, so they may be willing to loan funds at a relatively low rate because their preference is for future consumption. Other potential lenders may have young children to clothe and feed, so they may be willing to lend funds out of current income, and hence forgo consumption, only if the interest rate is very high. If the entire population of an economy is living at the subsistence level, time preferences for current consumption will necessarily be high, aggregate savings will be low, interest rates will be high, and capital formation will be difficult.

The *risk* inherent in the prospective medical practice, and thus in Mark's ability to repay the loan, would also affect the return lenders would require—the higher the perceived risk, the higher the interest rate. Investors would be unwilling to lend to high-risk businesses unless the interest rate was higher than on loans to low-risk businesses. Finally, because the value of money in the future is affected by *inflation*, the higher the expected rate of inflation, the higher the interest rate demanded by lenders.

Common Debt Instruments

There are many types of debt instruments, but in general they are broken down into *short-term debt*, having maturities of 1 year or less, and *long-term debt*, with maturities of more than 1 year.

Short-term Debt
Bank loans, the most common form of short-term debt, generally appear on a business's balance sheet as *notes payable*. Although banks do make longer-term loans, the bulk of their lending is on a short-term basis. Bank loans to businesses are often written as 90-day notes, so the loan must be repaid or renewed at the end of 90 days. When a bank loan is approved, the agreement is executed by signing a *promissory note*, which specifies such terms as the amount borrowed, the percentage interest rate, and the repayment schedule.

Banks sometimes require borrowers to maintain a checking account balance equal to 10–20% of the face amount of the loan. This is called a *compensating balance,* and it raises the effective interest rate on the loan.

A *line of credit*, sometimes called a *revolving credit agreement* or just *revolver*, is a formal understanding between a bank and a borrower that obligates the lender to supply some maximum amount of credit over some specified period of time, e.g., on December 31 a bank might indicate to Family Practice Associates that the bank regards the group as being good for up to $100,000 during the forthcoming year. If, on January 10, the group signs a promissory note for $20,000 for 90 days, this would be called *taking down* the credit line. This take-down would be credited to the group's checking account at the bank and, before repayment of the $20,000, the group could borrow additional amounts up to a total of $80,000 outstanding at any one time. Lines of credit are generally for 1 year or less, and borrowers typically have to pay an up-front commitment fee of about 0.5–1% of the total amount of the line.

Long-term Debt
The two primary types of long-term debt are term loans and bonds. Under a *term loan*, the borrower agrees to make a series of interest and principal payments, on specified dates, to the lender. Term loans generally are negotiated directly between a business and a lender, usually a financial institution such as a bank. Most term loans have maturities of 3–15 years.

Term loans typically are *amortized* in equal installments over the life of the loan, which means that part of the principal of the loan is retired with each payment. Term loans have three major advantages over bonds (which are discussed next): speed, flexibility, and low issuance costs. As term loans are negotiated directly between a lender and a borrower, formal documentation is minimized. The key provisions of the loan can be worked out much more quickly, and with more flexibility, than can those for a bond issue, because it is not necessary to go through the Securities and Exchange Commission (SEC) registration process. Also, after a term loan has been negotiated, changes can be renegotiated more easily than with bonds.

The interest rate on a term loan can be either fixed for the life of the loan or variable. If it is fixed, the rate used will be close to the rate on equivalent maturity bonds issued by businesses of comparable risk. If the rate is variable, it is usually set at a certain number of percentage points over an index rate such as the prime rate. When the index rate goes up or down, so does the interest rate that must be paid on the outstanding balance of the loan.

Similar to a term loan, a *bond* obligates the borrower to make payments of interest and principal on specific dates to the debtholder (bondholder). Although bonds are like term loans in many ways, a bond issue is generally registered with the SEC, offered to the public through investment bankers, and sold to many different investors, often thousands or more. As it is not practical to issue bonds in amounts less than $5 million, bond issues are used only by larger organizations.

Bonds generally are issued with maturities in the range of 15–30 years, but shorter maturities are occasionally used, as are longer maturities. (In the early 1990s, businesses, including Columbia/HCA Healthcare, issued 100-year bonds.) Unlike term loans, a bond's interest rate is generally fixed rather than variable. Also, unlike term loans, bonds typically pay interest only over the life of the bond, with the entire amount of the principal being repaid to bondholders at maturity. The most common types of bonds are mortgage bonds, debentures, and municipal bonds.

With a *mortgage bond*, the issuer pledges certain real property as security for the bond. To illustrate, Mid-Texas Healthcare System recently needed $30 million to build a new hospital. *First mortgage bonds* in the amount of $15 million, secured by a mortgage on the property, were issued. If Mid-Texas *defaults* on the bonds (i.e., fails to make a promised interest or principal payment), the bondholders could foreclose on the hospital and sell it to satisfy their claims. If it so chooses, Mid-Texas could also issue *second mortgage bonds* secured by the same $30 million hospital. In the event of bankruptcy and liquidation, the holders of these second mortgage bonds would have a claim against the property only after the first mortgage bondholders had been paid off in full. Thus, second mortgages are sometimes called *junior mortgages*, or *junior liens*, because they are junior in priority to claims of senior (first) mortgage bonds.

A *debenture* is an unsecured bond. As such, it has no lien against specific property as security for the obligation, e.g., in addition to its mortgage bonds, Mid-Texas Healthcare System has $5 million of debentures outstanding. These bonds are not secured by real property, but are backed instead by the revenue-producing power of the corporation. Therefore, debenture holders are general creditors whose claims are protected by property not otherwise pledged. In general, mortgage bonds carry lower interest rates than debentures issued by the same business, so businesses favor mortgage-backed debt. However, some businesses have only a small amount of assets suitable as collateral, so they must use debentures. In addition, companies that have used up their capacity to borrow in the lower-cost mortgage market may be forced to use higher-cost debentures.

Municipal ("muni") bonds are long-term debt obligations issued by states and their political subdivisions, such as counties and cities. Short-term municipal securities are used primarily to meet temporary cash needs, whereas municipal bonds are used to finance capital projects. Not-for-profit health care providers, through government-sponsored health care-financing authorities, have access to municipal bond financing.

Most municipal bonds are sold in *serial* form, i.e., a portion of the principal comes due periodically, anywhere from 6 months after issue to 30 years or more. Thus, a single issue actually consists of a series of subissues of different maturities. In effect, the bond issue is amortized, with a portion of the issue being retired every year. The purpose of structuring a bond issue in this way is to match the overall maturity of the issue to the maturity of the assets being financed, e.g., a new hospital wing having an estimated useful life of 30 years might be financed with a 30-year serial issue. Each year, some of the revenues associated with the new wing will be used to meet the *debt service requirements* (the interest and principal payments). At the end of 30 years, the entire issue will be paid off, and the issuer can plan for a replacement facility or major renovation that could be funded, at least in part, by another bond issue.

The primary attraction to investors (and issuers) of municipal bonds is their exemption from federal and state (in the state of issue) income taxes. To illustrate, the interest rate on long-term US Treasury bonds (T-bonds) recently was about 6%, whereas the rate on similar risk munis was about 4.6%. To an individual investor in the 40% federal-plus-state tax bracket, the T-bond's after-tax yield was 6% × (1 − 0.40) = 3.6%, whereas the muni's after-tax yield was the same as its before-tax yield—4.6%. This yield differential on otherwise similar securities illustrates why investors in high tax brackets are so enthusiastic about municipal bonds, and why such bonds carry relatively low interest rates.

Debt Contract Provisions

All debt agreements are formalized in a *debt contract*, called a *promissory note* for bank loans and an *indenture* for bond issues. The provisions of a debt contract affect not only the overall cost of the debt, including both the interest rate and issuance costs, but also may restrict the borrower's future flexibility.

A *prepayment provision*, or *call provision* for bond issues, gives the borrower the right to pre-pay (*call* or *redeem*) the debt before maturity. If a call provision is used, it generally states that the issuer must pay an amount greater than the initial amount borrowed. The additional sum required is defined as the *call premium*. Many callable bonds offer a period of call protection, which is referred to as a *deferred call*, that protects investors from a call just a short time after the bonds are issued, e.g., the 20-year callable bonds issued by Vanguard Healthcare in 1997 are not callable until 2007, which is 10 years after the original issue date.

The call privilege is valuable to the issuer but potentially detrimental to bondholders, especially if the bond is issued in a period when interest rates are cyclically high. In general, bonds are called when interest rates have fallen, because the issuer usually replaces the old issue with a new, lower-interest issue, and hence reduces annual interest expense. When this occurs, investors are forced to reinvest the principal returned in new securities at the then-current (lower) rate. The added risk to investors of a call provision causes the interest rate on a new issue of callable bonds to exceed that on a similar issue of noncallable bonds.

Restrictive covenants are provisions in debt agreements that place restrictions on the borrower. Most of the commonly used covenants focus on requiring the borrower to maintain some stated minimum financial condition over the life of the loan. Often, these minima are specified by ratios, such as a minimum current ratio (current assets/current liabilities) or a maximum debt ratio (total debt/total assets). The motivation for these restrictions is to ensure, to the extent that it is possible, that the creditworthiness of the borrower does not diminish during the life of the loan, which would increase the riskiness of the loan, and hence hurt the lender's position. If a borrower violates one of the restrictive covenants, but has not yet missed a payment, the borrower is said to be in *technical default*.

Debt Ratings

Since the early 1900s, bonds (and other types of debt) have been assigned quality ratings that reflect their probability of going into default. The three major rating agencies are Moody's Investors Service (Moody's), Standard & Poor's Corporation (S&P), and Fitch IBCA (Fitch's), which rate both corporate and municipal debt. These agencies' rating designations are somewhat different but, in general, they range from a high of triple-A (AAA), which signifies the highest quality (lowest default risk) debt, to D, which signifies that the debt is already in default. Debt with a BBB or higher rating is called *investment grade*, which is the lowest-rated debt that many institutional investors are permitted by law to hold. Double-B (BB) and lower debt, called *junk debt*, is more speculative in nature because it has a much higher probability of going into default than does higher-rated debt.

Debt ratings are important both to businesses and to investors. First, the rating has a direct influence on the interest rate required by investors, and hence on the borrower's cost of debt. Second, most taxable debt is purchased by institutional investors rather than by individuals. Many of these institutions are restricted to investment-grade securities. Also, buyers of municipal debt are highly conservative investors, and most are unwilling to assume much risk in their bond purchases. For these reasons, if an issuer's debt rating falls below BBB, the business will have a harder time trying to sell its debt, because the number of potential purchasers is reduced. As a result of its higher risk and more restricted market, low-grade debt typically carries much higher interest rates than does high-grade debt.

Credit Enhancement

Credit enhancement, or *bond insurance*, which is primarily used with municipal bonds, is a relatively recent development for upgrading a bond's rating to AAA. Credit enhancement is offered by several credit insurers, the three largest being the Municipal Bond Investors Assurance (MBIA) Corporation, AMBAC Indemnity Corporation, and Financial Guaranty Insurance Corporation, a subsidiary of General Electric Capital Corporation. Currently, almost 60% of all new health care municipal issues carry bond insurance.

Regardless of the inherent credit rating of the issuer, the bond insurer guarantees that bondholders will receive the interest and principal payments promised in the bond indenture, so bond insurance protects investors against default. As the insurer gives its guarantee that payments will be made, the bond carries the credit rating of the insurance company (AAA) rather than that of the issuer. Credit enhancement gives issuers access to the lowest possible interest rate, but not without a cost. Bond insurers typically charge an upfront fee of about 45–75 basis points of the total debt service requirement over the life of the bond. Most of the newly issued insured municipal bonds have an underlying credit rating of AA or A; the remainder are rated BBB.

Interest Rate Components

The interest rate set on individual debt securities reflects investors' required rates of return on those securities. The required rate of return on any debt issue has several components, so interest rates can change over time, differ among borrowers, and even differ on separate issues by the same borrower. The following are descriptions of the major components.

Real Risk-free Rate

The base on which all interest rates are built is the real risk-free rate (RRF). This is the rate that investors would demand on a debt security that is totally riskless when there is no inflation. Of course, inflation is rarely zero, and most debt securities have risk; thus, the actual interest rate on a debt security will typically be higher than the RRF.

Inflation Premium

Inflation has a major impact on interest rates because it erodes the purchasing power of the dollar and lowers the value of investment returns. Creditors build an inflation premium (IP) into the required interest rate that is equal to the average rate of inflation expected over the life of the security. Thus, the inflation rate built into a 1-year loan is the expected inflation rate for the next year, but the inflation rate built into a 30-year loan is the average rate of inflation expected over the next 30 years.

Default Risk Premium

The risk that a borrower will default has a significant impact on the interest rate set on a debt security. This risk, along with the expected consequences of default, is captured by a default risk premium. Treasury securities have no default risk; they carry the lowest interest rates on taxable securities in the US. For other bonds, the lower the bond rating, the greater the default risk premium.

Liquidity Premium

A *liquid* asset is one that can be sold quickly at a predictable fair market price, and thus can be converted to a known amount of cash on short notice. Active markets, which provide liquidity, exist for Treasury securities and for the debt of large businesses. Securities issued by small businesses, including health care providers that issue municipal bonds, are *illiquid*: they can be sold to raise cash, but not quickly and not at a predictable price. As a result of the difficulty in selling such securities, illiquid securities have relatively high *transactions costs*, which are the commissions, fees, and other expenses associated with selling a security. If a security is illiquid, investors will add a liquidity premium (LP) when they set their required interest rate.

Price Risk Premium

The market value (price) of a debt security declines when interest rates rise. This occurs because similar new securities provide a higher return to investors, and the only way to make existing lower interest rate securities attractive to buyers is to lower their prices. As interest rates can and do rise, all debt has an element of risk called *price risk*, and hence a price risk premium (PRP) is included in most interest rates. As a general rule, the longer the maturity of the debt, the greater the price risk, and hence the larger the PRP. PRPs tend to raise interest rates on long-term debt compared with short-term debt.

Call Risk Premium

As described earlier, bonds that are callable are riskier for investors than those that are non-callable, because callable bonds have uncertain maturities. To compensate for bearing call risk, investors charge a call risk premium on callable debt. The amount of this premium depends on such factors as the interest rate on the debt, current interest rate levels, and time to first call.

Combining the Components

When all the interest rate components are taken into account, the interest rate on any debt security can be expressed as follows:

$$\text{Interest rate} = RRF + IP + DRP + LP + PRP + CRP.$$

To illustrate, assume that RRF is 2%, and inflation is expected to average 3% in the coming year. As short-term treasury securities (called T-bills) have no default, liquidity, or call risk, and almost no price risk, the interest rate on a 1-year T-bill would be 5%:

$$\begin{aligned}\text{Interest rate}_{\text{T-bill}} &= RRF + IP + DRP + LP + PRP + CRP \\ &= 2\% + 3\% + 0 + 0 + 0 + 0 = 5\%.\end{aligned}$$

The combination of RRF and IP is called the *risk-free rate* (RF), so RF = 5% in this illustration. In general, the interest rate on T-bills is used as a proxy for the *short-term* risk-free rate, whereas the interest rate on long-term Treasury securities (T-bonds) is used as a proxy for the *long-term* risk-free rate.

For another example, consider the callable 30-year bonds issued by HCA. Assume that these bonds have an inflation premium of 4%, default risk, liquidity, and price risk premiums of 1%

each, and a call risk premium of 40 basis points. (A *basis point* is 1/100th of a percentage point.) Under these assumptions, the HCA bonds would have an interest rate of 9.4%:

$$\begin{aligned}\text{Interest rate}_{\text{30-year bonds}} &= RRF + IP + DRP + LP + PRP + CRP \\ &= 2\% + 4\% + 1\% + 1\% + 1\% + 0.4\% = 9.4\%.\end{aligned}$$

When interest rates are viewed as the sum of a base rate plus premiums for inflation and risk, it is easy to visualize the underlying economic forces that cause interest rates to vary among different issues and over time.

Equity Financing

The second primary source of capital to health care businesses is *equity financing*, which has different characteristics depending on whether the business is investor owned or not for profit.

Equity in Investor-owned Businesses

In for-profit businesses, equity financing is supplied by the owners of the business, either directly through the purchase of an equity interest in the business or indirectly through earnings retention. In a proprietorship there is a single owner (the *proprietor*); a partnership has just a few owners (the *partners*); and an investor-owned corporation usually has many owners (the *stockholders*). Business owners have certain rights and privileges. First and foremost, owners have the right to a proportionate share of the *residual earnings* of the firm. In effect, a business's net income, which is the residual earnings after all expenses have been paid, belongs to the owners. Some portion of net income will typically be paid out as *dividends* (perhaps in the form of bonuses). That portion of net income retained within the business will be invested in new assets, which presumably will increase the business's earnings, and hence dividends, over time. An increasing earnings and dividend stream means that the business will be more valuable in the future than it is today. Thus, owners typically expect to be able to sell their ownership rights at some time in the future at a higher price than they paid for it, and hence to realize a *capital gain*.

In addition to cash flow rights, owners have the right of control over a business. In proprietorships and partnerships, the owners typically are the managers of the business. In corporations, the stockholders elect the firm's directors, who in turn elect the officers who will manage the business. In small corporations, the major stockholder often assumes the senior management position. In large, publicly owned corporations, managers typically own some stock, but their personal holdings are insufficient to allow them to exercise voting control. Thus, stockholders can remove the management of most publicly owned firms if they decide a management team is ineffective.

Equity in Not-for-profit Businesses

Investor-owned businesses have two sources of equity financing: retained earnings and new equity sales (stock sales in corporations). Not-for-profit businesses, which must be organized as corporations, can and do retain earnings, but they do not have access to the equity markets, i.e., there are no owners to contribute new equity capital. Not-for-profit firms can, however, raise equity capital through government grants and charitable contributions.

On the surface, investor-owned businesses may appear to have a significant advantage in raising equity capital. In theory, new ownership capital can be raised at any time and in any reasonable amount. Conversely, charitable contributions and grants are much less certain. The planning, solicitation, and collection periods can take years, and pledges are not always collected. Therefore, charitable contributions that were counted on may not materialize. Also, the proceeds of new equity sales may be used for any purpose, but charitable contributions are often *restricted*, in which case they can be used only for designated purposes.

In reality, however, managers of investor-owned firms do not have complete freedom to raise equity capital. Small business owners often do not have the personal cash needed by the business, but they are usually reluctant to dilute their control by bringing in outside equity investors. For publicly held corporations, the issuance expenses associated with a new stock sale are not trivial. Furthermore, if market conditions are poor and the stock is selling at a low price, a new stock issue can dilute the value of existing shares and hence be harmful to current stockholders. Finally, new stock issues are often viewed by investors as a signal that the firm's stock is overvalued, and hence new issues often drive the stock price lower.

For all these reasons, owners (or managers) of investor-owned businesses generally would rather not sell new ownership rights. The key point here is that for-profit health care businesses do have greater access to equity capital than do not-for-profit corporations, but this may not be as great an advantage as it appears.

Capital Structure

The mix of debt and equity financing used by a business is called its *capital structure*, because it represents the structure of the capital (liabilities and equity) side of the balance sheet. One of the most perplexing issues facing health services managers is how much debt financing, as opposed to equity financing, should be used. Once the optimal proportion of debt financing has been determined, a second question arises. What is the appropriate mix of long- and short-term debt? Both of these decisions are discussed in this section.

The Capital Structure Decision

To gain some insights into the debt-versus-equity decision, commonly called the *capital structure decision*, consider the situation facing Super Practice, a for-profit medical practice that is just being formed. The practice requires $1,000,000 in assets to get into operation and, for simplicity, assume that there are only two financing alternatives available: all equity and 50% equity/50% debt.

Table 10-1 contains the business's projected first-year financial statements under the two financing alternatives. To begin, note that the practice will require $100,000 in current assets and $900,000 in fixed assets to get started. The asset requirement depends on the nature and size of the practice rather than on how the practice will be financed, so the asset side of the balance sheet is unaffected by the financing mix. However, the

Table 10-1. Super Practice Inc: Projected Financial Statements Under Two Financing Alternatives.

	All equity	Debt/Equity
Balance sheets		
Current assets ($)	100,000	100,000
Fixed assets ($)	900,000	900,000
Total assets ($)	1,000,000	1,000,000
Bank loan (10% cost) ($)	0	500,000
Common stock ($)	1,000,000	500,000
Total liabilities and equity ($)	1,000,000	1,000,000
Income statements		
Revenues ($)	1,500,000	1,500,000
Operating costs ($)	1,250,000	1,250,000
Operating income ($)	250,000	250,000
Interest expense ($)	0	50,000
Taxable income ($)	250,000	200,000
Taxes (40%) ($)	100,000	80,000
Net income ($)	150,000	120,000
ROE (%)	15	24
Total dollar return to investors ($)	150,000	170,000

ROE, return on equity.

type of financing used does affect the liabilities and equity side. Under the all-equity alternative, Super Practice's owners will put up the entire $1,000,000 needed to set up the business. If 50% debt financing is used, the owners will contribute only $500,000, with the remaining $500,000 obtained from creditors, say a bank loan with a 10% interest rate.

What is the impact of the financing mix on Super Practice's projected income statement? Revenues are projected to be $1,500,000 and operating costs are forecasted at $1,250,000, so the firm's operating income is expected to be $250,000. As a business's capital structure does not affect revenues and operating costs, the operating income projection is the same under both financing alternatives.

However, interest expense must be paid if debt financing is used. Thus, the debt/equity alternative results in a 0.10 × $500,000 = $50,000 annual interest charge, whereas no interest expense occurs if the practice is financed entirely with equity. The results are taxable income of $250,000 under the all-equity alternative and a lower taxable income of $200,000 under the debt/equity alternative. As the business will be taxed at a 40% federal-plus-state rate, expected tax liabilities are 0.40 × $250,000 = $100,000 under the all-equity alternative and 0.40 × $200,000 =

$80,000 for the debt/equity alternative. Finally, when taxes are deducted from the income stream, the projections are $150,000 in net income if the practice is all-equity financed and $120,000 in net income if 50% debt financing is used.

At first glance, the use of debt financing appears to be the inferior alternative. After all, if 50% debt financing is used, Super Practice's projected net income will fall by $30,000. But the conclusion that debt financing is bad requires closer examination. Super Practice's owners are more concerned with the return on their equity investment than in the practice's net income. One of the best measures of rate of return to owners is the *return on equity* (ROE), which is defined as net income divided by the book value of common equity. Under all-equity financing, projected ROE is $150,000/$1,000,000 = 0.15 = 15%, but with 50% debt financing, projected ROE increases to $120,000/$500,000 = 24%. The key to the increased ROE is that, although net income decreases when debt financing is used, so does the amount of equity capital needed, and this decrease is proportionally greater than the decrease in net income.

The bottom line of this illustration is that debt financing can increase the owners' expected rate of return. As the use of debt financing increases, or leverages up, the return to equity holders, such financing is referred to as *financial leverage*. Hence, the use of financial leverage is merely the use of debt financing.

To view the impact of financial leverage from a different perspective, take another look at the income statements in Table 10-1. The total dollar return to investors, including both the owners and the bank, is $150,000 in net income if all-equity financed, but $120,000 in net income plus $50,000 of interest = $170,000 when 50% debt financing is used. Where did the extra $20,000 come from? The answer is from the taxman. Taxes are $100,000 if the business is all-equity financed, but only $80,000 when debt financing is used, and $20,000 less in taxes means $20,000 more for investors. As the use of debt financing reduces taxes, more of a business's operating income is now available for distribution to investors.

At this point, it appears that Super Practice's financing decision is a "no brainer." Given only these two financing alternatives, 50% debt financing should be used, because it provides the owners with a higher rate of return. Unfortunately, like the proverbial no free lunch, there is a catch. The use of financial leverage not only increases owners' return; it also increases their risk. The risk increase occurs because (1) interest expense must be paid regardless of the level of operating income and (2) the level of operating income is not known with certainty. The addition of a fixed cost to a business's uncertain income stream increases the uncertainty of net income, and hence increases the owners' risk.

When risk is considered, the ultimate decision on which financing alternative is best for Super Practice is not so clear-cut. In fact, the decision is a classic *risk/return trade-off*; higher returns can be obtained only by assuming greater risk. What Super Practice's founders need to know is whether or not the higher expected return that comes with debt financing is enough to compensate them for the higher risk assumed. To complicate the decision even more, there are an almost unlimited number of debt level choices available, not just the 50/50 mix used in the illustration.

Finance theory is developed primarily to help managers grapple with difficult decisions. In the capital structure domain, the most widely used theory, the *trade-off theory*, recognizes that

the use of debt financing has both costs (associated with the higher probability of bankruptcy) and benefits (associated with the tax reduction) that increase with the amount of debt financing used. According to this theory, the optimal debt level is the amount that creates the largest *net* benefit. The bottom line here is that some debt is good, but too much debt is bad. Although the trade-off theory indicates that every business has an optimal capital structure consisting of some debt and some equity, it is of little value in helping managers to identify this structure for any given business, so a great deal of judgment is required. Some of the more important issues that managers consider in setting a firm's target capital structure include inherent business risk, lender/rating agency attitudes, reserve borrowing capacity, and industry averages.

Businesses face a certain amount of risk, called *business risk*, even when no debt financing is used. This risk is based on the uncertainty of future operating income: the greater the uncertainty, the greater the inherent (business) risk of the enterprise. When debt financing is used, owners must bear additional risk. In a capital structure context, the risk added when debt financing is used is called *financial risk*. As managers generally place some limit on the total amount of risk of a business, the greater the inherent business risk, the less "room" available for the use of financial leverage, and hence the lower the proportion of debt used.

Regardless of a manager's own views about a business's proper capital structure, there is no question that lender/rating agency attitudes are often important determinants of financial structures. In most cases, corporate managers discuss the business's financial structure with lenders and/or rating agencies and give much weight to their advice. Often, managers want to maintain some target debt rating, say, single A. Furthermore, rating agencies publish guidelines that link the capital structures of firms within an industry to specific bond ratings, so guidance is readily available.

Businesses generally maintain a *reserve borrowing capacity* that preserves access at all times to reasonably priced debt capital. This gives them *financial flexibility* to respond to changing market conditions. To maintain this flexibility, firms often use less debt than other factors might indicate should be used.

Managers usually act rationally, so the capital structures of similar businesses, particularly industry leaders, should provide insights about the optimal structure. In general, there is no reason to believe that the managers of one firm are better than the managers of any other firm. Thus, if one firm has a capital structure that is significantly different from other firms in its industry, the managers of that firm should identify the unique circumstances that contribute to the anomaly. If unique circumstances cannot be identified, then it is doubtful that the firm has identified the correct target structure.

The discussion of capital structure has focused on investor-owned businesses, but what about not-for-profit businesses? The same general concepts apply—namely, some debt financing is good, but too much is bad. However, not-for-profit corporations have a unique problem—they cannot go to the capital markets to raise equity capital. If an investor-owned firm has more capital investment opportunities than it can finance with retained earnings and debt financing, it can always raise the needed funds by a new stock issue. It may be costly, but it can be done. Also, it is relatively easy for investor-owned firms to adjust their capital structures. If a firm is underleveraged (i.e., using too little debt), it can simply issue more debt and use the proceeds to repurchase stock. On the other hand, if a firm is overleveraged (i.e., using too much debt), it can issue additional shares and use the proceeds to refund debt.

The Debt Maturity Decision

Most health care businesses experience seasonal and cyclical fluctuations in volume. As a result of the difficulties of changing the level of fixed assets, businesses usually carry enough to cover peak-volume demands. In addition, although the level of current assets fluctuates with volume, it never drops to zero, e.g., assume that seasonality causes Super Practice's total assets to fluctuate during the year between $1,000,000 and $1,050,000. Under these conditions, the practice has $1,000,000 in *permanent assets*, defined as the amount of total assets required to sustain opera-

tions during seasonal (or cyclical) lows. In addition, the practice carries *seasonal*, or *temporary*, *assets*, which fluctuate from zero to a maximum of $50,000.

The debt maturity policy followed by most businesses calls for the matching of asset and liability maturities, i.e., permanent assets are financed with permanent capital (equity and long-term debt) and temporary assets are financed with temporary capital (short-term debt). This strategy limits the risk that a business will be unable to pay off its maturing obligations. For Super Practice, the permanent asset level of $1,000,000 would be financed with $1,000,000 of permanent capital, say $500,000 of equity and $500,000 of long-term debt. The practice's temporary assets would be financed with short-term debt, probably a line of credit, which would vary from a high of $50,000 during peak volume periods to a low of zero during slack volume periods.

The critical point here is that, for debt maturity purposes, assets are not classified by their accounting definitions of current (short term) and long term, but rather by their finance definitions of permanent and temporary. Within this framework, maturity matching calls for the permanent portion of cash, receivables, and inventories (permanent current assets) along with fixed assets to be financed with *permanent capital* (long-term debt and equity).

Although maturity matching (in the finance sense) is the most commonly used debt maturity policy, there are alternatives. As with the capital structure decision, the choice among alternative debt maturity policies involves a risk/return trade-off. An aggressive policy, with a higher use of generally lower-cost short-term debt, has the highest expected return, but the highest risk. A conservative policy, with its higher use of generally higher-cost long-term debt, has the lowest expected return and lowest risk. The maturity matching policy followed by Super Practice falls between the extremes.

The Cost of Capital

The previous section focused on choosing between debt and equity financing. Once that decision has been made, the business will raise capital over time in accordance with its optimal (target) structure. Now, the discussion turns to estimating the cost of raising that capital.

The ultimate goal of cost-of-capital estimation is to estimate the business's *corporate cost of capital*, which represents the blended, or average, cost of a business's future financing. This cost, in turn, establishes the required rate of return, or hurdle rate, used when evaluating the business's capital investment opportunities, e.g., Pine Grove Hospital has a corporate cost of capital of 10%. If a new magnetic resonance imaging (MRI) investment is expected to return at least 10%, it is financially attractive to the hospital. If the MRI system is expected to return less than 10%, accepting it will have an adverse effect on the hospital's financial soundness.

Investor-owned Businesses

The first step in the cost-of-capital process is to estimate the business's cost of debt. It is unlikely that managers will know at the beginning of a planning period the exact types and amounts of debt that will be issued. However, they do know what types of debt the firm usually issues, e.g., Citrus Health System, an investor-owned company, typically uses bank debt to raise short-term funds to finance seasonal assets, and it uses 30-year corporate (taxable) bonds, along with equity, to finance permanent assets. As Citrus does not use short-term debt to finance permanent assets, its managers include only long-term debt in their corporate cost of capital estimate, and they assume that this debt will consist solely of 30-year bonds.

Suppose that Citrus's managers are developing the company's corporate cost of capital estimate. How should they estimate the cost of debt? Most managers would begin by discussing current and prospective interest rates with their firms' investment bankers, the institutions that help companies bring security issues to market. Assume that Citrus's investment banker states that a new 30-year bond issue would require a 9% interest rate. However, because interest expense is tax deductible for investor-owned businesses, the effective cost of debt is less than the stated interest rate. If Citrus's federal-plus-state tax rate

is 40%, its component cost of debt estimate is 5.4%:

$$\text{Cost of debt} = \text{Interest rate} \times (1-\text{T})$$
$$= 9.0\% \times (1-0.40) = 5.4\%.$$

By reducing the component cost of debt from 9% to 5.4%, the cost-of-debt estimate incorporates the benefit associated with interest payment tax deductibility.

What can smaller businesses without investment bankers do? If a business obtains the bulk of its debt financing from commercial banks, the firm's bankers can provide some insights on the cost of future debt financing. Managers can also look to marketplace activity for guidance, i.e., the interest rate currently being set on debt issues of similar-risk firms can be used to estimate the cost of debt. Here, similar risk can be judged either by debt rating or by subjective analysis (same industry, similar size, similar use of debt, etc.). An awareness of the current interest rate environment will provide a reasonable estimate for one's own cost of debt.

The cost of debt is based on the return that investors require on debt securities, and the *cost of equity* to investor-owned firms can be defined similarly: it is the rate of return that equity investors require to invest in the business. At first glance, it may appear that equity raised through retained earnings is a costless source of capital to investor-owned firms. After all, dividend payments must be paid on new shares that are sold, but no such payments are required on funds that are obtained by retaining earnings. The reason why a cost must be assigned to all forms of equity financing involves the *opportunity cost principle*. An investor-owned firm's net income belongs to its owners. Employees are compensated by wages, suppliers are compensated by cash payments for supplies, bondholders are compensated by interest payments, governments are compensated by tax payments, etc. The residual earnings of a firm, its net income, belongs to the owners and serves to "pay the rent" on owner-supplied capital.

Management can either pay out earnings in the form of dividends or retain earnings for reinvestment in the business. If part of the earnings are retained, an opportunity cost is incurred:

owners could have received these earnings as dividends and then invested this money in stocks, bonds, real estate, commodity futures, etc. Thus, the firm should earn on its retained earnings at least as much as its owners could earn on alternative investments of *similar risk*. If the firm cannot earn as much as owners can in similar-risk investments, a business's net income should be paid out as dividends rather than retained for reinvestment.

Whereas debt is a contractual obligation with an easily estimated cost, it is not nearly as easy to estimate the cost of equity, so we will not present the details here. Suffice it to say that for a given business the cost of equity is higher than the cost of debt, because investors consider equity investments to be riskier than debt investments. Assume that Citrus's managers estimate the firm's cost of equity to be 14%.

The final step in the cost-of-capital estimation process is to combine the debt and equity cost estimates to form the *corporate cost of capital*. The weights used in this calculation are the business's target capital structure weights. Citrus's optimal capital structure calls for 40% debt and 60% equity, so its corporate cost of capital (CCC) estimate is 10.6%:

$$CCC = (0.40 \times 5.4\%) + (0.60 \times 14\%) = 10.6\%.$$

The corporate cost of capital represents the percentage cost of each new dollar of capital raised in the future. It is not the average cost of all dollars that the firm has raised in the past. The primary interest here is in obtaining a cost of capital for use in capital investment analysis; for such purposes, a *marginal cost* is required. The corporate cost of capital formula implies that each new dollar of capital will consist of both debt and equity that is raised, at least conceptually, in proportion to the firm's target capital structure. Note that the corporate cost of capital is the correct hurdle rate for average-risk new investments regardless of the financing actually used.

Not-for-profit Businesses

The corporate cost of capital for not-for-profit businesses is developed in much the same way as

for investor-owned firms. The cost of debt for not-for-profit firms is estimated using the same techniques as for investor-owned businesses. The only difference is that not-for-profit firms have access to tax-exempt (municipal) debt, and hence pay a lower interest rate for debt financing. However, not-for-profit firms do not have the tax deductibility benefit. On net, the effective cost of debt is roughly comparable between investor-owned and not-for-profit firms of similar risk. Investor-owned firms have the benefit of tax deductibility of interest payments, whereas not-for-profit firms have the benefit of being able to issue tax-exempt debt.

A more meaningful difference occurs in the cost-of-equity estimate. There are at least two views on estimating the cost of equity (fund capital) in not-for-profit businesses. The first view—which might be called the *full opportunity cost method*—requires that the business's fund capital earn a return at least as high as the return available on security investments of similar risk. What return is available on securities with similar risk to health care assets? The answer is the return expected from investing in the stock of a similar investor-owned health care company. The premise here is that, instead of using fund capital to purchase real health care assets, a not-for-profit business could always use the funds to buy health care stock, and hence delay the real asset purchase until some time in the future. Under this view, the cost of fund capital to a not-for-profit business is an opportunity cost that is roughly the same as the cost of equity to a similar investor-owned business.

The second view does not recognize the opportunity cost concept when considering the cost of fund capital, because substituting securities ownership for real asset ownership is not consistent with the mission of a not-for-profit organization. However, this does not mean that the cost of fund capital is zero. To foster the orderly growth of a not-for-profit business, it is necessary for the business to grow its fund capital at the same rate as the business. Thus, the *sustainable growth rate method* assigns a cost of fund capital to the business that is equal to the business's expected growth rate. The concept here is that a firm's assets, and hence capital, will have to increase to support sales (volume) growth.

Unless a greater proportion of debt is taken on, the business will have to grow its fund capital at its growth rate.

Once the costs of debt and equity are estimated, a not-for-profit business combines these component costs to estimate its corporate cost of capital in the same way as investor-owned businesses, e.g., consider Pine Grove Hospital, a not-for-profit corporation. Its cost of long-term municipal debt is 4.8% and its cost of equity is 12.2%. Its target capital structure is 30% debt and 70% equity (fund) capital. These estimates result in a corporate cost of capital estimate for Pine Grove of 10.0%:

$$CCC = (0.30 \times 4.8\%) + (0.70 \times 12.2\%) = 10.0\%.$$

In general, there is not a large difference between the corporate costs of capital of similar investor-owned and not-for-profit businesses. The major capital acquisition advantage of not-for-profit status is the fact that income is not diluted by taxes, so all other things being equal, larger amounts of earnings are available for reinvestment in the business.

Using the Corporate Cost of Capital

From a purely financial perspective, if a business cannot earn its corporate cost of capital on new capital investments, no new investments should be made and no new capital should be raised. If existing investments are not earning the corporate cost of capital, they should be terminated, the assets liquidated, and the proceeds returned to investors for reinvestment elsewhere.

The primary purpose of estimating a business's corporate cost of capital is to help make capital investment decisions. The cost of capital is used as the benchmark *hurdle rate*, or minimum return necessary, for a new investment to be attractive. The best way to think about the corporate cost of capital is this: it is the rate of return that would be expected from securities investments of similar risk to the business, i.e., the corporate cost of capital is the opportunity cost rate for investment in the business.

However, the corporate cost of capital reflects the aggregate risk of the firm. Thus, the corporate cost of capital can be applied without

modification only to those projects under consideration that have average risk, where average is defined as that applicable to the firm's assets in the aggregate. If a project under consideration has risk that differs significantly from that of the firm's average asset, then the corporate cost of capital must be adjusted to account for the differential risk when the project is being evaluated. The key point here is that the corporate cost of capital is a benchmark. It is not a one-size-fits-all rate that can be used with abandon whenever an opportunity cost is needed in a financial analysis.

Capital Investment Decisions

Decisions to acquire new fixed assets are called *capital investment*, or *capital budgeting*, decisions. Capital budgeting decisions are of fundamental importance to the success or failure of any business, because a firm's capital budgeting decisions, more than anything else, shape its future.

The Role of Financial Analysis

For investor-owned firms, the role of financial analysis in investment decisions is clear. Those projects that contribute to owners' wealth should be undertaken, whereas those that do not should be ignored. However, what about not-for-profit firms, which do not have shareholder wealth maximization as a goal? In such firms, the appropriate goal is providing quality, cost-effective service to the communities served. (A strong argument could be made that this should also be the goal of investor-owned firms in the health services industry.) In this situation, capital budgeting decisions must consider many factors besides a project's financial implications, e.g., the needs of the medical staff and the good of the community must be taken into account. Indeed, in many situations, noneconomic factors will outweigh financial considerations.

Nevertheless, good decision-making, and hence the future viability of any organization, requires that the financial impact of capital investments be fully recognized. If a business takes on a series of highly unprofitable projects that meet nonfinancial goals, and such projects are not offset by profitable projects, the business's financial condition will deteriorate. If this situation persists over time, the business will eventually lose its financial viability and may even be forced into bankruptcy and closure.

As bankrupt firms cannot meet a community's needs, even managers of not-for-profit businesses must consider a project's potential impact on financial condition. Managers may make a conscious decision to accept a project with a poor financial prognosis because of its nonfinancial virtues, but it is important that managers know the financial impact up front, rather than be surprised when the project drains the firm's financial resources. Financial analysis provides managers with the relevant information about a project's financial impact, and hence helps managers make better decisions, including those decisions based primarily on nonfinancial considerations.

Time Value Analysis

The financial value of any asset, whether a *financial asset*, such as a stock or a bond, or a *real asset*, such as a piece of diagnostic equipment or an ambulatory surgery center, is based on future cash flows. However, a dollar to be received in the future is worth less than a current dollar, because a dollar in hand today can be invested, can earn interest, and hence can be worth more than a dollar in the future. As current dollars are worth more than future dollars, valuation analyses must account for cash flow timing differences. The process of assigning proper values to cash flows that occur at different points in time is called *time value analysis*. It is an important part of most finance decisions, because most financial analyses involve the valuation of future cash flows.

For capital budgeting purposes, cash flows expected to be received in the future must be converted into current dollars, a process called *discounting*. Mathematically, discounting is accomplished by dividing the future value by (1 + discount rate) some number of times, n, where n is the number of years in the future that the cash flow is expected to occur, e.g., the present value of $100 expected to be received 2 years from now, if the discount rate is 10%, is $100/(1.10)(1.10) = $100/(1.10)^2 = 82.64.

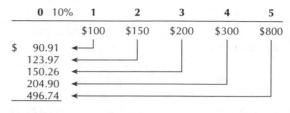

$1,066.78

Figure 10-1. Present value of an uneven cash flow stream.

In virtually all capital budgeting decisions, the cash flows expected from the project do not follow a regular pattern, and hence are referred to as an *uneven cash flow stream*. The present value of such a cash flow stream is found as the sum of the present values of the individual cash flows of the stream, e.g., the present value of the uneven cash flow stream shown in Fig. 10-1 is $1,066.78.

A key input into this time value analysis is the discount rate of 10%. Where does this value come from? The answer is that the *opportunity cost* concept is used to set the discount rate when investments are being analyzed. To illustrate, suppose that a person found the winning ticket for the Florida lottery and now has $1 million to invest. Should the person assign a cost to these funds? At first blush, it may appear that this money has zero cost because its acquisition was purely a matter of luck. However, as soon as the lucky person thinks about what to do with the money, he or she has to think in terms of the opportunity costs involved. By using the funds to invest in one alternative, e.g., UnitedHealth stock, the person forgoes the opportunity to make some other investment, e.g., buying US Treasury bonds. Thus, there is an opportunity cost associated with any investment planned for the $1 million even though the lottery winnings were "free."

As one investment decision automatically negates all other possible investments with the same funds, the cash flows expected to be earned from any investment must be discounted at a rate that reflects the return that could be earned on forgone opportunities, *regardless of the source of the investment funds*. The problem here is that the number of forgone opportunities is almost infinite, so which one should be used to establish the opportunity cost (discount) rate? It is the rate that could be earned on alternative investments of *similar risk*. Risk plays the key role in establishing the opportunity cost of capital because investors are *risk averse*. This means that higher-risk investments must offer higher expected rates of return to be attractive to investors.

Generally, opportunity cost rates are obtained by looking at rates that one could expect to earn on securities such as stocks or bonds. Securities are usually chosen to set opportunity cost rates because their expected returns are more easily estimated than rates of return on real assets such as group practices, hospital beds, MRI machines, and the like. Furthermore, securities generally provide the minimum return appropriate for the amount of risk assumed, so securities returns provide a good benchmark for other investments.

The bottom line here is that some opportunity cost rate has to be applied to discount future cash flows. The proper rate is the rate available on other investments with risk similar to the flows being discounted, and this rate normally is established by looking at expected returns on securities. Fortunately, for most capital investment decisions, a benchmark opportunity cost rate already exists. As explained earlier, that rate is the business's corporate cost of capital.

Cash Flow Estimation

The financial analysis of capital investment proposals typically involves the following five steps:

1. The capital outlay, or cost, of the project is estimated.
2. The operating and terminal cash flows of the project are forecasted. Steps 1 and 2 constitute the cash flow estimation process.
3. The riskiness of the estimated cash flows is assessed.
4. Given the riskiness of the project, the project's cost of capital is estimated. As discussed earlier, the business's corporate cost of capital reflects the aggregate risk of the enterprise. If the project being evaluated does not have average risk, the corporate cost of capital must be adjusted.

5. Finally, the financial impact (profitability) of the project is assessed. Several measures can be used for this purpose; two commonly used measures (NPV and IRR) are discussed here.

The most critical and most difficult step in evaluating capital investment proposals is *cash flow estimation*. This step involves estimating the investment outlays, the annual net operating flows expected when the project goes into operation, and the cash flows associated with project termination. Many variables are involved in cash flow estimation, and many individuals and departments participate in the process. Making accurate projections of the costs and revenues associated with a large, complex project is difficult, so forecast errors can be quite large. Neither the difficulty nor the importance of cash flow estimation can be overstated. Some of the key principles are contained in the following example.

Consider the situation faced by Pine Grove Hospital, a not-for-profit hospital, in its evaluation of a new MRI system. The system costs $1.5 million, and the hospital would have to spend another $1 million for site preparation and installation. As the system would be installed in the hospital, the space to be used has a very low, or zero, market value to outsiders. Furthermore, its value to Pine Grove for other projects is very difficult to estimate, so no opportunity cost has been assigned to account for the value of the site.

The MRI system is estimated to generate a weekly volume of 40 scans, and each scan on average would cost the hospital $15 in supplies. The system is expected to operate 50 weeks a year, with the remaining 2 weeks devoted to maintenance. The estimated average charge per scan is $500, but 25% of this amount, on average, is expected to be lost to indigent patients, contractual allowances, and bad debt losses.

The MRI system would require two technicians, resulting in an incremental increase in annual labor costs of $50,000, including fringe benefits. Cash overhead costs would increase by $10,000 annually if the MRI is activated. The equipment would require maintenance, which would be furnished by the manufacturer for an annual fee of $150,000, payable at the end of each year of operation. For book purposes, the MRI

Table 10-2. Pine Grove Hospital: MRI Cash Flow Analysis.

	Cash revenues and costs ($)					
	0	**1**	**2**	**3**	**4**	**5**
1	(1,500,000)					
2	(1,000,000)					
3		1,000,000	1,000,000	1,102,000	1,157,625	1,215,506
4		250,000	262,000	275,625	289,406	303,877
5		750,000	787,500	826,875	868,219	911,629
6		50,000	52,500	55,125	57,881	60,775
7		150,000	157,500	166,375	173,644	182,326
8		30,000	31,500	33,075	34,729	36,465
9		10,000	10,500	11,025	11,576	12,155
10		350,000	350,000	350,000	350,000	350,000
11		160,000	185,500	212,275	240,389	269,908
12		0	0	0	0	0
13		160,000	185,500	212,275	240,389	269,908
14		350,000	350,000	350,000	350,000	350,000
15						750,000
16	(2,500,000)	510,000	535,500	562,275	590,389	1,369,908

Here are the key points of the analysis by line number:

- *Line 1*: line 1 contains the estimated cost of the MRI system. In general, capital budgeting analyses assume that the first cash flow, normally an outflow, occurs today, or at the end of Year 0. Expenses, or cash outflows, are shown in parentheses.
- *Line 2*: the related site construction expense, $1,000,000, is also assumed to occur at Year 0.
- *Line 3*: annual gross revenues = weekly volume × weeks of operation per year × charge per scan = 40 × 50 × $500 = $1,000,000 in the first year. The 5% inflation rate is applied to all charges and costs that would likely be affected by inflation, so the gross revenue amount shown on line 3 increases by 5% over time. Although most of the operating revenues and costs would occur more or less evenly over the year, it is very difficult to forecast exactly when the flows would occur. Furthermore, there is significant potential for large errors in cash flow estimation. For these reasons, operating cash flows are often assumed to occur at the end of each year. Also, the assumption is that the MRI system could be put into operation quickly. If this were not the case, then the first year's operating flows would be reduced. In some situations, it might take several years from the first investment cash flow to the point when the project is operational and begins to generate revenues.
- *Line 4*: deductions from charges are estimated to average 25% of gross revenues, so in Year 1, 0.25 × $1,000,000 = $250,000 of gross revenues would be uncollected. This amount increases each year by the 5% inflation rate.
- *Line 5*: line 5 contains the net revenues in each year, line 3–line 4.
- *Line 6*: labor costs are forecasted to be $50,000 during the first year, but increase over time at the 5% inflation rate.
- *Line 7*: maintenance fees must be paid to the manufacturer at the end of each year of operation. These fees are assumed to increase at the 5% inflation rate.
- *Line 8*: each scan uses $15 of supplies, so supply costs in the first year total 40 × 50 × $15 = $30,000, and they are expected to increase each year by the inflation rate.
- *Line 9*: if the project is accepted, overhead cash costs will increase by $10,000 in the first year. Note that the $10,000 are cash costs that are related directly to the acceptance of the MRI project. Existing overhead costs that are arbitrarily allocated to the MRI project are not incremental cash flows, and thus should not be included in the analysis. Overhead costs are also assumed to increase over time at the inflation rate.
- *Line 10*: book depreciation in each year is calculated by the straight-line method, assuming a 5-year depreciable life. The depreciable basis is equal to the capitalized cost of the project, which includes the cost of the asset and related construction, less the estimated salvage value. Thus, the depreciable basis is ($1,500,000 + $1,000,000) − $750,000 = $1,750,000. Then, the straight-line depreciation in each year of the project's 5-year depreciable life is (1/5) × $1,750,000 = $350,000. Note that depreciation is based solely on acquisition costs, so it is unaffected by inflation. Also, note that the cash flows in Table 10-2 are presented in a generic format which can be used by both investor-owned and not-for-profit hospitals. Depreciation expense is not a cash flow, but rather an accounting convention that allocates the cost of fixed assets over time. As Pine Grove Hospital is tax exempt, and hence depreciation will not affect taxes, and because depreciation is added back to the cash flows on line 14, depreciation could be totally omitted from the analysis.
- *Line 11*: line 11 shows the project's operating income in each year, which is merely net revenues less all operating expenses.
- *Line 12*: line 12 contains zeros, because Pine Grove is not-for-profit, and hence does not pay taxes.
- *Line 13*: Pine Grove pays no taxes, so the project's net operating income equals its operating income.
- *Line 14*: because depreciation, a noncash expense, was included on line 10, it must be added back to the project's net operating income in each year to obtain each year's net cash flow.
- *Line 15*: the project is expected to be terminated after 5 years, at which time the MRI system would be sold for an estimated $750,000. This salvage value cash flow is shown as an inflow at the end of Year 5 on line 15. Note that for investor-owned businesses, the salvage value typically will have associated tax consequences.
- *Line 16*: the project's net cash flows are shown on line 16. The project requires a $2,500,000 investment at Year 0, but then generates cash inflows over its 5-year operating life.

will be depreciated by the straight-line method over a 5-year life.

The MRI system is expected to be in operation for 5 years, at which time the hospital's master plan calls for a new imaging facility. The hospital plans to sell the MRI at that time for an estimated $750,000 salvage value, net of removal costs. The inflation rate is estimated to average 5% over the period, and this rate is expected to affect all revenues and costs except depreciation. Pine Grove's managers assume at the start of an analysis that projects have average risk, and thus the hospital's 10% corporate cost of capital is used as the initial project cost of capital (opportunity cost discount rate).

Although the MRI project is expected to take away some patients from the hospital's other imaging systems, the new MRI patients are expected to generate revenue for some of the hospital's other departments. On net, the two effects are expected to balance out, i.e., the cash flow loss from other imaging systems is expected to be offset by the cash flow gain from other services used by new MRI patients. Also, the project is expected to have a negligible effect on the hospital's current asset and liability accounts, so changes in net working capital (current assets minus current liabilities) will be ignored in the analysis.

These data have been used to develop the flows listed in Table 10-2. The key to identifying the appropriate cash flows is to focus on *incremental cash flows*, which means the actual cash that flows into or out of an organization solely as a result of project acceptance, including opportunity costs.

Note that the cash flows in Table 10-2 do not include any allowance for interest expense. On average, Pine Grove Hospital will finance new projects in accordance with its target capital structure, which consists of 30% debt financing and 70% equity (fund) financing. The costs associated with this financing mix, including both interest costs and the opportunity cost of equity capital, are incorporated into the firm's 10% corporate cost of capital. As the cost of debt financing is included in the discount rate that will be applied to the cash flows, recognition of interest expense in the cash flows would be double counting.

Project Financial Measures

Now that the cash flows have been estimated, the next step is to estimate the MRI project's expected profitability. Like all investments, the expected profitability of proposed projects can be measured either in dollars or in percentage rate of return. In the next sections, a dollar measure—net present value (NPV)—and a rate of return measure—internal rate of return (IRR)—are discussed.

Net Present Value

Net present value is a dollar profitability measure that uses discounted cash flow (DCF) techniques, so it is often referred to as a *DCF measure*. The following two steps are used to calculate NPV:

1. Find the present (time 0) value of each net cash flow, including both inflows and outflows, when discounted at the project's cost of capital.
2. Sum the present values. This sum is defined as the project's net present value.

Applying these steps, we find the NPV of the MRI project to be $82,493 (Fig. 10-2). Financial calculators and spreadsheets have NPV functions

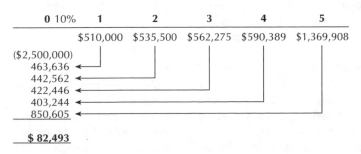

Figure 10-2. MRI project NPV.

that easily perform the mathematics if given the cash flows and cost of capital (discount rate).

The rationale behind the NPV method is straightforward. An NPV of 0 signifies that the project's cash inflows are just sufficient to return the capital invested in the project and to provide the required rate of return (opportunity cost rate) on that capital. If a project has a positive NPV, it is creating value that can be reinvested in the business and, for investor-owned firms, used to pay dividends. If a project has a negative NPV, its cash inflows are insufficient to compensate the business for the opportunity costs associated with the capital invested or even to recover the dollar value of the investment. For investor-owned firms, NPV is a direct measure of the contribution of the project to shareholder wealth, so NPV is usually considered to be the best measure of project profitability.

The NPV of the MRI project is $82,493; on a present value basis, the project is expected to generate a cash flow excess of over $80,000 after all costs, including capital costs, have been considered. Thus, without considering its riskiness, the project is profitable and its acceptance would have a positive impact on the hospital's financial condition.

Internal Rate of Return

As for NPV, internal rate of return is also a DCF measure of profitability. However, whereas NPV measures a project's dollar profitability, IRR measures a project's percentage profitability (i.e., its expected rate of return). Mathematically, the IRR is defined as the discount rate that equates the present value of the project's expected cash inflows to the present value of the project's expected cash outflows, so the IRR is simply the discount rate that forces the NPV of the project to equal 0. As for NPV, financial calculators and spreadsheets have IRR functions that calculate IRRs very rapidly.

The IRR of the MRI project is 11.1%. When all of the project's cash flows are discounted at 11.1%, the NPV of the project is 0. Put another way, the project is expected to generate an 11.1% rate of return on its $2,500,000 investment.

If the IRR exceeds the project's cost of capital, a surplus is projected to remain after recovering the invested capital and paying for its use, and this surplus accrues to the firm's stockholders (or to the business). If the IRR is less than the project's cost of capital, however, taking on the project imposes an expected financial cost (loss) to the business. The MRI project's 11.1% IRR exceeds the project's 10% cost of capital. Thus, as measured by IRR, the project is profitable and its acceptance would enhance the hospital's financial condition.

Comparison of the NPV and IRR Methods

Consider a project with a 0 NPV. In this situation, the project's IRR must equal its cost of capital. The project has 0 expected profitability, and acceptance would neither enhance nor diminish the firm's financial condition. To have a positive NPV, the project's IRR must exceed its cost of capital, and a negative NPV signifies a project with an IRR less than its cost of capital. Thus, projects that are deemed profitable by the NPV method will also be deemed profitable by the IRR method. In the MRI example, the project would have a positive NPV for all costs of capital less than 11.1%. If the cost of capital were greater than 11.1%, the project would have a negative NPV. In effect, the NPV and IRR are perfect substitutes for each other in measuring whether or not a project is profitable.

Project Risk Analysis

Previous sections covered the basics of capital budgeting, including cash flow estimation and profitability measures. This section extends the discussion of capital budgeting to include risk analysis, which is composed of two elements: assessing the project's risk and incorporating that risk assessment into the capital budgeting decision process.

Assessing Risk

Why are projects risky? The answer is simple. Many of the variables that determine a project's cash flows are uncertain, sometimes highly uncertain. If the realized value of such a variable is different from its expected value, the project's realized profitability will differ from that expected. As there is some chance of realizing less profit than expected, risk is present. The two

Table 10-3. MRI project sensitivity analysis. Parentheses indicate negative values.

Change from Base case level (%)	Net present value ($)	
	Volume	Salvage value
−30	(814,053)	(57,215)
−20	(515,193)	10,646
−10	(216,350)	35,923
0	82,493	82,493
+10	381,335	129,062
+20	380,178	175,361
+30	979,020	222,200

primary tools used to assess project risk are sensitivity analysis and scenario analysis.

Sensitivity analysis indicates exactly how much a project's profitability (NPV or IRR) will change in response to a given change in a single input variable, other things being held constant. It begins with a *base case* developed using *expected values* (in the statistical sense) for all uncertain variables. To illustrate, assume that Pine Grove's managers believe that all of the MRI project's cash flows are known with certainty except for weekly volume and salvage value. The expected values for these variables (volume = 40 and salvage value = $750,000) were used in Table 10-2 to obtain the base case NPV of $82,493. Sensitivity analysis is designed to provide managers the answers to such questions as these: What if volume is more or less than the expected level? What if salvage value is more or less than expected?

In a sensitivity analysis, each uncertain variable is usually changed by a fixed percentage amount above and below its expected value, whereas all other variables are held constant at their expected values. Thus, all input variables except one are held at their base case values. Table 10-3 contains the NPV sensitivity analysis for the MRI project, assuming only two uncertain variables: volume and salvage value. Note that the NPV is a constant $82,493 when there is no change in either variable from its base case value.

Managers can examine the values in Table 10-3 to get a feel for which input variable has the greatest impact on the MRI project's NPV—the larger the NPV change for a given percentage input change, the greater the impact. The

sensitivity analysis indicates that the MRI project's NPV is very sensitive to volume, but only mildly sensitive to salvage value. If two projects were being compared, the one with the most input value sensitivity would be regarded as riskier because a relatively small error in estimating a variable, e.g., volume, would produce a large error in the project's projected NPV.

Although sensitivity analysis is widely used in project risk analysis, it does have severe limitations, e.g., suppose that Pine Grove Hospital had a contract with a health maintenance organization (HMO) that guaranteed a minimum MRI usage at a fixed reimbursement rate. In that situation, the project would not be very risky at all, in spite of the fact that the sensitivity analysis showed NPV to be highly sensitive to changes in volume. In general, a project's risk depends on both the sensitivity of its profitability to changes in key input variables and the ranges of likely values of these variables. As sensitivity analysis considers only the first factor, it can give misleading results. Furthermore, sensitivity analysis does not consider any interactions among the uncertain input variables; it considers each variable independently of the others.

Despite the shortcomings of sensitivity analysis as a risk measure, it does provide managers with valuable information. First, it provides breakeven information for the project's uncertain variables, e.g., Table 10-3 shows that just a small percentage decrease in expected volume makes the project unprofitable, whereas the project remains profitable even if salvage value falls by more than 10%. Although somewhat rough, this breakeven information is clearly of value to Pine Grove's managers.

Second, sensitivity analysis tells managers which input variables are most critical to the project's profitability, and hence to the project's financial success. In this example, volume is clearly the key input variable of the two that were examined, so Pine Grove's managers should ensure that the volume estimate is the best possible. The concept here is that the hospital's managers have a limited amount of time to spend on analyzing the MRI project, so the resources expended should be as productive as possible. Also, if Pine Grove's managers could reduce the uncertainty in volume, say through a managed

Table 10-4. MRI Project Scenario Analysis.

Scenario	Probability of outcome	Volume	Salvage value ($)	Net present value ($)
Worst case	0.20	30	500,000	(819,844)
Most likely case	0.60	40	750,000	82,493
Best case	0.20	50	1,000,000	984,829
Expected value		40	750,000	82,493
Standard deviation				570,688

care contract, they could influence the riskiness of the MRI project rather than merely assess it.

Often, the results of sensitivity analyses are shown in graphical form. Then, the slope of each line shows how sensitive the project's profitability is to changes in each of the uncertain input variables. The steeper the slope, the more sensitive profitability is to a change in that variable. Spreadsheet models are ideally suited for performing sensitivity analyses, because such models both automatically recalculate NPV when an input value is changed and facilitate graphing.

Scenario Analysis

Scenario analysis is a risk analysis technique that considers the sensitivity of NPV to changes in key variables, the likely range of variable values, and the interactions among variables. To conduct a scenario analysis, managers pick a "bad" set of circumstances (low volume, low reimbursement rates, high costs, etc.), a "most likely" (average) set, and a "good" set. The resulting input values are then used to create three different profitability scenarios for the project.

To illustrate scenario analysis, assume that Pine Grove's managers regard a drop in weekly volume below 30 scans as very unlikely, and a volume above 50 is also improbable. On the other hand, salvage value could be as low as $500,000 or as high as $1 million. The most likely values are 40 scans per week for volume and $750,000 for salvage value. Thus, volume of 30 and a $500,000 salvage value define the lower bound (worst case) scenario, whereas volume of 50 and a salvage value of $1 million define the upper bound (best case) scenario.

The input values are used to obtain each scenario's NPV. Pine Grove's managers used a spreadsheet model to conduct the analysis, and

Table 10-4 summarizes the results. The most likely case results in a positive NPV; the worst case produces a large negative NPV; and the best case results in a large positive NPV. These results can be used to determine the expected NPV and standard deviation of NPV if an estimate is made for the probabilities of occurrence of each scenario. Suppose Pine Grove's managers estimate a 20% chance for the worst case occurring, a 60% chance for the most likely case, and a 20% chance for the best case. Of course, it is very difficult to estimate scenario probabilities with any confidence.

The expected NPV in the scenario analysis is the same as the base case NPV—$82,493. The consistency of results occurs because the input values used in the scenario analysis, along with the assigned probabilities, produce the same expected input values that were used in Table 10-2 base case analysis. The standard deviation of NPV is $570,688. As standard deviation is a measure of the dispersion of a distribution about its mean, it measures the MRI project's risk. Pine Grove's managers can compare the standard deviation of NPV of this project with the uncertainty inherent in the hospital's aggregate profitability. On the basis of this judgmental comparison of risk, Pine Grove's managers concluded that the MRI project is riskier than the firm's average project, so it was classified as a high-risk project.

Scenario analysis can also be interpreted in a less mathematical way. The worst-case NPV, a loss of about $800,000 for the MRI project, represents an estimate of the worst possible financial consequences of the project. If Pine Grove can absorb such a loss without much impact on its financial condition (which it can), the project does not represent a significant financial danger.

Conversely, if such a loss would mean financial ruin for the hospital, its managers might be unwilling to undertake the project, regardless of its profitability under the most likely and best-case scenarios.

Although scenario analysis provides useful information about a project's risk, it is limited in two ways. First, it considers only a few discreet states of the economy, and hence provides information on only a small number of potential outcomes, whereas an almost infinite number of possibilities actually exist. Although the scenario analysis could be expanded to include more states of the economy, say five or seven, there is a practical limit on how many scenarios can be included.*

Second, scenario analysis—at least as normally conducted—implies a very definite relationship among the uncertain variables, i.e., the analysis assumed that the worst value for volume (30 scans per week) would occur at the same time as the worst value for salvage ($500,000), because the worst case scenario was defined by combining the worst possible value of each uncertain variable. Although this relationship (all worst values occurring together) may hold for some projects, it does not hold for most.

Project Risk Incorporation

The most common method for incorporating project risk into the capital budgeting decision process is the *risk-adjusted discount rate method*. In this method, the base-case (expected) cash flows remain unchanged, and the risk adjustment is made to the discount rate (the opportunity cost of capital). All average-risk projects are discounted at the business's corporate cost of capital, which represents the opportunity cost of capital for such projects; high-risk projects are assigned a higher cost of capital and low-risk projects are discounted at a lower cost of capital.

The good news here is that the process has a starting benchmark, the firm's corporate cost of capital. This discount rate reflects the riskiness of the business in the aggregate or of the firm's average project. The bad news is that typically there is no theoretical basis for setting the size of the adjustment, so the amount of adjustment remains a matter of judgment.

Pine Grove's standard procedure is to add four percentage points to its 10% corporate cost of capital when evaluating high-risk projects, and to subtract two percentage points when evaluating low-risk projects. Thus, to estimate the high-risk MRI project's differential risk-adjusted NPV, the project's expected (base case) cash flows are discounted at 10% + 4% = 14%. This rate is called the *project cost of capital*, as opposed to the corporate cost of capital, because it reflects the risk characteristics of a specific project rather than the aggregate risk characteristics of the business. The resultant NPV is –$200,017, so the MRI project becomes unprofitable when the analysis is adjusted to reflect its high risk. Pine Grove's managers may still decide to go ahead with the MRI project, but at least they know that its expected profitability is not enough to make up for its riskiness, and hence it is likely to be a financial drain on the hospital.

At this point, you might believe that the entire process of capital budgeting analysis is one big shot in the dark. If so, you are probably right. Nevertheless, health care managers need to have some feel, even if it is not very precise, for the financial consequences of new projects. In hindsight, some will work out well and some will work out poorly, but good capital budgeting analyses give managers an edge in picking the good ones and passing on the poor ones.

References
1. Gapenski LC. *Healthcare Finance: An Introduction to Accounting and Financial Management*. Chicago: Health Administration Press, 2002.
2. Gapenski LC. *Understanding Health Care Financial Management*. Chicago: Health Administration Press, 2001.

---

* *Monte Carlo simulation* is a risk analysis technique that overcomes many of the deficiencies of scenario analysis. For more information see Gapenski [1,2].

11

Fundamentals of Biostatistics

David L. DeMets and Marian R. Fisher

Introduction

Progress in medical research and health care delivery has partly resulted from careful research that has led to better treatments and their appropriate application. A critical part of this process is proper experimental design and statistical analysis of the resulting data. In this chapter, we explore some of the fundamental concepts that are central to good experimental design and data analysis. We do not try to explore these concepts in great technical detail because it would not be feasible in a single chapter. Some excellent texts for further detail are Armitage, Brown and Hollander, and Fisher and Van Belle [1–3]. There is also an excellent series of journal articles that we recommend by Gore *et al.*, which go through many of these issues in greater detail [4–26].

Basic Research Design

There are many examples of individual researchers using astute observation and anecdotal evidence to create medical breakthroughs. However, we cannot rely on this as a research strategy. Instead, we need to collect data and summarize the results to make some conclusions and proceed on to the next study, using the results from the last study to guide us. We consider two basic types of research designs: observational studies and experimental designs.

Observational Studies

Observational studies involve careful observation of a laboratory or clinical population. No manipulation or treatment of the population is performed. One of the best uses of observational studies is to identify factors that might influence or predict subject outcome. In some instances, treatment effect can be inferred from such data, when several required assumptions are fulfilled. In this setting, it will be important to distinguish between association and causation. Observational studies are helpful in identifying factors that might be associated with disease occurrence. However, it is not usually possible to infer disease causation unless the associations are quite dramatic and repeated with several populations. Causation implies a direct link between a risk factor and disease outcome. Association means that a factor and a disease occur together, but it does not mean that the factor causes the disease. We briefly describe three basic observational designs.

Retrospective or Case–Control Studies

Epidemiologists often use the case–control design to identify risk factors for diseases, especially diseases that are rare. The case–control design looks at a group of individuals (designated as cases) who have a disease, such as lung cancer, and compares that group with another group (designated as controls) who do not have the disease. The goal of the case–control design is to identify one or more factors that differ between the groups and use them to predict an increased risk of the disease. This type of design is retrospective in that information is collected looking backward in time, e.g., the association of lung cancer with cigarette smoking came initially from this type of data. Patients with lung cancer were compared with those who did not have clinically diagnosed lung cancer. Data on many variables of exposure and lifestyle were collected. Researchers observed that many more lung cancer patients were or had been smokers than in the control population. This increase can be quantified using a statistic called the odds ratio, which we define later in this chapter. An odds ratio of 1 would indicate no increased risk as a result of the factor under review. As the odds ratio increases or decreases from 1, the strength of the associated risk increases. The estimate of risk in a case–control study, however, depends heavily on the selection of the control series of participants.

Cross-sectional Studies

In contrast to case–control studies that look backward in time, cross-sectional designs look at a population (designated as a cohort) at one point in time, or as a cross-sectional snapshot. Typically, researchers choose populations that can be thoroughly evaluated and are considered to be at risk for the disease in which the researcher is interested. Some members of the cohort will have the disease of interest and others will not. By examining the prevalence of the disease over various measured factors, researchers may identify some factors as being more strongly associated with the presence or absence of the disease than others are. These associated factors are thus identified as possible risk factors, some of which may be modifiable to reduce the risk of the disease.

An example of this type of design is the Wisconsin Epidemiological Study of Diabetic Retinopathy (WESDR), which carefully examined a cohort of patients with diabetes in southwestern Wisconsin. The presence of diabetic retinopathy was recorded in each member. The frequency of diabetic retinopathy was examined across a large number of factors. One result was the increase in diabetic retinopathy in individuals with high levels of glycated hemoglobin [27], making this a candidate for risk factor modification. This, in fact, was examined in a prospective trial, the Diabetes Control and Complications Trial (DCCT Research Group), which established that tight control of glycated hemoglobin reduced the incidence of retinopathy or disease progression [28]. Risk can be estimated in these studies with an odds ratio or a relative risk estimator,

defined later. Although the cross-sectional study can be useful, important risk factors could be missed, because this type of study can evaluate only those who have the disease and are still living.

Prospective Studies

When feasible, the prospective observational study provides the most effective way to identify possible risk factors. A cohort is identified, as in the cross-sectional study, but the cohort is followed forward or prospectively over time. The cross-sectional study provides the prevalence, and the prospective follow-up provides the incidence or development of the disease. In the prospective study, disease occurrence is recorded over time, the length of time depending on the frequency of the disease, i.e., the less frequent the disease, the longer the follow-up period required to accumulate enough events to establish the risk factor association. Relative risk or odds ratio can also be estimated from this type of design. Although the prospective study can take more time and be more costly, it is less subject to the bias of observing only living participants, as in the cross-sectional design, or the bias resulting from control group choice, as in the case–control design. One of the earliest and most successful prospective studies in medical research is the Framingham Heart Study, which followed a population in Framingham, Massachusetts for heart disease incidence over four decades [29]. From this study, researchers found that smoking, high blood pressures, elevated cholesterol and lipids, and diabetes were associated with the incidence of heart disease and mortality [29]. However, identifying these associations did not necessarily infer causation. Later, clinical studies demonstrated that lowering blood pressure, for example, resulted in a lowering of cardiovascular mortality and morbidity.

Experimental Designs

By experimental designs, we mean clinical or laboratory studies in which some factor is manipulated and participants are followed over time to evaluate the impact of that change. An essential feature of this approach is that, except for the factor being modified, the two or more groups must be comparable in all important risk factors. There are three basic experimental designs for clinical research.

Historical Control
The historical control design compares patients treated currently with a new drug, device, or procedure with patients treated previously or historically with another established treatment. As with the case–control design, the choice of the historical control is critical for the validity of this approach, and comparability is not easy to demonstrate. The disease process itself may have changed, or background therapy may have improved such that the historical control is not relevant. Data for the control taken from the literature or historical databases may not be comparable to data collected for the current treatment group. Thus, this is the least reliable of the three approaches.

Concurrent Control
The concurrent control group approach compares all patients treated currently by one method to all patients currently treated in another way. In contrast to the historical control approach, the concurrent control approach means that many factors may be similar in data collection and time trends. The biggest challenge is making sure that the two patient groups are comparable in all important risk factors. Patients may self-select into one or another group as a result of hospital or clinic preferences or geographic factors, which might also affect risk levels. Patients may be treated differently because of clinical preferences or decisions based on clinical assessment of risk. For these reasons, the concurrent control is not as reliable as the third method, the randomized controlled clinical trial.

Randomized Controlled Trial
The randomized controlled clinical trial is a basic experimental design in which patients or participants are randomly assigned to receive either the new experimental treatment or the standard control treatment. For reasonably sized studies, the process of randomization produces comparability between the two or more arms of the clinical trial. The randomized controlled trial (RCT) has become the standard research tool for clin-

ical research and for laboratory studies as well. As both control and experimental arms are being followed concurrently, the data should be of the same quality and completeness. There are many excellent references for more details concerning clinical trials [30–33].

Data Description and Summary

Once an experimental design has been selected and the experiment completed, the data collected must be summarized in a way that allows the information to be communicated easily to other scientists. There are both simple graphical and statistical measures that summarize the data. We comment on only a few of these methods, and standard introductory texts should be consulted for more details. We shall focus on three types of data: (1) continuous measures, such as weight or intraocular pressure, (2) dichotomous or binary outcomes, such as success or failure, and (3) time to an event or time to failure.

Graphical Methods
These include frequency plots, histograms, and box-and-whisker plots. All of these summarize the distribution of the observed data. For illustration, consider the data for intraocular pressure (IOP in mm/Hg). The data are 20, 16, 18, 21, 23, 25, 23, 18, 19, 23, 17, 14, 18, 19, 21, 18, 20, 17, 16, 17, 20, 18, 15, 18, 16, and 24. These data can be used to create a *histogram* (Fig. 11-1). The histogram plots the data as the number of observations that occurred for each value shown on the bottom axis and illustrates the smallest and largest values, as well as the most common or frequent observations. The 50th percentile is the value at which half of the observations fall below that value. The 25th percentile is the value beneath which a quarter of the observations fall. Similarly, the 75th percentile is the value at which three-quarters of the observed values are less.

Let the first 10 observations be group 1 and the remaining observations group 2. A *box-and-whisker plot* shows the 25th percentile and the 75th percentile points at the ends of the box that is plotted, with the 50th percentile inside the box. The ends of the whiskers are the 5th and 95th percentile points. Figure 11-2 is a side-by-side

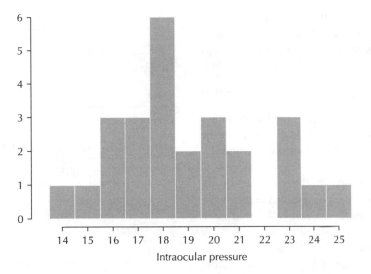

Figure 11-1. Histogram.

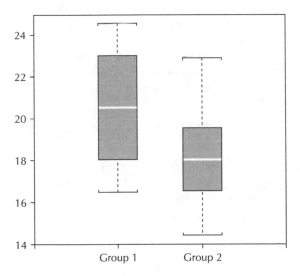

Figure 11-2. Box-and-whisker plot.

box-and-whisker plot for groups 1 and 2. From Fig. 11-2, we get information on the differences and similarities of the results from each group.

Summary Statistics
These provide some of the same information that the graphical methods present. A few summary statistics can identify important features of the distribution. The difference between the largest and smallest observed values is the *range* of the data. The *median* value is the 50th percentile, i.e., the value for which 50% of observed values lie on either side. Another measure of central tendency is the *mean value* or *average value*. The mean is the sum of the observations divided by the number of observations. For these data, the range is 11, the median is 18, and the mean value is 19.

For distributions of data that are *symmetric*, the mean and median are the same. However, if the distribution of the data is not symmetric, the distribution is *skewed*. The frequency distribution or histogram would have a longer tail on one side of the median than on the other. The skewness is in the direction of the longer tail. The mean value will be on same side of the median as the tail of the distribution. The mean value is sensitive to extreme values in the data. Extremely small or large values relative to the median will pull the mean value in that direction. The median is not affected by a few extreme values. Figure 11-1 illustrates that the distribution is slightly skewed, with a longer tail for higher values and the mean value of 19 compared to the median of 18.

If we let the observation be denoted by x_i, then, for n total observations, the mean value μ can be estimated by summing all the observations and dividing this sum by n. We define this as the *sample mean*, $\bar{x}$ where $\bar{x} = \sum_{i=i}^{n} x_i/n$.

Another descriptive statistic for continuous-type data is a measure of variability. The range of the data is one simple measure. However, we also use the variance of the data to give a measure of variability. The variance s^2, denoted σ^2, can be estimated by the *sample variance* s^2 which is computed by $s^2 = \sum_{i=i}^{n} (x_i - \bar{x})^2/(n - 1)$. The square root of the variance is the *standard deviation*, denoted by σ. The standard deviation is estimated by the square root of the sample variance, denoted by s.

There is variability in the estimate of the mean value, i.e., from experiment to experiment, each with n samples, the mean value will vary. We can quantify the variability of the sample mean by the quantity σ^2/n. This is estimated by using the sample variance s^2, so that our estimate of the variability of the sample mean is s^2/n. The square root of this quantity is the *standard error of the mean* $s/\sqrt{n}$. For these data, we can calculate the sample mean, the sample variance, the sample standard deviation, and the standard error of the mean as 19, 8.24, 2.87, and 0.56, respectively.

For binary data, we can estimate the response frequency or success rate p by $\hat{p}$, which is computed by the number of success divided by the number of subjects or experimental units. $\hat{p} = \sum_{i=i}^{n} x_i/n$, where $x_i = 1$ for a success and 0 for a failure. We can also reverse this and consider the failure rate, recognizing that the success rate is just 1 minus the failure rate. The estimated variance of the success rate is the sample variance $\hat{p}(1 - \hat{p})/n$. As before, the standard error is the square root of the sample variance $\sqrt{\hat{p}(1 - \hat{p})/n}$. From the mean response and the variance, we can construct statistics that give some indication of the deviation of the observed data from what is expected. This is described in the next section.

Two other summary statistics already mentioned are the odds ratio and relative risk. If there are two treatment groups, we can summarize the risk of the event in one group $\hat{p}_1$ to the risk of the event in the second group $\hat{p}_2$ by the ratio or relative risk (RR) of $\hat{p}_1/\hat{p}_2$. An RR of 1 means that the same level of risk exists in each group. An RR > 1 suggests the risk is greater in group 1 than in group 2. An RR < 1 would mean the risk is greater in group 2 than in group 1. For our study the

Table 11-1. Events by group.

	Event	No event	Total
Group 1	a	b	$a+b$
Group 2	c	d	$c+d$
Total	$a+c$	$b+d$	n

Table 11-2. Events by intraocular pressure.

	IOP (mmHg)		
	> 22	≤ 21	Total
Group 1	4	6	10
Group 2	1	15	16
Total	5	21	26

event rate $\hat{p}_1$ in group 1 is $a/(a + b)$ and the event rate $\hat{p}_2$ in group 2 is $c/(c + d)$. Then the relative risk $\hat{p}_1/\hat{p}_2$ is the ratio of $a/(a + b)$ to $c/(c + d)$ (Table 11-1).

As an illustration, consider the data in group 1 and group 2 and define the event as an intraocular pressure (IOP) greater than 22 mm/Hg (Table 11-2).

Group 1 data are: 20, 16, 18, 21, 23, 25, 23, 18, 19, 23

Group 1 events are: 0, 0, 0, 0, 1, 1, 1, 0, 0, 1

Group 2 data are: 17, 14, 18, 19, 21, 18, 20, 17, 16, 17, 20, 18, 15, 18, 16, 25

Group 2 events are: 0, 0, 0, 0, 0, 0, 0, 0, 0, 0, 0, 0, 0, 0, 0, 1.

The odds ratio is related to the relative risk and is estimated by the ratio ad/bc. For small or low event rates, the odds ratio is very close to the relative risk. Researchers sometimes interchange these two quantities, but they are actually different. For the data shown in Table 11-2, the relative risk is 6.4 and the odds ratio 10.0.

Test Statistics

Once we have summarized the observed data using graphical methods as well as summary statistics, we often want to evaluate whether the observed data agree with what we expected

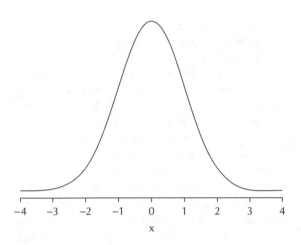

Figure 11-3. Normal distribution.

based on some prior experience or theoretical assumptions. Fortunately, many of the summary statistics can be rescaled according to the expected values of the summary response using a particular distribution, the *normal distribution* with mean 0 and variance 1, which we denote as normal(0,1). The normal distribution is shown in Fig. 11-3. The normal distribution has 2.5% of the distribution above the value 1.96 and 2.5% below −1.96. Approximately 63% of the distribution is between −1.0 and +1.0; 50% is below 0. The mean and median values are both 0.0. This classic distribution can sometimes be used to summarize observed data, but that is not our interest here. Many test statistics have a standard form obtained by subtracting the expected value of the mean or proportion from the observed value, and dividing by the square root of the variance of the estimated summary statistic. These statistics often have a normal(0,1) distribution, so it is relatively easy to describe the test statistics results.

One Sample Case

For a single experimental group with a continuous response outcome, we can form a test statistic of the general form described. Suppose $\bar{x}$ represents our summary statistic. We expect the sample mean to have a value of μ. For a large enough sample, say $n > 20$, we can rescale the sample mean as $Z = (\bar{x} - \mu)/(\sigma/\sqrt{n})$.

This rescaled statistic can be used to test whether the observed data are consistent with the theoretical value μ expected under the usual experimental conditions. Perhaps we would like to show that the new treatment gives a response better than what has been observed previously, or that there is a response at all. If the value of the rescaled test statistic were 0, then the sample mean would be exactly as expected from the previous assumption. However, this would be unlikely to happen as a result of variation in the sample obtained. The new statistic is likely to vary some from 0, even if the assumed value is the true value. If Z has a large absolute value, the observed sample mean is different from that expected. We can quantify the variation in the rescaled statistic Z though the normal distribution. The rescaled statistic has a normal distribution with mean 0 and variance 1. Thus, if the statistic is larger than +1.96 or less than −1.96, we know that this would happen with a probability of 0.05. If the rescaled statistic were larger, with an absolute value of 2.58, this would happen with a probability of 0.01. Thus, we can quantify how unusual or different the observed results are from what we expected or assumed.

Hypothesis Testing

This discussion for the one-sample continuous-outcome measure has, in an informal way, introduced the concept of hypothesis testing. The rescaled statistic Z is formally referred to as the *test statistic*. We assume that there is some hypothesis we would like to reject, from which we can claim the observed response is different. We might assume that the true mean response μ is equal to 0. This is referred to as the *null hypothesis*, although the assumed value does not have to be 0. We may hope to reject the null hypothesized value so that we can claim that our new treatment has a response better than what we assumed from previous results, for example. This would be referred to as the *alternative hypothesis*. If we observe a sample mean that is quite different from the assumed mean value μ_0, such that the test statistic Z is larger in absolute value than, say, 1.96, we would begin to disbelieve that the real response is in fact μ_0 and thus reject that hypothesis.

However, it is possible, with probability of 0.05, that a test statistic of that size could be observed even if the true mean response were μ_0. If that were to happen, we would incorrectly reject the null hypothesis, and this is referred to as a *type I error*. The probability of a type I error is the *significance level*, i.e., the probability of incorrectly rejecting the null hypothesis or of a false-positive claim. We want to keep the probability of a type I error small. We have traditionally set the significance level at either 0.05 or 0.01. The values of the test statistic must be larger than the corresponding *critical value*, which in this case are 1.96 and 2.58, respectively. The *p*-value is the probability, assuming the null hypothesis to be true, that we would observe a sample mean this large or larger. If the *p*-value is less than the significance level, say 0.05, we would reject the null hypothesis and claim that the underlying true response is different from what was assumed.

Using the example from our data where $\bar{x} = 19$ and the standard error is 0.56, we can test the null hypothesis that the true mean response μ_0 is 21 and calculate $Z = (19 - 21)/0.56 = -3.57$. We reject the null hypothesis of the true mean response as 21 with $p < 0.05$ (in this case $p < 0.01$).

For a binary response from a single group, we can test the hypothesis that the true response rate is p_0 and try to see if we can reject that hypothesis in favor of a better response rate. Again, for a sufficiently large sample (say $n > 20$), we can rescale the observed $\hat{p}$ as follows:

$$z = (\hat{p} - p_0)/\sqrt{\hat{p}(1 - \hat{p})/n}$$

This test statistic also has a normal(0,1) distribution. We can follow the same procedure as described earlier to test whether the observed response rate is consistent with the assumed value. Using the data, we can test the null hypothesis that the true portion, p_0 with an IOP greater than 22 is 40% and calculate $Z = (0.19 - 0.40)/(0.19 \times 0.81 \div 26) = -3.56$. We can reject the null hypothesis that the true portion is 40% with $p < 0.05$ (in this case $p < 0.01$).

Two Sample Case

For many research designs, we may want to compare responses between the experimental arm and the control arm. The response variable could be either continuous or binary. We briefly illustrate both cases.

If we have continuous outcome variables for an experimental arm and a control arm, with sample means $\bar{x}_1$ and $\bar{x}_2$, we would like to compare the differences between them, $\bar{x}_1 - \bar{x}_2$. The null hypothesis is that there is no difference between the true responses, $\mu_1 - \mu_2 = 0$. If an observed difference in the sample means $\bar{x}_1 - \bar{x}_2$ is large, then the null hypothesis may not be true. We can formulate a test statistic for comparing two sample means as follows:

$$Z = (\bar{x}_1 - \bar{x}_2)/\sqrt{s_1^2/n_1 + s_2^2/n_2}$$

Using the data, we can test the null hypothesis of no difference between group 1 and group 2 as $Z = (20.6 - 18.0)/(0.909) = 2.86$. We can reject the null the hypothesis of no difference in the true means of group 1 and group 2 with $p < 0.05$.

For comparing two binomial response rates, we can follow an analogous procedure. The null hypothesis is that the true response rates are equal, i.e., $p_1 - p_2 = 0$. If $\hat{p}_1 - \hat{p}_2$ is sufficiently large, we may be able to reject the null hypothesis.

The test statistic is $(\hat{p}_1 - \hat{p}_2)/\sqrt{\hat{p}(1 - \hat{p})\left(\dfrac{1}{n_1} + \dfrac{1}{n_2}\right)}$

where $\hat{p} = (n_1\hat{p}_1 + n_2\hat{p}_2)/(n_1 + n_2)$. This test statistic has a normal distribution. For these data, we can test whether the two response rates are equal and calculate $Z = (0.40 - 0.06)/(0.158) = 2.15$. We can reject the null hypothesis that the true event rates are equal with $p < 0.05$.

Correlation and Regression

Some experiments may have two continuous variables, say X and Y, and the investigator's goal is to understand the relationship between these two variables, e.g., X might be age and Y bone density. A researcher may want to understand the relationship between the aging process and the decline or loss of bone density. We can quantify the relationship or *association* between these two. This may also be referred to as the *correlation* between X and Y. As indicated earlier,

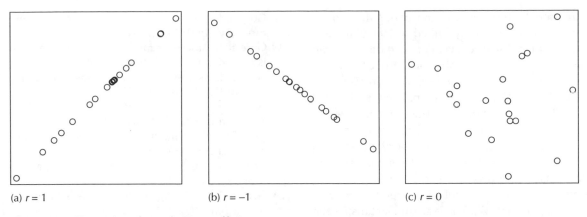

(a) *r* = 1 (b) *r* = −1 (c) *r* = 0

Figure 11-4. Examples of correlation coefficients.

a high degree of association or correlation does not imply causation. If we obtained data about the number of home personal computers purchased and the rise of the stock market during the 1990s, we would get a strong association or correlation. However, we should not infer that one causes the other, but rather that both are caused by some other factor, such as the national economy.

We can quantify the correlation by using Pearson's correlation coefficient ρ [2]. We can estimate the correlation ρ from the observed data as follows:

$$\sum (x_i - \bar{x})(y_i - \bar{y}) / \sqrt{\sum (x_i - \bar{x})^2 \sum (y_i - \bar{y})^2}$$

The estimated correlation coefficient lies between −1.0 and +1.0. A perfect linear correlation would yield a correlation coefficient of +1.0, and a perfect negative correlation would give −1.0. For no correlation, ρ = 0.0. Examples of data for these correlation coefficients are given in Fig. 11-4.

In some circumstances, we would like to summarize the relationship as a linear regression. In this situation, we can express the dependent response *Y* as a function of the independent variable *X* by the relationship *Y* = *a* + *bX*.

The parameters *a* and *b* can be estimated from the observed *n* pairs of data, x_i and y_i. However, even if the correlation coefficient is close to 1, we cannot assume that a change in the value *x*(Δ*x*) will cause a change in *y* (Δ*y*) by an amount *a* + *b*Δ*x*. We can say only that the value of *x* will be predictive of the value *y*.

Survival Analysis

One of the common outcomes in clinical or laboratory research is time to response or time to failure. The goal is to identify the probability of surviving to a specific time point free of the event or failure. The method for estimating this survival curve is the Kaplan–Meier method [34]. Although we do not go through the details of this method, we give the basic motivation. The Kaplan–Meier method divides the follow-up time into smaller intervals, each defined by the time of a failure or event. For each interval, the probability of surviving that specific interval is computed, based on the cohort of patients who survived to begin that interval of follow-up. From those probabilities, the Kaplan–Meier estimate can be computed. The probability of surviving through the second time interval is the product of two probabilities: the probability of surviving the first interval times the probability of surviving the second interval, given that the first interval had been survived. By repeating this process, we can estimate the survival curve for the entire follow-up time. It is important to keep track of the number of patients at risk at the beginning of each interval, the number of events at each time point, and the number of patients lost to follow-up during the interval. With these data elements, the probabilities of surviving each interval can be computed [35].

A second issue is to compare two survival curves to test, for example, whether a new treatment affects the survival of a cohort compared with another cohort given the standard or control treatment. The process of comparing the two survival curves is closely linked to the elements of the Kaplan–Meier curve. For each distinct event or failure time, the status of the two cohorts is summarized in a 2×2 table. Each cohort is represented with the number of patients still at risk just before the event and the number of events recorded at that time point. Completing this process for each event time, a series of 2×2 tables are generated. These tables are often summarized by a statistic proposed for survival analysis that is referred to as the Mantel–Haenszel statistic or the logrank test [36,37]. There are other statistics that compare two or more survival curves, but the logrank test is the most common.

References

1. Armitage P. *Statistical Methods in Medical Research*, 2nd edn. New York: John Wiley & Sons, 1975.
2. Brown BW Jr, Hollander M. *Statistics—A Biomedical Introduction*. New York: John Wiley & Sons, 1977.
3. Fisher L, Van Belle G. *Biostatistics—A Methodology for the Health Sciences*. New York: John Wiley & Sons, 1993.
4. Gore SM. Assessing clinical trials—between-observer variation. *BMJ* 1981; **283**: 40–3.
5. Gore SM. Assessing clinical trials—protocol and monitoring. *BMJ* 1981; **283**: 369–71.
6. Gore SM. Assessing methods—many variables. *BMJ* 1981; **283**: 901–5.
7. Gore SM. Assessing methods–critical comment. *BMJ* 1981; **283**: 966–9.
8. Gore SM. Assessing clinical trials—first steps. *BMJ* 1981; **282**: 1605–7.
9. Gore SM. Assessing clinical trials—trial size. *BMJ* 1981; **282**: 1687–9.
10. Gore SM. Assessing clinical trials—design I. *BMJ* 1981; **282**: 1780–1.
11. Gore SM. Assessing clinical trials—design II. *BMJ* 1981; **282**: 1861–3.
12. Gore SM. Assessing clinical trials—why randomise? *BMJ* 1981; **282**: 1958–60.
13. Gore SM. Assessing clinical trials—simple randomisation. *BMJ* 1981; **282**: 2036–9.
14. Gore SM. Assessing clinical trials—restricted randomisation. *BMJ* 1981; **282**: 2114–7.
15. Gore SM. Assessing clinical trials—double blind trials. *BMJ* 1981; **283**: 122–4.
16. Gore SM. Assessing clinical trials—trial discipline. *BMJ* 1981; **283**: 211–3.
17. Gore SM. Assessing clinical trials—record sheets. *BMJ* 1981; **283**: 296–8.
18. Gore SM. Assessing clinical trials—rash adventures. *BMJ* 1981; **283**: 426–8.
19. Gore SM. Assessing methods—descriptive statistics and graphs. *BMJ* 1981; **283**: 486–8.
20. Gore SM. Assessing methods—transforming the data. *BMJ* 1981; **283**: 548–50.
21. Gore SM. Assessing methods—art of significance testing. *BMJ* 1981; **283**: 600–2.
22. Gore SM. Assessing methods—confidence intervals. *BMJ* 1981; **283**: 660–2.
23. Gore SM. Assessing methods—recognising linearity. *BMJ* 1981; **283**: 711–3.
24. Gore SM. Assessing methods—a feel for other things. *BMJ* 1981; **283**: 775–8.
25. Gore SM. Assessing methods—survival. *BMJ* 1981; **283**: 840–3.
26. Gore SM, Jones IG, Rytter EC. Misuse of statistical methods: critical assessment of articles in BMJ from January to March, 1976. *BMJ* 1977; **i**: 85–7.
27. Klein R, Klein BE, Moss SE, Davis MD, DeMets DL. Glycosylated hemoglobin predicts the incidence and progression of diabetic retinopathy. *JAMA* 1988; **260**: 2864–71.
28. Diabetes Control and Complications Trial Research Group. Progression of retinopathy with intensive versus conventional treatment in the Diabetes Control and Complications Trial. *Ophthalmology* 1995; **102**: 647–61.
29. National Heart Lung and Blood Institute. *Research Milestones*. www.nhlbi.nih.gov/about/framingham/timeline.htm January 2000.
30. Peto R, Pike MC, Armitage P *et al*. Design and analysis of randomized clinical trials requiring prolonged observations of each patient. I. Introduction and design. *Br J Cancer* 1976; **34**: 1976.
31. Armitage P. The analysis of data from clinical trials. *Statistician* 1980; **28**: 171–83.
32. Pocock S. *Clinical Trials: a Practical Approach*. New York: John Wiley & Sons, 1984.
33. Friedman LM, Furberg CD, DeMets DL. *Fundamentals of Clinical Trials*, 3rd edn. New York: Springer-Verlag, 1998.
34. Kaplan E, Meier P. Nonparametric estimation from incomplete observations. *J Am Statist Assoc* 1958; **53**: 457–81.
35. Perkins T, Fisher M. When is "final"? *Ophthalmology* 1998; **105**: 395–6.
36. Mantel N. Evaluation of survival data and two new rank order statistics arising in its consideration. *Cancer Chemotherapy Report* 1966; **50**: 163–70.
37. Mantel N, Haenszel W. Statistical aspects of the analysis of data from retrospective studies of disease. *J Natl Cancer Inst* 1959; **22**: 719–48.

12

Epidemiology and Health Outcomes

Karen J. Cruickshanks

Epidemiology and Medical Practice

Few physicians are taught epidemiology in medical school, yet we expect physicians to be able to critically evaluate the plethora of new scientific information published monthly on treatments and preventive measures and apply this knowledge to patient care. Although it is beyond the scope of this chapter to provide a solid foundation in epidemiology, we provide an overview of epidemiologic concepts important in evaluating the medical literature. Readers who want more in-depth material are referred to one of the many excellent introductory texts available [1–3].

Epidemiology is the study of patterns of disease in people. The questions epidemiologists pose sound simple: What are the characteristics (genes, behaviors, socioeconomic conditions, exposures, etc.) of people who develop the disease, the place (environment) where disease is prevalent, and the time when the disease occurs (seasonality, cohort effects, temporal change, etc.)? Epidemiologists seek to interpret these patterns in the context of what we know from basic science and clinical observation in order to learn how best to reduce the burden of disease in the population.

Epidemiology can often contribute to the prevention of morbidity and mortality before we know the true underlying causal pathway or agent, e.g., John Snow's investigation of a cholera epidemic in England in the mid-1800s is hailed as an example of an early success story in epidemiology [4]. Without knowing what pathogen was responsible for cholera, he was able, through careful documentation of the characteristics of people and their environment, to recognize that more deaths were occurring in households with water service from a particular company that drew its water from a polluted part of the Thames than in households that were served by a less polluted water source. Through his efforts to discontinue water usage from the Broad Street pump, he implemented a means of preventing disease without understanding the disease agent and without substantiating clinical trial data. For a parallel in the modern world of chronic disease, consider our present view of smoking's effects on cardiovascular mortality, even without evidence clearly indicting a specific chemical component of cigarette smoke or a definition of the underlying mechanism [5].

Epidemiologic methodology provides guidelines for conducting scientific investigations of biomedical research questions that minimize bias and misleading results. Through its focus on collaborative research with basic scientists and clinical specialists, epidemiology can serve as a translator of basic science findings into clinical practice. It is the foundation on which much of preventive medicine rests [6].

Evaluating the Evidence

Although medicine continues to use the apprenticeship model of training with its reliance on clinical experience, there is increasing emphasis on the need for evidence-based decisions. Beginning in 1993, one group has published a series of articles to guide practicing physicians through the difficulties of translating research findings into their own clinical practices [7–31]. From an epidemiologic perspective, we seek to accomplish the same goal by describing how research methods and statistical analyses help us to interpret risk factor associations and possible prevention strategies.

The Impact of Study Design

In medical research, study designs vary from reports of observations by astute clinicians to randomized controlled clinical trials. When evaluating the medical literature, it is important to understand the strengths and limitations of each design in order to appropriately judge its relative contribution. Table 12-1 summarizes the strengths and weaknesses of the various designs.

Case Reports and Case Series

Although not generally included when discussing epidemiology, these reports account for a large proportion of the medical literature. They can provide important insights into rare conditions, generate hypotheses to be tested in well-designed studies, or report new surgical procedures that may become generally accepted after rigorous evaluation. Patients are usually selected because they were seen in the author's clinic or practice group, and therefore these papers report experiences, not scientific evidence. The patients who attend a particular clinic or seek a physician's care may differ from the average patient in important ways, such as severity of disease, co-morbidity from other disorders, compliance, age, or sex, which may have influenced the clinical outcome. In addition, treatment outcomes may be specific to the skills of the surgeon performing the procedure.

Ecologic Studies

Another type of epidemiologic study is the ecologic study. In this design, individuals are not studied; comparisons are made at a region or country level. Generally, areas with greatly different rates of disease are compared to discover possible explanations for the risk differential, e.g., early evidence of the possible link between high-fat diet and breast cancer was obtained by comparing the dietary patterns in Western countries, where breast cancer rates are high, with countries such as Japan where breast cancer rates are low [32]. This type of study can be useful in sorting out the role of genes, the environment, and lifestyle factors, but is limited by the lack of individual measures of exposures. Ecologic studies can easily produce misleading associations, but they are useful for generating hypotheses.

Case–Control Studies

In case–control studies, people are selected for study on the basis of disease status, i.e., cases are people with the disease of interest and controls are people without the disease. Information is obtained about past exposures to determine which factors differed between those with and those without the disease, and which might therefore be related to developing the disease. This design is very useful when diseases are rare, because the investigator can select the sources for cases and controls to ensure the numbers needed for adequate statistical power. Sampling strategies to enroll more controls than cases can also increase the analytic power.

Eligible subjects can be identified through hospital or clinical records, disease registries, death certificates, or a community. Studies based on community samples are called population based and are considered stronger methodologically because there is less potential for selection bias. As in case series, when participants are selected from a hospital or clinic, their experience may differ from that of the "average" patient. They may be sicker or may have different lifestyles and exposures because of the characteristics of the hospital or clinic's patient population. Identifying all people with the disease who live in a community or region means that the entire spectrum of disease is studied.

There are similar problems when trying to select appropriate controls. Some studies choose patients seen at the same facility as the cases but who have other diagnoses. Some use friends or neighbors, others rely on people found through random-digit telephone dialing, and others select comparable people through household censuses. Although the goal is to have controls who are similar to the cases in age, sex, and perhaps socioeconomic factors, to ensure that they had an equal chance of developing the disease, it is easy to end up with a biased group of controls as the result of the difficulties of persuading healthy people to take part in medical research.

Table 12.1. Overview of study designs.

Design	Selection of participants	Strengths	Limitations
Case series	Consecutive patients	May generate hypotheses or techniques for evaluation	Describes clinical experience; not scientific evidence
Ecologic	Compare countries or regions with different rates of disease	Generates hypotheses about factors that may explain the risk differential	Lacks individual measures of exposures Uncertainty that exposures of people with disease are reflected by the region as a whole
Case–control	Select people on the basis of disease presence and absence	Inexpensive Good for generating hypotheses Good for rare diseases	Susceptible to selection bias, recall bias, etc Difficult to choose appropriate controls Retrospective assessment of exposures; no information on temporal sequence Cannot measure relative risk or incidence
Cohort	Select people without the disease—follow to monitor for the development of disease	Measures incidence and relative risk Establishes temporal sequence Good for rare exposures Less subject to bias	Expensive Large numbers of subjects Long follow-up time Poor for rare diseases
Clinical trials	Randomize people to treatments or placebo	Measures cause and effect Reduces bias if masking employed	Not always ethical Expensive Size Loss to follow-up Compliance problems
Community-based trials	Assign a community to each intervention arm	When risk factor/behavior is common Environmental exposure	Cost Size Changing exposure at the population level

Other limitations of this design are substantial. The most important is that ascertainment of exposures or characteristics is done after the disease developed. Therefore, the researcher cannot be sure that the exposure preceded, or led to, development of the disease. The patterns observed may reflect some impact of the disease process or its treatment, e.g., in early studies of cholesterol and coronary heart disease, people with heart disease had higher cholesterol levels than those without heart disease [33]. It was not known whether having a heart attack somehow resulted in a subsequent rise in cholesterol or whether high cholesterol was a risk factor for heart disease. Only longitudinal studies that study people before the development of the disease can establish the temporal sequence of events.

Much of the information about exposures and potential risk factors in case–control studies is obtained from medical records or questionnaires. Medical records are often incomplete or unavailable, and they may be limited further because test methods vary by facility and doctors differ in practices, leading to nonuniform information. Questionnaire data rely on participant recall, which may differ between cases and controls. *Recall bias* is the term used to describe the phenomenon that people with a disease are more likely than controls to report adverse exposures and behaviors in their efforts to understand why they were afflicted [34].

Cohort Studies

Cohort, longitudinal, or prospective studies are all terms used to describe studies in which participants who are free of the disease of interest are selected for study. In this design, exposures, behaviors, and other characteristics are measured when people are healthy, so the chance for recall bias is minimized. Testing, examination, and questionnaire methods can all be standardized so there is less measurement error. As measurement error is nondifferential—i.e., randomly distributed among those who will develop the disease later and those who will remain disease free—it does not bias the risk association estimate.

Participants are recontacted or reexamined periodically to monitor for the development of disease. At specified intervals, data are analyzed to determine whether baseline measurements of exposures and other factors predicted who developed the disease during the follow-up period. Cohorts can be population based, drawing participants from a defined geopolitical area, or be based on volunteers, occupational groups, or other sampling frames. The cohort study is the only study design that permits the measurement of the incidence or absolute risk of disease and therefore the evaluation of the relative contributions of various risk factors. It establishes measures of risk factors before the outcome is known and so ensures that the exposure preceded the disease.

Sampling frames can be established to permit studies of rare exposures that may be missed in case–control studies. The quality of the study depends on the source of the cohort, completeness of participation, completeness of follow-up, and the accuracy of the measurements of risk and outcomes. Although cohort studies have many design strengths, they are costly and require large numbers of participants and long periods of observation. For rare diseases, they may be very inefficient as a result of the sample size requirements. The Framingham Heart Study is an example of a population-based cohort study that has enriched our understanding of risk factors for heart disease and has contributed clinically useful methods for predicting heart disease risk [35].

Two special types of cohort studies are the natural history study and the cross-sectional study. In the first, people with the disease are selected for study in order to determine the long-term sequelae and their risk factors, e.g., much has been learned about preventing diabetic retinopathy through a cohort study of people diagnosed with type 1 and type 2 diabetes [36,37]. Unlike a traditional cohort study, the Wisconsin Epidemiologic Study of Diabetic Retinopathy included only people who all had a diagnosis of diabetes at the time of enrollment [36,37]. Participants were followed with periodic eye examinations to determine the development of retinopathy and, more specifically, of proliferative retinopathy, the major vision-threatening endpoint.

In cross-sectional cohort studies, the entire target group or population is examined to determine the prevalence of the disease and, similar to case–control studies, comparisons are made between those with and without the disease to identify potential risk factors. Usually, disease-free participants are followed with periodic reexaminations to determine the incidence of disease. Cross-sectional studies can generate many useful insights while follow-up time is being accrued to check the consistency of the initial findings with longitudinal data.

Clinical Trials

The previously described study designs are classified as observational epidemiology. Experimental epidemiologic study designs include randomized clinical trials and community-based trials. In either design, the investigator controls the exposure or intervention by assigning eligible individuals or groups into exposure/treatment or placebo/usual care groups. Trials may be aimed at primary prevention (intervening before the disease develops to reduce risk), secondary prevention (treating and curing the disease once it has occurred), or tertiary prevention (reducing subsequent morbidity associated with having the disorder) [34]. Participants for randomized clinical trials may be recruited from hospitals, clinics, volunteers, or population-based sampling frames, whereas in community-based trials similar towns or regions may be allocated to the treatment arms. Important features of well-designed trials are the methods used to ensure random assignment to the various treatment options, the methods used to mask the participants (and investigators in a double-blind or doubly masked trial) to the treatment assignment, the methods used to determine compliance with the protocol (pill counts, laboratory measures of medication metabolites, etc.), and the standardized follow-up, the completeness of the follow-up, and the length of follow-up.

Measuring Risk

Prevalence and incidence are the basic measures of disease burden in epidemiologic studies. The *prevalence rate*, the percentage of a population with the disease at a point (or during a short interval) in time, provides a measure of how many people have the disease [34]. This measure can be used to predict health service needs and the relative importance of a disease. However, it depends on the duration of the disease as well as its incidence, and so may underestimate the burden if mortality is high.

The *incidence rate* is a measure of the risk of developing a disease during a specified time. It is defined as the number of new cases occurring in a population during a specified period of time divided by the number of people at risk during that time interval [34]. It is useful for projecting how many new cases will need health care services in a period of time and for determining absolute risk. Incidence rates in those with and those without the exposure are used to calculate the *relative risk* associated with an exposure or other risk factor [34]. Only longitudinal cohort studies directly produce these estimates of risk. Case–control studies cannot measure the relative risk because disease incidence is not measured. They can be used to calculate the *odds ratio*, which is an estimate of the relative risk when certain assumptions are met. The odds ratio represents the likelihood of being exposed to the risk factor among cases compared with controls [34].

As outlined in Chapter 11, many statistical techniques are available to calculate relative risks and odds ratios and to determine their statistical significance. Most studies use methods such as logistic regression to adjust for the influence of other factors when focusing on the relationship between a particular factor and the likelihood of developing the disease. Measurement error, or

the inability to accurately and precisely assess exposure or the outcome, can result in misleading estimates of the association (either over- or underestimating the true risk). Small sample sizes can lead to statistically insignificant findings, and large sample sizes can make small, clinically insignificant effects statistically significant. Epidemiologists evaluate both the size of the odds ratio and the relative risk to understand the magnitude of the association, and they evaluate the confidence interval to judge the precision of that estimate.

It is also important to consider other explanations for the findings. Some misleading or spurious results may result from poorly constructed sampling frames, low participation rates, or other forms of selection bias that result in cases and controls differing in some important way or in a cohort that does not represent the general population.

An important source of error comes from the confounding effects of other factors. Epidemiologists recognize that apparent associations between a risk factor and a disease may be the result of the effects of another factor, called a confounder, e.g., a hypothetical association between coffee drinking and oral cancer may be found in a study. Unless the researcher has included cigarette smoking in the analytic model or verified that the coffee drinking–cancer association is similar for people who smoke and those who do not, the results may stem from an association between coffee drinking and cigarette smoking, i.e., if coffee drinkers are more likely to smoke than nondrinkers, and if smoking is associated with oral cancer, coffee drinkers might appear to have more oral cancers than nondrinkers when the true underlying etiologic factor is the exposure to tobacco-related carcinogens. Similarly, uncontrolled confounding may mask a real association.

When evaluating the literature, it is important to consider whether other factors that might be important in the etiologic pathway and those that might differ between exposed and unexposed participants, or cases and controls, have been measured and included in the analytic approach. Multivariate analytic techniques are important tools for assessing the effects of confounding if the investigator considered the possibility of confounding during the study design phase and obtained the necessary data. When interpreting the significance of the findings, it is important to remember Occam's razor—"the assumptions introduced to explain a thing must not be multiplied beyond necessity"—which teaches that the simplest explanation that fits the data is probably the best [34].

When is a Risk Factor an Etiologic Factor?

Epidemiology has been criticized for the confusing and conflicting results sometimes generated by epidemiologic studies [38]. This confusion is caused, in part, by the misleading lay press coverage of the findings reported in individual papers. Epidemiology teaches the careful consideration of the body of scientific evidence before assuming a cause-and-effect relationship between an "exposure" and a disease outcome. Before accepting the findings of a study, epidemiologists evaluate it for design flaws, adequate measurement of risk factors and outcomes, appropriateness of analyses, and the consideration of confounding effects. The next step is to place that report in perspective by considering the body of scientific evidence before accepting a causal link. The guidelines generally used to evaluate the evidence of causality stem from standards first formulated by Henle and Koch in the infectious disease arena and modified over time to broaden their applicability to chronic diseases [39,40]. The five areas to be considered are: consistency, strength, specificity, temporal relationship, and coherence. Systematically considering the evidence for each of these tenets can help to make sense of the enormous volume of literature.

First, one should evaluate whether the studies are consistent, i.e., has the same association been demonstrated in case–control studies, cohort studies, clinical trials? Has it been found in studies conducted in different populations or groups of subjects? Studies with strong designs and thorough analyses should be weighted more heavily than flawed studies.

Strength refers to the size of the association and the precision of its estimate. Published studies should demonstrate a similar effect size, with the effect large enough to be of clinical significance. Confidence intervals should be small enough to suggest a reasonable degree of certainty. Evidence of a dose–response relationship is an important aspect.

Specificity requires that the exposure be associated with only one disease. This condition is often not met because of systemic effects. Instead, it is likely that many exposures will have multiple adverse health effects if the exposure reaches a variety of target tissues, affects molecular structures, or is a heterogeneous exposure. If specificity of effect is demonstrated, it strengthens the evidence for a causal effect, but it should not be considered an essential condition.

A temporal relationship requires that there be evidence that the exposure precedes the development of the disease. As discussed earlier, this type of evidence requires data from longitudinal studies. This can be difficult to establish because of long latency periods, as is often seen with cancers. A long subclinical phase may make it difficult to establish the order of events as well. Diagnostically, we are used to thinking of diseases as present or absent. However, many conditions, such as hypertension, cataract, and diabetes, are measured on continuous scales and may represent a gradual decline in function. In these cases it may be difficult to establish the event order because of the arbitrary nature of clinically relevant cut points.

Assessing coherence, or biologic plausibility, asks the fundamental question: "Does the association make sense from what we already know about the basic biology of the organ system and the action of the agent? Is there a sound reason for thinking a link might exist?"

Most epidemiologists are extremely cautious about concluding that there is a causal link between an exposure and a disease. Yet concerns about public health sometimes require making policy before obtaining adequate scientific evidence. This can lead to changes in recommendations as new information comes in. The translation of epidemiologic evidence into clinical practice and public health policy remains a challenge that is complicated by today's hunger for health information. Clinicians must make difficult judgments when applying research findings to the care of individual patients.

Epidemiologic studies measure risk at the population level, not the individual level. Risk models may not be applicable to individuals in a given practice because they predict the average or typical experience. Clearly, there remains an important role for sound clinical judgment and experience in providing the best patient care.

Health Outcomes from an Epidemiologic Perspective

After the advent of antibiotics, there was a paradigm shift or transition period as investigators changed their focus from infectious disease to chronic disease. Some believe that another paradigm shift is occurring today as we become more concerned about the morbidity and quality-of-life costs of disease than mortality. The term "health outcomes" is used by researchers and policymakers in many contexts. From an epidemiologic point of view, health outcomes encompass all aspects of the disease burden from the cost in lost lives (mortality) to morbidity and the decreased quality of life that many disorders can cause. For epidemiologists, the focus remains on measuring the impact of disease at the population level.

Epidemiology has helped to advance our understanding of diseases through the application of standardized, objective measures of diseases and exposures. There has been an emphasis on replacing "soft" assessment techniques, such as self-reported or self-assessed measures, with objective or performance-based measures to reduce measurement variability and error. Recently there has been growing interest in considering the individual's perspective as a valid and important measure of health or disability, particularly in evaluating health care.

Clinicians have begun to include measures of treatment or care outcomes as a way to evaluate practice groups. In this context, the focus often becomes individual satisfaction with health status [41,42]. Although incorporating this aspect of disease burden may broaden our understanding of the total picture or cost of disease, there is a danger that such subjective measures will vary between people as a result of coping styles, willingness to complain, and competing illnesses

or social problems. There remains important methodological work to be done to fully understand the disparities between objective and subjective measures of health and to develop a comprehensive model for quantifying the total burden of disease in order to effectively allocate health care resources and implement prevention strategies.

Acknowledgment This research is supported by the Lew R. Wasserman Award from the Research to Prevent Blindness.

References

1. Lilienfeld DE, Stolley PD. *Foundations of Epidemiology*, 3rd edn. New York.: Oxford University Press, 1994.
2. Gordis L. *Epidemiology* Philadelphia: WB Saunders Co., 1996.
3. Mausner JS, Kramer S. *Mausner and Bahn Epidemiology – An Introductory Text*, 2nd edn. Philadelphia: WB Saunders Co., 1985.
4. Snow J. On the mode of communication of cholera. In: *Snow on Cholera*. New York: The Commonwealth Fund, 1936: 1–175.
5. Simpson D, Ball K. From observation to policy: Smoking. In: Marmot M, Elliott P, eds. *Coronary Heart Disease Epidemiology: from aetiology to public health*. New York: Oxford University Press, 1996: 451–62.
6. Rose G. *The Strategy of Preventive Medicine*. New York: Oxford University Press, 1992.
7. Oxman AD, Sackett DL, Guyatt GH, for the Evidence-Based Medicine Working Group. Users' guides to the medical literature. I. How to get started. *JAMA* 1993; **270**: 2093–5.
8. Guyatt GH, Sackett DL, Cook DJ, for the Evidence-Based Medicine Working Group. Users' guides to the medical literature. II. How to use an article about therapy or prevention. A. Are the results of the study valid? *JAMA* 1993; **270**: 2598–601.
9. Guyatt GH, Sackett DL, Cook DJ, for the Evidence-Based Medicine Working Group. Users' guides to the medical literature. II. How to use an article about therapy or prevention. B. What were the results and will they help me in caring for my patients? *JAMA* 1994; **271**: 59–63.
10. Jaeschke R, Guyatt G, Sackett DL, for the Evidence-Based Medicine Working Group. Users' guides to the medical literature. III. How to use an article about a diagnostic test. A. Are

the results of the study valid? *JAMA* 1994; **271**: 389–91.

11. Jaeschke R, Guyatt G, Sackett DL, for the Evidence-Based Medicine Working Group. Users' guides to the medical literature. III. How to use an article about a diagnostic test. B. What are the results and will they help me in caring for my patients? *JAMA* 1994; **271**: 703–7.

12. Levine M, Walter S, Lee H, Haines T, Holbrook A, Moyer V, for the Evidence-Based Medicine Working Group. Users' guides to the medical literature. IV. How to use an article about harm. *JAMA* 1994; **271**: 1615–19.

13. Laupacis A, Wells G, Richardson S, Tugwell P, for the Evidence-Based Medicine Working Group. Users' guides to the medical literature. V. How to use an article about prognosis. *JAMA* 1994; **272**: 234–7.

14. Oxman AD, Cook DJ, Guyatt GH, for the Evidence-Based Medicine Working Group. Users' guides to the medical literature. VI. How to use an overview. *JAMA* 1994; **272**: 1367–71.

15. Richardson WS, Detsky AS, for the Evidence-Based Medicine Working Group. Users' guides to the medical literature. VII. How to use a clinical decision analysis. A. Are the results of the study valid? *JAMA* 1995; **273**: 1292–5.

16. Richardson WS, Detsky AS, for the Evidence-Based Medicine Working Group. Users' guides to the medical literature. VII. How to use a clinical decision analysis. B. What are the results and will they help me in caring for my patients? *JAMA* 1995; **273**: 1610–13.

17. Hayward RSA, Wilson MC, Tunis SR, Bass EB, Guyatt G, for the Evidence-Based Medicine Working Group. Users' guides to the medical literature. VIII. How to use clinical practice guidelines. A. Are the recommendations valid? *JAMA* 1995; **274**: 570–4.

18. Wilson MC, Hayward RSA, Tunis SR, Bass EB, Guyatt G, for the Evidence-Based Medicine Working Group. Users' guides to the medical literature. VIII. How to use clinical practice guidelines. B. What are the recommendations and will they help you in caring for your patients? *JAMA* 1995; **274**: 1630–2.

19. Guyatt GH, Sackett DL, Sinclair JC, Hayward R, Cook DJ, Cook RJ, for the Evidence-Based Medicine Working Group. Users' guides to the medical literature. IX. A method for grading health care recommendations. *JAMA* 1995; **274**: 1800–4.

20. Naylor CD, Guyatt GH, for the Evidence-Based Medicine Working Group. Users' guides to the medical literature. X. How to use an article reporting variations in the outcomes of health services. *JAMA* 1996; **275**: 554–8.

21. Naylor CD, Guyatt GH, for the Evidence-Based Medicine Working Group. Users' guides to the medical literature. XI. How to use an article about a clinical utilization review. *JAMA* 1996; **275**: 1435–9.

22. Guyatt GH, Naylor CD, Juniper E, Heyland DK, Jaeschke R, Cook DJ, for the Evidence-Based Medicine Working Group. Users' guides to the medical literature. XII. How to use articles about health-related quality of life. *JAMA* 1997; **277**: 1232–7.

23. Drummond MF, Richardson WS, O'Brien BJ, Levine M, Heyland D, for the Evidence-Based Medicine Working Group. User's guides to the medical literature. XIII. How to use an article on economic analysis of clinical practice. A. Are the results of the study valid? *JAMA* 1997; **277**: 1552–7.

24. O'Brien BJ, Heyland D, Richardson WS, Levine M, Drummond MF, for the Evidence-Based Medicine Working Group. User's guides to the medical literature. XIII. How to use an article on economic analysis of clinical practice. B. What are the results and will they help me in caring for my patients? *JAMA* 1997; **277**: 1802–6.

25. Dans AL, Dans LF, Guyatt GH, Richardson S, for the Evidence-Based Medicine Working Group. Users' guides to the medical literature. XIV. How to decide on the applicability of clinical trial results to your patient. *JAMA* 1998; **279**: 545–9.

26. Richardson WS, Wilson MC, Guyatt GH, Cook DJ, Nishikawa J, for the Evidence-Based Medicine Working Group. Users' guides to the medical literature. XV. How to use an article about disease probability for differential diagnosis. *JAMA* 1999; **281**: 1214–19.

27. Guyatt GH, Sinclair J, Cook DJ, Glasziou P, for the Evidence-Based Medicine Working Group and the Cochrane Applicability Methods Working Group. Users' guides to the medical literature. XVI. How to use a treatment recommendation. *JAMA* 1999; **281**: 1836–43.

28. Barratt A, Irwig L, Glasziou P *et al.*, for the Evidence-Based Medicine Working Group. Users' guides to the medical literature XVII. How to use guidelines and recommendations about screening. *JAMA* 1999; **281**: 2029–34.

29. Randolph AG, Haynes RB, Wyatt JC, Cook DJ, Guyatt GH. Users' guides to the medical literature XVIII. How to use an article evaluating the clinical impact of a computer-based clinical decision support system. *JAMA* 1999; **282**: 67–74.

30. Bucher HC, Guyatt GH, Cook DJ, Holbrook A, McAlister FA, for the Evidence-Based Medicine Working Group. Users' guides to the medical literature XIX. Applying clinical trial results. A. How to use an article measuring the effect of an intervention on surrogate end points. *JAMA* 1999; **282**: 771–8.

31. McAlister FA, Laupacis A, Wells GA, Sackett DL, for the Evidence-Based Medicine Working Group. Users' guides to the medical literature XIX. Applying clinical trial results. B. Guidelines for determining whether a drug is exerting (more than) a class effect. *JAMA* 1999; **282**: 1371–7.

32. Carroll KK. Experimental evidence of dietary factors and hormone-dependent cancers. *Cancer Res* 1975; **35**: 3374–83.

33. Lawry EY, Mann GV, Peterson A, Wysocki AP, O'Connell R, Stare FJ. Cholesterol and β-lipoproteins in the serum of Americans: well persons and those without coronary heart disease. *Am J Med* 1957; **22**: 605–23.

34. Last JM. *A Dictionary of Epidemiology*, 2nd edn. New York: Oxford University Press, 1988.

35. Kannel WB. The Framingham experience. In: Marmot M, Elliott P, eds. *Coronary Heart Disease Epidemiology: from Aetiology to Public Health*. New York: Oxford University Press, 1996: 67–82.

36. Klein R, Klein BEK, Moss SE, Cruickshanks KJ. The Wisconsin Epidemiologic Study of Diabetic Retinopathy. XVII. The 14-year incidence and progression of diabetic retinopathy and associated risk factors in Type 1 diabetes. *Ophthalmology* 1998; **105**: 1801–15.

37. Klein R, Klein BEK. Vision disorders in diabetes. In: Harris MI, Cowie CC, Stern MP, Boyko EJ, Reiber GE, Bennett PH, eds. *Diabetes in America*, 2nd edn. Bethesda: US Public Health Service, NIH-NIDDK Publication no. 95–1468, 1995: 293–338.

38. Taubes G. Epidemiology faces its limits. *Science* 1995; **269**: 164–9.

39. Evans AS. Causation and disease: a chronological journey. Thomas Parran Lecture. *Am J Epidemiol* 1995; **142**: 1126–35.

40. Susser M. What is a cause and how do we know one? A grammar for pragmatic epidemiology. *Am J Epidemiol* 1991; **133**: 635–48.

41. Ware J, Snow K, Kosinski M, Gandek B. *SF-36 Health Survey Manual and Interpretation Guide*. Boston: The Health Institute, New England Medical Center, 1993.

42. Fryback DG, Dasbach EJ, Klein R *et al.* The Beaver Dam health outcomes study. Initial Catalog Health-State Quality Factors. *Med Decis Making* 1993; **13**: 89–102.

13

Health Law

Burton Wagner

This chapter provides a basic overview of legal issues that may affect a physician's practice in a managed-care relationship, and it will help you to understand the lawyer's perspective of that practice. Although the physician/patient relationship is at the heart of providing care, the relationship is both surrounded and influenced by legal concepts and requirements. The role of the law is often confusing and appears counterproductive. However, from a physician's point of view, understanding certain basic legal issues is essential to the successful practice of medicine.

Contracts

Contracts are pertinent to the physician–patient relationship and are especially important in managed-care organizational situations. The legal theory of contract is founded on the concept of mutual assent, i.e., that both parties know and understand the bargain they are making. Contract law is a basic concept within the law, and the elements of a contract are well settled. For there to be a valid contract, there must be an offer from one party to the other, an acceptance, and an exchange of consideration. Consideration may be a thing, such as money, or an action, such as performing a service, or a promise to do something in the future. In the health care setting, consideration is usually an exchange of money for the provision of medical services. Although many contracts are enforceable even if they are not in writing, contracts should be written to confirm the intent of the parties, to avoid mistakes, and to provide evidence at a future time.

As contracts depend on mutual assent and agreement, going to the contract for legal enforcement is usually a last resort. However, legal enforcement is necessary when one party does not live up to the terms of the contract. In this situation, a clear written expression of the terms is essential for enforcement. Usually, the parties seeking enforcement must have fulfilled their part of the agreement and have 'clean hands.' In the health care context, a disparity of power or knowledge between the parties can make contracts unenforceable because of *unconscionability*. This means that the contract terms are so unreasonably favorable to one party that the other party lacks a meaningful choice. In health care, contracts can be found to be unconscionable because of the timing of a contract or because specific terms relieve the more powerful contracting party of liability, e.g., if a practitioner refuses to serve a patient in dire need without a contract that limits liability or charges excessive fees, enforcement of that contract could be challenged because the terms may be regarded as unconscionable.

Some contracts are void and not enforceable because they violate public policy. Contracts that violate the Medicaid and Medicare fraud and abuse laws by requiring referrals or kickbacks will not be enforced by the courts, because they violate public policy. In a Texas case, *Polk County v Peters*, 800 F. Supp. 1451 (E.D. Texas 1992), the US District Court in Texas held that a physician recruitment agreement that required the physician to refer patients to the hospital and absent exceptional circumstances violated the federal fraud and abuse statute. The agreement was illegal and therefore void and not enforceable.

Contracts are essential in the physician–patient relationship, the facility–patient relationship, and the facility or managed care–physician relationship.

Torts

Torts are civil wrongs. The law classifies torts as intentional or unintentional, normally referred to as negligence. To prosecute a negligence case, one must show that there was a duty, a breach of that duty, harm, and a causal connection between the breach of duty and the harm.

A key issue in dealing with torts involving physicians in managed-care settings is the allocation of responsibility. In a typical employment setting, the concept of respondeat superior—"let the master answer"—generally applies. In the case of a resident within a hospital or a staff model health maintenance organization (HMO), this legal concept and the allocation of responsibility are relatively straightforward. However, in most managed-care organizations, the physician is an independent contractor. This relationship is similar to that of the independent physician who has clinical privileges at a hospital but is not employed by the hospital. In these cases, the physician retains professional control of the services to be provided and how they are performed. Therefore, the allocation of responsibility between the organization or facility and the physician becomes an issue.

Until recently, managed-care organizations have been able to insulate themselves from the negligent actions of providers. Several early cases* affirmed the specific obligation of the provider to do what is needed and relieved the managed-care organizations of responsibility. More recent cases have focused on policies, procedures, and limitations required by the managed-care organizations being a basis for liability equal to or greater than that of the physician. In *Petrovich v Share Health Plan of Illinois, Inc.*, 719 NE. 2d 756, 764 (Ill. 1999), the court concluded that:

[t]he principle that organizations are accountable for their tortious actions and those of their agents is fundamental to our justice system. There is no exception to this principle for HMOs. To the extent that HMOs are profit-making entities, accountability is also needed to counterbalance the inherent drive to achieve a larger and ever-increasing profit margin.

The allocation of responsibility when a patient is injured is an important issue in tort/negligence law. At present, this is a very unsettled area, and it will continue to change as managed-care organizations become more selective in regard to who may provide services under their auspices. Just as hospitals were required to assume responsibility for unfortunate events, even when they involved physician error, so will managed-care organizations be responsible for events when their policies and procedures and the actions of their employees are contributing factors.

Patient Information

Patient information is a critical element in providing care and treatment. How this information is obtained, protected, and disclosed affects the patient–doctor relationship. The following are some basic concepts and guidelines useful in working with patient information.

The patient record is a compilation of information related to the care and treatment of a particular patient. This information may be obtained directly from the patient in the form of historical information or from laboratory or other diagnostic tests performed on the patient. Information that is unrelated to the care and treatment of the patient should not be maintained in the patient's record.

As the patient record concerns the care and treatment of an individual, the custodian of that record is responsible for the entries made into the record, the maintenance of the record, and the protection of the record. Usually, entries in a patient record are made by the physician, but other health care providers working under the physician's direction can make entries and record laboratory and diagnostic test data. Protection

* *Wickline v State* 727 P.2d 753 (Cal. 1986); *Wilson v Blue Cross of So. Cal.*, 222 Cal. App. 3d 660, 271 Cal. Rptr. 876 (Cal. Ct. App. 1990).

of the record itself, as well as protection of the confidential information contained within it, is the responsibility of the custodian. Therefore, records should be properly secured and maintained at all times.

The patient's record, in addition to providing information for patient care, is also a formal legal document. As such, the information contained in the document is often the basis for inferring whether or not a procedure was performed, whether negligence was committed, and whether all appropriate consents were obtained. An incomplete or inaccurate patient care record is not only a hindrance to those intending to provide care, but it is harmful in a legal sense.

There are no strict guidelines for how long any health care record should be maintained. Although regulations such as those for Medicare specify a minimum time for retention of records (5 years), the record custodian should make decisions on retention based on sound medical judgment, facility policies, and applicable state and/or federal regulations. A simple guideline is to retain records of patients who have been discharged for a time that is equal to the minimum statute of limitations for the purposes of bringing a lawsuit.

Most of the information in a patient health care record is obtained directly from the patient. As a result of the patient–provider relationship, patients expect any information that they provide to be necessary for their care and treatment, and they expect providers to hold this information in confidence. This expectation of confidentiality has both legal and ethical origins. The ethical origin dates back to the Hippocratic Oath. The legal origin is based primarily in case law and is derived from issues relating to breach of privacy and professional misconduct. Confidentiality is also protected by statute. Most state statutes relating to health care records assert that the patient information in a health care record is confidential and may not be disclosed. These statutes often include penalties for violation.

Notwithstanding the obligation of the health care provider to protect patient information, most state statutes specifically authorize the release of some or all of the information for certain designated purposes: to other health care providers who need the information, to researchers, to pub-

lic health officers, for purposes of billing and collection, and for similar reasons.

Information about the patient may, of course, be released to anyone, including the patient, with the informed consent of the patient. Federal and state regulations usually specify how and to whom information may be released with the consent of the patient.

Although confidentiality and the concept of physician–patient privilege are related, they are distinct concepts. Although we usually refer to information as privileged, what is usually meant is that the information is confidential and is intended to be protected by the physician. Privilege, on the other hand, addresses situations where a physician may not be compelled to testify in a legal proceeding. If a privilege exists, it exists because the state has enacted a statute to protect information derived from a bona fide physician–patient relationship. Even statutory privileges often have exceptions, e.g., information relating to child abuse and neglect, or information about the patient's condition when it is the subject of a lawsuit or when there is a court-ordered examination. The privilege belongs to the patient. A patient may waive the privilege, in which case the physician can testify about information obtained in the care and treatment of that person.

Two areas relating to patient confidentiality are of particular concern. First, most states have a specific statutory provision relating to the release of information about HIV test results and the diagnosis of AIDS. Although greater confidentiality protections are usually afforded to this problem, the limitations differ so widely that it is important to determine what your state requires. The second area of concern relates to alcohol and other substance abuse records. Special federal rules apply to information about patients who are being treated or have been treated for substance abuse. These protective regulations are more specific and extensive than are state regulations. The federal regulations supersede any lesser state requirement (42 C.F.R. Pt 2).

There may be times when patient-related information must be disclosed to protect the public's health or the health and safety of a particular person. Most health care record statutes provide exceptions to the general duty of confidentiality where the public's health is concerned. Generally, these statutes permit the release of information to the public health officer. Again, these rules differ state-by-state, so you must know the requirements for your state, e.g., most states require you to report communicable diseases, but as in the case of HIV, the kind of report may be limited.

There is also a growing body of cases that assert an obligation to disclose patient-care information to a person who is at risk. The leading case in this area is *Tarasoff v Regents of the University of California*, 17 Cal. 3d 425, 131 Cal. Rptr. 14, 551 P. 2d 334 (Cal. 1976). In that case, the patient made a believable threat to kill a young woman, and the California Supreme Court determined that the patient's psychiatrist should have either warned the victim or advised others able to warn the victim of the danger from this particular patient. Although not all states have adopted the *Tarasoff* doctrine, the duty to warn when there is a readily identifiable victim should be taken very seriously.

Health care providers owe a duty of confidentiality to their patients, because of the special relationship that exists and the expectations of the patient. The health care provider is obligated to obtain information from the patient, maintain and protect that information, and disclose that information only under prescribed circumstances. The duty of confidentiality is critical to the physician–patient relationship.

Two provisions of the Health Insurance Portability and Accountability Act of 1996 relate to standards for electronic transmission of health care data (45 C.F.R. Part 162) and patient privacy (45 C.F.R. Parts 160 and 164). Regulations pertaining to both these areas were published in 2000. The regulations affecting Electronic Transactions and Code Sets were published in 65 Fed. Reg., p. 5,031 (August 17, 2000). The standards for Privacy of Individually Identifiable Information were published in 65 Fed. Reg., p. 82,462 (December 28, 2000).

Patient Consent

The right of a patient to participate in decisions about his or her care is, in today's health care environment, a given. The regulatory agencies, the providers of care, and the patients all agree that it is appropriate for the patient to be directly involved in care decisions. This is evidenced by state statutes and various patients' bills of rights promulgated by governmental and private agencies.

To enable a patient to participate in his or her own decisions, enough information must be provided so that participation can be informed. In a very general sense, this requires that the patient be made aware of the inherent risks related to the test, procedure, or therapy to be performed, the benefits to be derived, and whether there are any alternatives to achieving the same result. Although there is a general consensus on this aspect of informed consent, there is no consensus on most other aspects.

First, there are differing views in regard to whether an informed consent must be in writing, on a particular form, and obtained by or witnessed by a particular person. An informed consent need not be in writing in order to be valid. However, from a legal perspective, the written document provides evidence of the information provided, the date, the parties involved, etc. As a document to be used to recollect events of the past, the written informed consent is an excellent tool. An unwritten consent may also be valid, but proof of such consent is much more difficult.

A second issue related to the consent document is the amount and type of information to be provided. Typically, a consent form for a particular procedure/test/examination includes certain basic elements and allows space for the person obtaining the consent to include specific information. Such a form is much preferred over a preprinted form that is expected to address all possible alternatives. In the end, however, negligence in the performance of the procedure will not be saved by a valid written informed consent. On the other hand, a well-executed informed consent will lessen the likelihood of a negligence action, based not on a bad procedure but on a bad informed consent.

There are two approaches to the question of how much and what kind of information must be included in the informed consent form. One is called the professional standard and the other the material risk standard. States that follow the professional standard generally require that the information provided to a patient conform to the information that a "reasonable" practitioner in that community would provide to a patient in order to ensure informed consent. Typically, in professional standards situations, proof of what a reasonable physician would provide requires direct testimony, primarily from other physicians or experts.

The other approach is the material risk standard or the reasonable patient standard. In states that have adopted this approach, the information to be provided must be relevant to the patient's decision-making process. This means that the information must be tailored to the ability of the patient to make a decision, e.g., the amount of information provided to a health professional, such as a nurse, would likely differ from the information provided to a person with a high school education not working in health care. Similarly, information that is critical to the patient's ability to make a decision—i.e., information that is *material*—must be provided in order for consent to be informed. Whether such information is material, and is appropriate, does not require "expert" testimony. Lay people can determine whether the information would be understood and was critical to a reasonable patient.*

Whether the professional standard or the material risk standard is applied, any action based on the failure to provide sufficient information must show that the failure to provide the necessary information was directly related to the unfortunate result. Failure to provide information about a risk that never occurs, or one that would not have deterred the patient from proceeding anyway, is not a basis for a finding of negligence against the physician.

The right of a patient to participate in the decision-making process includes the right of the patient to reject his or her participation. The general rule in this area is that a competent adult may

refuse health care and treatment services even if that refusal would hasten or cause death.[†] This concept has also been extended to people who are unable to actively participate in the decision-making process when there is enough evidence that the individual would have made the proposed decision if he or she was able to do so.

Unfortunately, in those cases where an individual has not declared his or her intent and becomes incompetent before expressing such an intent, there may be very little that the health care provider can do other than continuing to maintain the status quo or providing additional care.

To enable people to have a way to direct their health care when they are incapable of making decisions, the federal government and most states have enacted advance directive provisions. The Federal Patient Self-Determination Act; 42 U.S.C. § 1395CC (1990); Omnibus Budget Reconciliation Act of 1990, Pub. no. 101–508 §§ 4206, 4751 requires health care providers to advise people of their right to make such advance directives. This federal law, however, does not prescribe the format, nor does it require uniformity between states. The states themselves have enacted various forms of advance directives, usually taking the form of a living will—a declaration by the patient regarding care and treatment at a point where he or she is unable to participate in the process—or a power of attorney or agent document, which permits a third party to make decisions on behalf of a person who is unable to make those decisions. Unfortunately, because of the lack of uniformity throughout the US, it is essential for you, as a health care provider, to confirm whether your state has specific regulations and whether the state provides protection if you act pursuant to the advanced directive.

Fraud and Abuse

Fraud and abuse are probably the last issue that any physician wishes to know about. Unfortunately, understanding what is meant by fraud and abuse and how to comply with the various

---

* In *Canterbury v Spence*, 150 DC App. 263, 464 F.2d 772, *cert. denied* 409 U.S. 1064 (1972), the court stated that a risk is material "when a reasonable person, in what the physician knows or should know to be the patient's position, would be likely to attach significance to the risk or cluster of risks in deciding whether or not to forgo the proposed therapy".

[†] In *Cruzan v Director, Mo. Dept. of Health*, 497 U.S. 261 (1990) the Supreme Court stated that "A competent person has a liberty interest under the Due Process Clause in refusing unwanted medical treatment".

requirements related to it is an essential component of every physician's practice. The general reference to fraud and abuse arises from the Social Security Act, § 1128(b). These provisions in the Social Security Act are not new. They originated shortly after the introduction of Medicaid and Medicare. Since that time, this portion of the act has been modified several times to strengthen it. This statute is a criminal statute, i.e., violation carries with it the possibility of a fine and/or imprisonment. As a result of the criminal nature of fraud and abuse law, one should be especially careful to comply.

The statute is divided into two major sections. The first prohibits false claims regarding seeking or obtaining benefits, false statements regarding institutional qualifications and provider status, charging for or receiving payments from eligible recipients or others that exceed the rates approved by the programs, and limitations on violating assignments. The second section prohibits kickbacks and rebates. The provisions of this section prohibit both the knowing and willful solicitation or receipt, and the payment of any remuneration (including any kickback, bribe, or rebate) directly or indirectly, in cash or in kind, in return for or in order to induce:

> The referral of an individual to a provider for the furnishing of, or arranging for the furnishing of, any item or service, or ... the purchase, lease, order, arrangement or recommendation to purchase, lease or order of any good, facility, service or item for which payment may be made in whole or in part under a Federal health care program.

The prohibition on kickbacks and rebates is two-pronged. The statute not only prohibits knowingly and willfully accepting a kickback or rebate for providing a patient referral, but also for the offering or giving of a kickback or rebate. Therefore, not only are health-care services provided by health care providers directly implicated by this statute, but also the acceptance of goods or services that are used by health care providers. Violation of either section of the statute is punishable by up to 5 years in prison and/or fines of up to $25,000. In addition, the Medicare program has the authority to exclude violators from continued participation.

Those who enforce this statute look at fraud and abuse from a perspective that may differ from what is common in the business world. In the context of the Medicaid and Medicare programs, fraud is defined as:

> An intentional deception or misrepresentation made by a person with the knowledge that the deception could result in some unauthorized benefit to himself or some other person. It includes any act that constitutes fraud under application federal or state law. (42 C.F.R. 455)

Abuse is defined as:

> Provider practices that are inconsistent with sound fiscal, business, or medical practices, and result in an unnecessary cost to the Medicaid program, or in reimbursement for services that are not medically necessary or that fail to meet professionally recognized standards for health care. It also includes recipient practices that result in unnecessary cost of the Medicaid program. (42 C.F.R. 455)

Briefly, any practice that the provider knows is inappropriate and is intended to gain something from the program is actionable as fraud. Any practice that encourages unnecessary utilization or has the potential to increase cost to the program or ties remuneration to referrals or volume of a business is considered abusive. If there are other legitimate health care and/or business reasons for the practice, these reasons may mitigate.

As a result of the breadth of the fraud and abuse statutes, Congress has tried to provide guidance to the provider community. This guidance has taken various forms. Initially, Congress directed the Department of Health and Human Services to develop "safe harbors" intended to clarify the anti-kickback provisions.*

---

* The original 11 safe harbors were published in 1991 Fed. Regulation Vol. 56, no. 145, p. 35984, July 29, 1991 and included the following: (1) investment interests, (2) space rental, (3) equipment rental, (4) personal services and management contracts, (5) sale of a practice, (6) referral services, (7) warranties, (8) employees, (9) discounts, (10) good purchasing organizations, (11) waiver of coinsurance and deductibles.

Several of the initial safe harbors paralleled exceptions that were already in the fraud and abuse statute, specifically certain discounts, payments to employees, and payments made by vendors to group purchasing organizations. Since that time, Congress has added additional safe harbors, the latest in November 1999.*†

Although the safe harbors are intended to provide guidance to focus the practices of physicians, their scope is considered so narrow that the vast majority of health care practices fall beyond the "bright line" defined by the safe harbors. None the less, they do provide some guidance and direction.

In addition to the Medicare and Medicaid fraud and abuse provisions, Congress also enacted what has come to be known as the Stark Law [42 U.S.C. § 1345(nn)]. The Stark Law, initially passed in 1989 and expanded in January 1995, prohibits physicians from owning an interest in various entities to which the physician may make a referral. The Stark Law was initially directed at ownership interests in clinical laboratory services, but it was expanded in 1995 to include the following:

1. Physical therapy
2. Occupational therapy
3. Radiology or other diagnostic services
4. Radiation therapy
5. Durable medical equipment
6. Parenteral and enteral nutritional nutrients, supplies and equipment
7. Prosthetics, and orthotic and prosthetic devices
8. Home health services
9. Outpatient prescription drug services
10. Inpatient and outpatient hospital services.

---

* The 1992 interim safe harbors finalized in 1996 in Fed. Reg. Vol. 61, no. 17, Thursday, January 25, 1996, p. 2122 included: (1) increase coverage, reduce costs or premiums offered by a health plan, (2) price reductions offered to health plans. 42 C.F.R. 1001.
† The 1999 additional safe harbors published in 64 Fed. Reg. 63518 (to be codified in 42 C.F.R. 1001) included: (1) investment interests in underserved areas, (2) investment interests in ambulatory surgery centers, (3) investment interests in group practices, (4) practitioner recruitment, (5) obstetrical malpractice subsidies, (6) referral agreements for specialty services, (7) cooperative hospital service organizations, (8) share risks.

Regulations applicable to the Stark designated health services were published in 66 Fed. Reg., p. 856 (January 4, 2001).

There are, of course, exceptions for physicians primarily in group practices or for physicians who invest in large, publicly traded organizations that happen to provide any of the included services. As in the case of the fraud and abuse provisions, guidance has been limited. Moreover, the government enforcers view the Stark Law and the fraud and abuse laws as significantly different. When the Department of Health and Human Services published its most recent rules and regulations relating to fraud and abuse, it made the following comment:

> The Stark Law is a civil statute that generally (i) prohibits physicians from making referrals for clinical laboratory or other designated health services to entities in which the physicians have ownership or other financial interests and (ii) prohibits entities from presenting or causing to be presented claims or bills to any individual, third-party payor, where other entity for designated health services furnish pursuant to a prohibited referral. The antikickback statute, on the other hand, is a criminal statute that prohibits the knowing and willful offer, payment, solicitation, or receipt of the remuneration to induce federal health care program business. A transaction must fall entirely within an exception to be lawful under the Stark Law. The antikickback statute, on the other hand, establishes an intent based criminal prohibition with optional statutory and regulatory "safe harbors" that do not purport to define the full range of lawful activity. (Fed. Reg. Vol. 64, no. 223, Friday, November 19, 1999, p. 63518)

As a result of the difference in approach and interpretation, case law under the fraud-and-abuse statute has had a significant role in interpreting the law. The initial case defining what was intended under the fraud-and-abuse statute is *United States v Greber*, 760 F.2d 68 (3rd Cir. 1985), *cert. denied* 474 US. 988 (1985). In that case, the court held that, if a payment is intended to "induce" a physician to use a particular service, the fraud-and-abuse statute is violated even if the payments are also intended to compensate for other professional services. This concept of inducement has been the primary thrust of enforcement under the fraud-and-abuse statutes. However, in 1995 the court in the case of *Hanlester Network v Shalala*, 51 F.3d 1390 (9th Cir. 1995), held that, because the fraud-and-abuse statute is a criminal statute, it requires knowing and willful intent to violate the statute. The person in violation must know that the intended act is wrong and still commit it.

Although the fraud-and-abuse laws have generally been applied to governmental programs, the Health Insurance Portability and Accountability Act of 1996* (HIPPA) created a new federal law. HIPPA makes it a federal crime to perpetrate a fraud not only on government programs, but on any health benefit program. In addition, the HIPA law created a national fraud data collection program intended to gather a database of adverse actions taken against health

care providers and suppliers, which may indicate fraud.

Conclusion

Legal issues arise in many health care contexts. The involvement of physicians in managed care complicate many basic health law interactions because of the involvement of the managed-care entity. Allocating responsibility for care decisions affects negligence and the contractual responsibilities between the physician and patient, the physician and managed-care entity, and the patient and managed-care entity. Medical record entries, ownership, and requirements for disclosure often result in competing issues and values. Practices that are considered to be routine, or even customary, may result in violation of the fraud-and-abuse laws, especially with overlapping and undefined responsibilities for purchases, referrals, etc. The overlay of a managed-care relationship with a physician's practice simply raises more legal issues and requires further analysis.

---

* Publ. L. no. 104–191, 110 Stat. 1936 (codified as amended in scattered sections of 42 U.S.C.).

14

Medical Ethics

Daniel M. Albert

Introduction

What is Medical Ethics?

Medical ethics refers to the collective values, principles, and methods that determine the resolution of moral dilemmas in health care. Medical ethics has been inevitably preoccupied with the conflicting dictates of altruism and self-interest.

The Nature of Medical Ethics

Physicians have a long tradition of ethical discourse that goes back to the ancient Greeks. Traditional medical ethics are viewed within the profession as embodying a lofty moral philosophy. Contemporary bioethicists, however, claim that physicians' ethics are remarkably insular and self-serving [1,2].

Until the 1960s, physicians developed and maintained the ethical principles followed in health and medicine. The classic corpus of medical ethics focused on physicians' rights and responsibilities—how they should behave toward their patients and interact with their colleagues [3]. Contemporary bioethicists hold that traditional medical ethics has limited relevance to the complex and unresolved ethical problems created by the advances of medical and scientific technology, socioeconomic factors, and social change that we face today.

For physicians who seek to understand and deal with issues of medical ethics, the first key is history, and specifically a knowledge of the long tradition of medical ethics in Western culture. The manner in which health services in the US are now organized and carried out arose directly out of the history and culture of the medical profes-

sion [4]. Even doctors who ignore or denigrate history still have its events and traditions playing a central role in how they practice medicine.

The second key to understanding and dealing with the modern problems of medical ethics is a knowledge of philosophy. Philosophy is preoccupied with meaning and value, with raising the normative questions and seeking the preferred ends. Albert Jonsen, Professor of Medical History and Ethics at the University of Washington, points out that physicians can think and talk and perform excellent science and competent clinical medicine without hearing a word of philosophy. Yet when dealing with medical ethics—and trying to understand what is happening, or what has gone wrong, or what ought to be done—philosophical principles are constantly at work [5].

The Influence of Modern Medical Practice on Medical Ethics

Since 1960, medical issues have become embedded in the social and political fabric of the country. The proliferation of medical knowledge and advances in technology have revolutionized both the effectiveness and the cost of medicine. The health care system has been modified to respond to federal and state financing and market forces. There has been rapid growth of managed care, initiation of vast public health programs, growth of the for-profit nursing home industry, growth of investor-owned hospital chains, and mergers and affiliations in the not-for-profit sector. There is now increased social democracy, which has led to an emphasis on patients' rights and an abhorrence of paternalism. Ethical problems in patient research, the selection of patients for organ transplantation, neonatal care, genetic therapy, the use of fetal tissues, and unwanted prolongation of life have been in the limelight. These changes have resulted in the erosion of medicine's autonomy and independence as a profession. Physicians have seen nonphysicians take an ever-increasing role in decision-making and in the intellectual discourse about medical ethics.

All of this has had a profound impact on the ethical decisions of physicians. In this chapter we examine how we arrived at this point and then consider how physicians can meet the new challenges.

History of Medical Ethics
The Code of Hammurabi

A good starting point for a review of the origins of Western medical ethics is the Hammurabi Code (about 2000 BC). Our knowledge of this important commentary on Babylonian medicine is derived from a black diorite block, eight feet high, containing 2540 lines of writing, and decorated with the figure of the king receiving a law from the Sun God. Carved into this stone was a body of laws many of which relate to the medical profession. Copies of this monument were set up in Babylon "in order that anyone oppressed or injured, who had a tale of woe to tell, might come and stand before his image, that of a king of righteousness, and there be the priceless orders of the King, and from the written monument solve his problem" [6]. Encoded among these laws were the following [6]:

> If a doctor has treated a man for a severe wound with a bronze lancet and has cured the man, or has opened an abscess of the eye for a man with the bronze lancet and has cured the eye of the man, he shall take 10 shekels of silver. (Paragraph 215)

> If a doctor has treated a man for a severe wound with a lancet of bronze and has caused the man to die, or has opened an abscess of the eye for a man and has caused the loss of a man's eye, one shall cut off his hands. (Paragraph 218)

This may be the first recognition of patients' rights and physicians' rights.

Greek Medicine—First Do No Harm

Hippocrates: The Man and His Writings

The tradition of medical ethics that Western physicians share goes back to Hippocrates and the ancient Greeks. Hippocrates (about 460–375 BC) is a shadowy figure about whom we have little firsthand knowledge. Aristotle, who was the son of a physician and whose own philosophical writings are relevant to medicine, referred to him as "the Great Hippocrates," but we know little about his life. Many writings have been attributed to Hippocrates, but it is difficult to determine which are really the work of the Father of Medicine himself. As with the books of the Bible, different Hippocratic writings seem to have been composed by different scribes at different times, setting down a permanent record of what had previously been an oral tradition of belief and practice [7]. A central theme of Hippocratic medicine was the recognition that: "All disease has a nature and arises from a natural cause, and is capable of cure" [8]. These writings are the cornerstone of modern Western medicine.

According to Sir William Osler (1849–1919), two particular features of the Hippocratic writings have influenced the evolution of medical ethics. The first of these is the note of humanity. This can be seen in the Hippocratic phrase: "Where there is love of humanity, there will be a love of the profession". The second feature is the directness with which Hippocrates addressed medical and ethical issues. Osler notes: "Everywhere one finds a strong clear common sense, which refused to be entangled either in theology or in philosophical speculation" [9].

The Oath of Hippocrates

This was probably written between 450 and 370 BC, and it establishes a code of ethics separate from the laws of the state. It consists of both a pledge to uphold a high ethical standard of practice and an indenture in which the candidate agrees to share the earnings produced with the teacher, to help the teacher financially when necessary, and to teach student signatories of the

Oath in the manner that one would teach one's own child [10]. The physician is to help the sick and respect the art of medicine and, in addition, to refrain from poisoning, gossip, and sexual misconduct. There is a clear implication that the healer who practices ethically will have a return on his moral investment. Even in ancient times it was recognized that good ethics was good business. It is clearly indicated that adherence to medical ethics differentiates the good healer from the bad.

Galen

Hippocrates' medical ethics were emphasized by Galen (AD 131–201), who was the greatest Greek physician after Hippocrates. He also stressed the close association between morality and technical competence. Galen's writings exerted a tremendous influence up to the time of Vesalius in the sixteenth century, and during this period his views on anatomy, physiology, disease, and medical ethics were regarded as definitive [11].

The Late Middle Ages Through the Fifteenth Century

Compassion and Self-sacrifice in the Care of the Sick

The Greek origins of our medical ethics assume that medical care is neither a right nor a privilege, but rather a service provided by doctors who must be competent and do no harm. The importance of altruism was not stressed. It was during the late medieval period (1096–1438) that medicine became infused with Judeo-Christian values, and altruism in medical care was incorporated into the moral foundation of medicine [12,13].

Medicine Becomes a University Discipline

Early in the medieval period, the pope and emperor generated legislation for chartering and building universities. During this period, medicine was transformed into a university discipline. The Hippocratic concept of competence was retained as the foundation for medical practice (a notable virtue). However, in addition to personal adherence to an accepted code of behavior, licensure came into being in the late Middle Ages and represented the state's permission to practice medicine. By the end of the fifteenth century,

there were well-organized hospitals and medical schools. Laws regulated the practice of medicine and included harsh penalties for those who practiced without the required license. Medicine emerged as a guild activity, and, as with other guilds, enjoyed a social tolerance for its monopoly in return for a promise of social benefit. In medicine this took the form of competent and dedicated medical care [14].

The Medical Hierarchy: Medical Doctors, Surgeons, Barbers, and Quacks

The university-trained medical physicians, known as Masters or Doctors in Medicine, were by and large a contentious and arrogant lot [15]. These physicians were regarded as academicians and occupied university chairs. Their services were sought by the hierarchy of the church and the nobility. Although these physicians on occasion would give written surgical advice, they did not practice surgery. Medical doctors viewed the skills of the surgeon as an inferior art, unworthy of scholars. Indeed, in the fourteenth century the practice of surgery was considered so demeaning that medical students in Paris were required to swear that they would not perform any operations.

The surgeons evolved as an order of professionals lower than the physicians. These individuals rarely knew Latin. They were for the most part itinerants who traveled from town to town operating for urinary calculi, hernias, and cataracts, and extracting diseased teeth. But within surgery there developed a hierarchy based largely on skill and dedication. At the top were men who—although ignorant of the works of Hippocrates, Galen, and Celsius—were gifted in the art of surgery. They maintained rooms where they treated patients and trained their apprentices in the surgical arts. Beneath the surgeons in skill were the barbers, important figures in medicine from medieval times into the eighteenth century. They gained importance in about 1100 when the monks who required their haircutting services also used them for bloodletting. Eventually they were charged with the treatment of boils, lumps, and open wounds. In addition the barbers did cupping and pulled teeth, and gave enemas.

At the bottom of the hierarchy were quacks, traveling from city to city and disappearing before the results of their treatment became apparent. Treatment of cataract and other eye diseases tended to be relegated to the more irregularly trained practitioners. By the sixteenth and seventeenth centuries, the skills of regularly trained physicians and surgeons were so deficient that these irregular practitioners were countenanced and legitimized in the so-called Quack's Charter of Henry VIII [16]. Thus, in the Middle Ages we see the rights and privileges of physicians, surgeons, and even quacks acknowledged in return for their services to the towns. For physicians and surgeons the medieval guilds evolved into the profession of medicine.

The Renaissance

The Renaissance (1453–1600) was a remarkable transition period from medieval to modern civilization. It is connected with a number of major events, including the discovery of America, the invention of gunpowder, Magellan's circumnavigation of the globe, the establishment of heliocentrism by Copernicus, the Reformation, and the invention of the printing press by Gutenberg about 1454.

The Renaissance brought with it a spirit of scientific investigation and was highlighted by Vesalius' great work that put anatomy on a scientific basis. Medical societies such as the Royal College of Physicians were founded in the sixteenth century, and medical oaths began to be sworn by medical students. It is thought that the Hippocratic Oath gained primacy because of its ethical compatibility with Christianity.

The Seventeenth Century

The Beginnings of Scientific Medicine and the Concept of Rights
The spirit of medical discovery continued into the seventeenth century with Harvey's study of the circulation and Boyle's wide-ranging physiological observations. Thomas Sydenham, "the English Hippocrates," contributed to medicine an empirically based classification of diseases in which individual diseases were identified by their discreet signs and symptoms. Thus, by the close of the seventeenth century, we see a more scientific medicine forming, which had at its moral base commitments to competency and

avoidance of harm to one's patients, as well as compassion and self-sacrifice in the care of the sick.

John Locke: Natural Law
John Locke (1632–1704), the British philosopher, was the most articulate and influential proponent of the modern concept of "rights". As we have seen, the concept of rights has antecedents in the Code of Hammurabi as well as in Roman law and medieval political theology. The modern concept of "rights" was formulated in the seventeenth and eighteenth centuries. The political philosopher Ernest Barker summarized Locke's philosophy of "rights" as follows [17]:

> There is, Locke taught, a Natural Law rooted and grounded in the reasonable nature of man; there are natural rights to life, liberty, and health, and property, existing in virtue of such law. Among these, the right of property, and things with which men have mixed their labor, is cardinal.

Locke believed that men entered into contracts to distribute both their liberty and their property in certain ways [17]. Until the second half of the twentieth century, solo practice on a fee-for-service basis was considered to be the best social and economic arrangement for such a contract for physicians [18]. In today's world we are moving from "the possessive individualism of physicians as proprietors of their skill to the cooperative, contractual relationship between autonomous physicians and autonomous patients" [19].

The Eighteenth Century

Evolution of Medicine and Medical Ethics
During the eighteenth century, traditional medicine evolved and with it most of our traditional code of medical ethics. During this century medicine was still relatively ineffective in changing the course of most diseases or in prolonging life. As the century dawned, the physicians and surgeons in Europe and America remained, on the whole, a "disreputable lot" [15]. Regular practitioners were for the most part still poorly educated and often dishonest. Medicine's governing bodies, such as the Royal College of Physicians,

were composed of squabbling, egotistical members. As the century progressed, however, the status and training of doctors showed improvement. The distinctions between the physician and the surgeon became blurred, and the image of the gentleman physician and surgeon began to take shape [15]. In the writings and practice of these physicians one can recognize their ideal of "the nobility of service."

Medical Guilds

Also during the eighteenth century in Europe, medical ethics became inseparably connected with guilds. Codes or regulations evolved that reflected the influence and power of the guilds. In England, these codes of ethics were influenced by the Royal College of Physicians. There was by now a firmly established contractual relationship between the King and the physicians. The physicians received a charter granting a strict monopoly on defined goods and services, while the sovereign received a guarantee of a high standard of service. Much of the impetus for the development of modern medical ethics arose from the conflict between those who were protected by the guild and those who were not. The latter included surgeons, apothecaries, midwives, various "irregulars," and quacks. It was during this time that the guild made the claim that only those who subscribed to certain orthodox systems of medical science should be recognized as physicians and permitted to practice. This enabled physicians to stake claim to a special relationship with their patients, a relationship over which the physician exercised strong authority [20]. During the eighteenth and nineteenth centuries, legislation was passed in both England and America granting licenses and licensing power to societies of practitioners representing, almost exclusively, the medical orthodoxies.

John Gregory: The Doctor as a Man of Learning and Feeling

Two British physicians were responsible for shaping medical ethics in England and America for the next 200 years, and their influence remains strong today. These were John Gregory (1724–73) and Thomas Percival (1740–1804). John Gregory was a Scottish physician who spent his life in Aberdeen and Edinburgh. In 1770, Gregory

published a work entitled *Observations on the Duties and Offices of a Physician*. In 1772, this was expanded into a new work entitled *Lectures on the Duties and Qualifications of a Physician*. In these works, Gregory applied the norms of moral philosophy to the practice and character of physicians. Gregory's goal was to "advance the art of medicine by freeing its practice of *imposture* and its science of *conjecture*" [21]. Haakonssen states: "[Gregory's] task, as he saw it, was to convince a new generation of physicians that it was indeed in their own interest, as well as in their profession's best interest, that they should 'labor to be wise'" [21].

At the core of Gregory's medical ethics was the belief that a physician must combine the virtues of the "rational" doctor with those of "the man of feeling." Gregory wrote [22]:

> Physicians require that sensibility of heart which makes us feel for the distresses of our fellow-creatures, and which of consequence incites in us the most powerful manner to relieve them. Sympathy produces an anxious attention to a thousand little circumstances that tend to relieve a patient; an attention which money can never purchase: hence the inexpressible comfort of having a friend for a physician.

Thomas Percival: "Espirt de Corps" and "Noblesse Oblige"

Thomas Percival is best remembered by medical historians for his pioneering work as an epidemiologist in the field of communicable diseases and as a pioneer in population medicine. He also provided the most important work on medical ethics in England during the eighteenth century, *Medical Jurisprudence* (1794). His role in the development of modern medicine is explained by Haakonssen as follows [23]:

> From Bacon's epigrammatic statements to Gregory's ethics we have found the idea that every man who takes up the office of a profession owes a debt to the body of men making up this profession as well as to the society which they jointly are professing to serve. A profession was thus primarily a voluntary association characterized by a set of duties and rights. For Percival such an association

could be understood in terms of its *esprit de corps*, which like honor could be either honest or dishonest. If the former, it was "a principle of action founded in human nature, and when duly regulated, is both rational and laudable".

Percival summarized this concept of *esprit de corps* as follows [24]:

Every man who enters into a fraternity engages, by a *tacit compact*, not only to submit to the laws, but to promote the honor and interest of the association, so far as they are consistent with morality, and the general good of mankind.

In addition, Percival described the paradigm of *noblesse oblige* that was expanded upon in the writings and lectures of Sir William Osler in the nineteenth century. Percival wrote [25]:

Physicians and surgeons should minister to the sick, reflecting that the ease, health, and lives of those committed to their charge depend on their skill, attention, and fidelity. They should study, in their deportment, so to unite tenderness with steadiness, and condescension with authority, as to inspire the minds of their patients with gratitude, respect, and confidence.

These words were incorporated into the Code of Ethics of the American Medical Association and stood unchanged from 1847 to 1912.

Jeremy Bentham: The "Greatest Good"
Jeremy Bentham (1748–1832) enunciated the principle of the "greatest happiness to the greatest number". Bentham was a strong advocate during the industrial revolution of rational social planning based on facts, to make government, economics, and education produce the "greatest good" for the public [26]. With the input of Bentham's colleagues and followers, particularly John Stuart Mill and Henry Sidgwick, the philosophical system of utilitarianism evolved. Although utilitarianism is well established among philosophical systems, its application to health care is recent. Many bioethicists and economists now apply the utilitarian position for problems facing modern medicine, particularly the allocation of scarce resources.

Benjamin Rush: The Importance of Sympathy
Benjamin Rush (1745–1813) had a profound impact on the formative medical ethics of the US. Rush was a signer of the Declaration of Independence and, for a period, surgeon general during the American Revolution. Garrison characterizes him as [27]:

a man of highly original mind, well-read, well-trained in his profession, an attractive straight-forward teacher of wide human interests, sometimes wrong-headed as well as strong-headed.

Rush studied medicine in Edinburgh, London, and Paris before returning to Philadelphia. He carried back with him the ideas of John Gregory and Thomas Percival and gave to them the stamp of his own country's culture. The *pursuit of happiness*, a right guaranteed in the new constitution, meant to Rush the moral, intellectual, and physical well-being of the individual in society. He believed it was the responsibility of the physician to encourage a culture of morals and to undertake experiments for their improvement.

In 1805, in an introductory lecture to his students at the University of Pennsylvania entitled "On the Utility of the Knowledge of the Faculties and Operations of the Human Mind, to a Physician," he stated the following [28]:

In feeling the pulse, inspecting the eyes and tongue, examining the state of excretions, and afterwards prescribing according to their different conditions, [the physician] performs but half his duty in a sick room. To render his prescription successful, he should pry into the state of his patient's mind and so regulate his conduct and conversation, as to aid the operation of the physical remedies.

In an earlier lecture delivered in 1801, entitled: "The Importance of Sympathy, or the Capacity to Suffer with Sufferings of Others in the Conduct of a Physician," Rush stated [29]:

This noble sympathy in physicians is sometimes so powerful as to predominate over the

fear of death; hence we observe them to expose, and frequently sacrifice, their lives in
contending with mortal epidemics.

In the same lecture he addressed the guilds so
coveted by most Edinburgh-trained physicians,
and denounced them as anathema to the enlightened man of science [30]:

> Conferring exclusive privileges upon bodies
> of physicians, and forbidding men, of equal
> talent and knowledge, under severe penalties,
> from practising medicine within certain dis-
> tricts of cities and counties . . . however, sanc-
> tioned by ancient charters and names, are the
> bastiles [*sic*] of our science.

The Nineteenth Century

Effective Physicians and Nobility of Service

During most of the nineteenth century, medicine was a relatively low-cost and relatively
low-profile occupation [31]. Most nineteenth century American physicians were independent
general practitioners, many of whom performed
surgery. Patients were acquired through a lay
referral network. The social and financial status
of nineteenth century physicians was insecure
and ambiguous. Physicians were a heterogeneous group: those at the top of the profession had
graduated from recognized medical schools and
had often received at least part of their training in
Europe. In the middle were the vast majority,
who had served apprenticeships often combined
with a formal course of lectures, or obtained a
two- or three-semester medical degree; they had
received little general education. The lowest
ranks were practitioners who had attended small
proprietary schools with ungraded curricula and
were largely self-taught [32].

The view of the nineteenth century American physician became somewhat sentimental-
ized in the following century. Dr Richard Cabot
(1868–1939), the distinguished Harvard physician and ethicist, described the general practitioner of the nineteenth century as "a Christian
gentleman of intrinsic goodness, law abiding and
loyal to the codified rules of one's professional
society" [33].

"Heroes" of Medicine in the Nineteenth Century

The prototype of the great nineteenth century
physician for both the public and his contemporary physicians was Sir William Osler. Jonsen
notes [34]:

> [Osler's] entry into the titled nobility is more a
> symbol than a significant fact about Osler's
> life and thought. Sir William was a peer of
> medicine rather than a peer of the realm.

A number of Osler's colleagues and contempor-
aries also attained hero status among their colleagues and the public, including David Hayes
Agnew, Silas Wier Mitchell, Samuel Gross,
William Stewart Halsted, Oliver Wendell Holmes,
William and Charles Mayo, Walter Reed, William Henry Welch, and Harvey Cushing. These
men brought to the medical profession in
America a respect it had not previously known
by virtue of their abilities as well as their character and personalities. Their lives and writings
demonstrate that foremost among their medical
ethics was the concept of *noblesse oblige*. Jonsen
defines this as "the attitude of persons brought
up in a definite tradition, enjoying privileges of
social status, wealth, and education and endowed
with a strong sense of their own worth and
dignity. . . . The privileges are not earned but
bestowed" [15]. The flaw of *noblesse oblige* is [35]:

> . . . the strong tendency of the nobility to
> defend itself and its privileges when under
> attack. Even the most generous and benevol-
> ent noble can withdraw into the manor under
> the onslaught of the "ungrateful".

Advances in Epidemiology, Germ Theory, and Aseptic Technique

The increasing trust and respect for physicians as
the nineteenth century progressed were closely
related to the progress made in many fields of
medicine. Foremost among these advances was
the containment of epidemic disease and its prevention by immunization. Related to this was
the development of statistics and the science of
epidemiology. These advances benefited public
health in general, and the individual clinical

practice of medicine as well. Statistics had its beginnings in the 1830s when the French physician Pierre Louis developed his "numerical method" of determining the efficacy of a procedure. The science of epidemiology followed from the work of Percival and even more importantly from the studies of incidence, prevalence, and periodicity of disease by Dr William Farr, a leader of the Sanitary Movement [36]. By the nineteenth century, common law recognized both the vital role of human experimentation and the need for physicians to obtain patients' consent [37]. Claude Bernard and Louis Pasteur in France carried out some of the most dramatic clinical investigations. Bernard wrote in 1865 [38]:

> The principle of the medical and surgical morality consists in never performing on man an experiment which might be harmful to him to any extent, even though the result might be highly advantageous to science, i.e., to the health of others.

The development of the germ theory and the adoption of aseptic technique in surgery were monumental achievements, as was the introduction of local and general anesthesia. The development of cellular pathology by Rudolph Virchow was an additional milestone that strengthened public faith in scientific medicine. Organized medicine laid claim to the possession of true science and emphasized the ability to use this science for the benefit of the public. The advances medicine made convinced legislatures to reenact licensure laws reinforcing orthodox physicians' monopoly on the practice of medicine. The medical establishment also became more expansive in its definition of medical problems, "medicalizing" areas that had previously been largely outside the physician's realm such as reproduction, childbirth, and sexuality.

The American Medical Association

Most of the major American medical organizations emerged during the nineteenth century, and paramount among these was the AMA. This society was formed in 1847 following a convention of delegates for medical societies and colleges in New York who met to plan a national medical association for the US. The organization was founded largely through the efforts of Nathan Smith Davis, who later recalled the composition to be "of the younger, more active, and perhaps more ambitious members of the profession". These physicians wanted to establish formal examinations and formal standards for American doctors. During its first 50 years, the AMA was a voluntary organization without any chartered privileges and with no authority to enforce its own edicts. The AMA became embroiled in political squabbles, and its inability to command deference reflected the profession's difficulties [32].

Struggles with the Homeopaths and Eclectics

The AMA engaged in the second half of the nineteenth century in a long struggle against two formidable challengers of "regular" physicians— the homeopaths and the eclectics. These alternative groups found wide acceptance among the public and politicians. Adherents of homeopathy saw disease fundamentally as a matter of spirit and believed that what occurred inside the body did not follow physical laws. Homeopaths maintained that diseases could be cured by drugs that produced the same disease symptoms when given to a healthy person, and that the effectiveness of drugs could be heightened by administering them in minute doses. The second alternative medical group, the eclectics, agreed with most conventions of the orthodox medical profession, but campaigned against the excessive "drugging and bleeding" done by the regular doctors. This prolonged battle absorbed much of the attention and energy of the AMA during this period.

Medical Specialization

Also during the second half of the nineteenth century a strong movement toward medical specialization arose in the US. Medical specialization was already advanced in Europe but was strongly resisted in America. Until well into the twentieth century, the AMA continued to resist this trend. The general membership regarded as anathema all attempts to grant specialists exclusive privileges over any kind of medical work that might limit the scope of practice of the general practitioner and surgeon. The AMA was able to obscure and suppress the distinction between better-trained and less-trained medical practitioners. Stevens notes: "Posed by opponents in terms of elitism vs. democracy, these attempts consistently failed" [39].

In 1901, at the meeting in St Paul, the AMA was reorganized into its present structure based on membership in the state medical societies, which in turn is based on membership in the county societies. Both state and national organizations have an elected House of Delegates that transacts business in a reasonable, efficient, and organized manner [32].

AMA Code of Ethics

The AMA's first code of ethics was published in 1847 and was based on the Hippocratic Corpus and on the writings of Thomas Percival. After several revisions it was rewritten as the *Principles of Medical Ethics* in 1912, and was last modified in 1980. During its earlier years the organization focused on promoting competency, and exposing and censuring quackery, patent nostrums, and other frauds. It stressed the importance of physicians having access to current developments in the field in order to provide ethical medical care. Its early code of ethics also emphasized that it is the duty of physicians to stamp out quackery: "Physicians as conservators of public health are bound to bear emphatic testimony against quackery in all forms" [40]. What the American medical profession did achieve during the nineteenth century was to establish a distinction between regular and irregular practitioners and lay claim to a professional monopoly on the practice of medicine.

The First Half of the Twentieth Century: The Golden Age of American Medicine

Medical Practice at the Start of the Twentieth Century

Doctors of this period remained almost exclusively solo practitioners and depended on their fees for service for their livelihood. Physicians' authority at the bedside was unquestioned and the necessity of withholding bad news and engendering hope was accepted by doctor and patient. The physicians' armamentarium was

sufficiently ineffective to make any concern about the patient's "right to death" in hopeless cases a nonissue. During the early decades of the twentieth century physicians were still overwhelmingly generalists who had had difficulty distinguishing themselves from each other on purely professional grounds [41]. Patients' rights were exercised primarily in having the option to select the physician of their choice. For middle-class and wealthy patients, the selection was made on the basis of personality and bedside manner, education, religion, and family background. Rothman notes [42]:

> The majority of the poor did not have a doctor, but they had doctors who were integral to their communities.

The ability to obtain a complete medical history and carry out a thorough physical examination was paramount in making the correct diagnosis. To maintain a successful practice, doctors had to be reasonably sensitive, able to listen, available, and responsive to crises, or their patients would go elsewhere. Physicians were very much involved in the social life of their communities and occupied the same social space as their patients [43]. Rothman concludes:

> The critical element in their relationship was not silence, but a shared outlook. Under these circumstances the degree of mutual trust was great enough to keep strangers away from the bedside, and to give bedside ethics standing not only with the profession but with the lay public.

Doctor–patient encounters took place primarily in the patient's home [41]. There was a pace and rhythm to a doctor's practice that included house calls, office hours, and bedside contact with hospitalized patients. The successful physician worked hard, and myocardial infarction was known in the profession as "the doctor's disease".

Medical Competency

The greatest concern to responsible leaders of American medicine at the start of the twentieth century was the lack of competence of many practicing physicians. What they looked for in a practitioner was the ability to diagnose and treat specific diseases and understand their causes, signs, symptoms, courses, and prognoses [33]. This was especially important in the absence of advanced diagnostic technologies. Medical competency was effectively improved as a result of the Flexner report. In 1910, the Carnegie Foundation commissioned a study by Dr Abraham Flexner of the conditions in 155 medical schools in the US. His report brought to the public's attention the appalling conditions in many medical schools, which were at the root of the competency problem. The Flexner report had an immediate and lasting impact on medical education in the US. Many of the severely criticized schools undertook extensive revision of their programs, facilities, and faculties; others closed. The AMA's council on medical education's concern extended from undergraduate education preparatory to medical education and continuing medical education. The medical curriculum became standardized. The president of the AMA, Dr Ray Lyman Wilbur, declared, "The doctor who stops learning goes backward". State and federal governments took action as well. Uniform licensing examinations for physicians were adopted, and physicians could initiate practice only after successfully passing state board examinations or national examinations through the National Board of Medical Examiners [44].

Medical Specialties
Largely because of technological advances in the medical and surgical specialties, attempts at forming specialty societies were finally successful in the early twentieth century. These early societies, such as the American College of Surgeons and the American College of Physicians, were much more like voluntary specialist societies than the complex network of influence that characterized the British Royal Colleges [39]. The AMA finally conceded the need for more adequate training and higher standards for specialists. The creation of specialty sections was now permitted within this organization. The medical specialties themselves moved toward board examination and certification. The first board was the American Board of Ophthalmic Examinations (now the American Board of Ophthalmology),

which was formally created in 1916 and incorporated the following year. The first examinations were held in December 1916 [45].

Sectarian Hospitals
In the twentieth century the two great "rites of passage," birth and death, both moved from the home into the hospital, the first occurring by the 1920s and the second by the 1950s [46]. Well into the twentieth century, the norm for patients was to enter their own ethnic institutions. Rothman notes:

> To be a patient at a St. Vincent's or a Beth Israel, or a Mt. Sinai, or a Sisters of Mercy was to be in familiar surroundings at a time of crisis.

He further observes that in New York City from 1925 to 1945, 60% of the 58 general hospitals had religious sponsorship [46].

Rothman explains this phenomenon as follows [47]:

> There were many reasons why religious and ethnic communities built and frequented their own hospitals. They were, for example, self-consciously offering a gift to American society, paying tribute and demonstrating allegiance to American values. Immediate self-interest operated as well. For minorities, each hospital represented a place in which a group's members could learn and practice medicine, and in an era when prejudice against Jewish and Catholic applicants to medical schools and residency programs at major hospitals was widespread, this opportunity was critical. The sectarian hospital, then, was an investment in professional careers for those who might otherwise be excluded from medicine, which meant of course, that in these hospitals the sick were most likely to be treated by fellow ethnic or co-religionists, that patients and doctors would share a language, tradition, and values.

Medical Research
In terms of advances in medicine during the first half of the twentieth century, research involving cellular pathology represented the cutting edge of medical investigation, and impressive progress

was made in the understanding of disease processes. The introduction of the sulfonamides
in 1935 represented a major breakthrough, and
the two world wars led to the more effective
treatment of trauma. Therapy for most diseases
was still limited to random intervention. The
statistical methods necessary for controlled clinical trials were developed in the 1930s by Sir
A. Bradford Hill and Sir Roland Fischer [36]. The
seeds for future controversy were also sown in
the mid-1930s when the US Public Health Service
(PHS) began its ill-conceived study of the natural
history of syphilis in a poor, rural black population in Tuskegee, Alabama.

The focus of medicine was still on doing
everything possible for the individual patient.
The inequalities in medicine between the social
prestige, knowledge, and training of the physician and the physical and psychological disability, financial difficulties, and ignorance of health
care on the part of the patients was accepted.
Motivated by nobility of service, physicians tried
to serve the poor, but there were emerging concerns about access to health care related to its
rising costs. The traditional ethics stressing competence, avoidance of harm for one's patients,
compassion, and self-sacrifice in the care of the
sick remained an effective moral basis for the
doctor–patient relationship. Doctors were trusted
and respected, though their increasing financial
success was resented. Rothman, for example,
notes that at midcentury "The public's hostility
rested, perhaps unfairly, on an image of the
doctor in his Cadillac and his wife in a mink
coat" [48].

The Second Half of the Twentieth Century and into the New Millennium: Medicine and Medical Ethics Redefined

Setting the Scene
The practice of medicine in the second half of
the twentieth century, and particularly the last
three decades, has been shaped by powerful and
sometimes contradictory forces. These include a
vastly expanded interest by the public in what
doctors do; the growing power of managed-care
organizations, insurers, and employers; the asser-
tion of consumer rights in the health system; the

required sharing of decision-making with other
groups; the loss of jurisdiction over the workplace and the establishment of new relationships
with ancillary caregivers; an increasing demand
for specialists and related technology; and the
opportunity and enticement of entrepreneurial
activities in medicine. This has caused the medical profession to redefine how it practices medicine and has radically altered the relationship of
the doctor and patient.

How the Practice of Medicine Has Changed: Specialists and Chronic Disease
Beginning in the decades preceding the middle
of the century, the solo general practitioner, who
had been the prototype of the American physician, was progressively replaced by specialists
trained for acute, interventionist, high-technology
medical care targeted to focused problem areas
[49]. These physicians with their new armamentarium enabled patients to survive illnesses that
in the earlier decades of the century would have
killed them, and this resulted in the creation of
a population of older patients with chronic illnesses. In fact, by 1995, it was estimated that 99
million people in the US had chronic conditions,
characterized by "persistent and recurrent health
consequences lasting for years" [50].

Restructuring of Medical Economics
Federal payment for health care radically altered
medical practice. There was a precipitous rise in
health costs in the 1960s. Economists soon recognized that it was not the patients seeking care
who were primarily responsible for the volume
of care given. Rather it was the doctors, who
determined the need for treatment, prescribed
medicines, referred patients for surgery, and
ordered hospital tests and hospital admissions,
who created the volume and, to a large extent, the
cost of medical care [51].

The Transition from Individual to Population Medicine
These social and economic factors have resulted
in a realignment of human resources among the
primary care and specialty groups as determined
by the job market. Primary care physicians have
been assigned the role of gatekeeper or "resource
allocator". Both primary care physicians and spe-

cialists have been forced to shift their concerns from the well-being of the individual patient to the care of groups of patients (i.e., population medicine). The doctor–patient encounter tends to be impersonal. The patient is no longer seen in his home or in a doctor's private office with its familiar and supportive receptionist and nurse. The ethnic hospital has ceased to have real meaning and exists in name only. The diagnostic and treatment methods are highly technical, and a bewildering number of individuals can be involved. Physicians are increasingly viewed by their patients as technicians with less status and authority than was the case in earlier decades. Doctors are remote from their patients and are often strangers. Rothman notes that conversations with patients have become "add-ons"—something physicians do as a moral, not medical, obligation [52].

A Multitude of Changes

Patients regard their medical care as a right or a privilege, and as a result of the great expansion of medical information in the press and on the Internet they are often extremely well informed. But as Friedson points out [53]:

> The professions...continue to possess a monopoly over at least some important segment of formal knowledge that does not shrink over time.

The physician is limited in the care that he or she is permitted to give; overtreatment is now a mark of incompetence, and instead of doing "everything possible" physicians must do "everything reasonable". Compassion, care, and restraint must complement competence. Also, the allocation of resources must be borne in mind. The physician is under pressure to reduce inpatient cases, to shorten the length of hospitalization, to bear cost in mind when selecting medications. Finally, physicians move to a different rhythm than their predecessors in earlier decades. They follow a template with an increased patient load often determined by a managed-care or health maintenance organization.

Let us examine how the traditional medical ethics have been extended and superseded to meet these new situations.

Medical Decision-making Redefined from Outside the Profession

To understand the new forces controlling the practice of medicine, let us consider some of the major decisions, regulations, and definitions from legal bodies, regulatory agencies, and commissions that deal with the definition of life and death, professional obligations, patients' rights, informed consent, confidentiality, and many other issues. This is an extensive topic that can be reviewed here only briefly. Table 14-1 includes 13 decisions, regulations, and definitions that have had a major impact on the practice of modern medicine and medical ethics. We will discuss these in chronological order.

The Definition of Health

Physicians accept the fact that medical science is dedicated to the maintenance of health and the treatment and prevention of disease. Obviously, the definitions of health and disease have important implications for medical care, health policy, and medical ethics. In 1946, representatives of 61 countries met under the auspices of a World Health Organization (WHO). They drafted a preamble to the constitution of the WHO that formulated principles for the purposes of cooperation among these countries and for the promotion and protection of the health of all peoples. They presented the broadest possible definition of health, defining it as follows:

> Health is a state of complete physical, mental, and social well being and not merely the absence of disease or infirmity.

This definition proved both controversial and influential and has been repeatedly cited by physicians and bioethicists in consideration of medical care as a right rather than a privilege [54].

Establishment of IRBs

In the 1960s public attention focused on several research projects that involved the unethical use of human subjects. These included the Tuskegee study and the study of the natural history of hepatitis at Willowbrook State Hospital in New York. Congressional hearings were held, and gradually

Table 14-1. Legal and Regulatory Rulings Reshaping the Practice of Medicine and Medical Ethics.

Year	Decision, Act or Regulation	Importance
1946	Preamble to the Constitution of the World Health Organization	The concept of health; led to acceptance of health care as a "right"
1962	Javits' Amendment: investigators required to obtain the consent of patients taking experimental drugs	Established IRBs to protect safety of subjects in clinical research
1965	Title XVIII and XIX of the Social Security Amendments of 1965	Introduction of national health insurance (Medicare and Medicaid)
1966	United States Public Health Service Guidelines	Set up institutional review boards to approve all federally funded research involving human experimentation
1966	Food and Drug Administration Statement on Policy Concerning Consent for Use of Investigational New Drugs on Humans	Established comprehensive rules regarding patient consent and clinical drug trials
1969	Down's syndrome baby allowed to die from a digestive disorder at Johns Hopkins University Hospital	Focused public attention on who makes decisions and principles of individual ethics in the newborn nursery
1972	*Canterbury v Spence*	Reinforced the premise that every human being of adult age and sound mind has a right to determine what shall be done with his or her own body
1975	*Goldfarb v Virginia State Bar*	Stated that law—and by extension medicine—is a *trade* subject to the rules of the Federal Trade Commission
1976	*Quinlan* decision by Supreme Court of New Jersey	Seminal case of judicial involvement in medical decision-making; reinforced patients' autonomy to make decisions
1976	*Superintendent of Belchertown State School v Saikewicz*	Permitted withholding of chemotherapy from a mentally retarded adult suffering from leukemia; diminished authority of physicians and ethics committees
1976	*Tarasoff v Regents of the University of California*	Stated that confidentiality is a *prima facie* duty but not an absolute duty of the physician
1977	*Bates v Arizona State Bar*	Stipulated that advertising by the legal profession—and by extension, physicians—could not be proscribed unless false or misleading
1981	President's Commission for the Study of Ethical Problems in Medicine and Biomedical Behavioral Research	Established criteria for brain death
1990	*Cruzan* decision by US Supreme Court	Competent patients have the right to make their own decisions about life-sustaining treatment

legislation was passed and regulations issued providing for the safety of patients participating in medical research. These laws and regulations recognized patients' rights, including the right to informed consent. In 1962, in the aftermath of the thalidomide tragedy, Senator Estes Kefauver introduced legislation for more stringent regulation of experimental drugs. Included in this proposal was an amendment by Senator Jacob Javits

requiring the Secretary of Health Education and Welfare (HEW) to issue regulations for the safety of participants in clinical investigations. After this, the Food and Drugs Agency (FDA) required investigators to obtain the consent of patients taking experimental drugs. In February 1966, the USPHS issued guidelines dealing with all federally funded research involving human investigation. This resulted in the establishment of

Institutional Review Boards (IRBs) to review and approve investigators' procedures. In August 1966, the FDA issued a "Statement on Policy Concerning Consent of the Use of Investigational New Drugs on Humans," which contained comprehensive rules regarding patient consent in clinical drug trials.

Decisions in the Newborn Nursery

In 1969, a Down's syndrome baby suffering from a digestive abnormality was moved to a corner of the nursery at Johns Hopkins University Hospital and allowed to starve to death over a period of 15 days. This became known as the "Johns Hopkins Case," and it came to graphically illustrate the moral dilemmas that existed in the neonatal nursery. The questions of who makes decisions and what constitutes a "hopeless case" became the focus of academic and popular discourse. During the Reagan administration, the federal government tried to set standards for legally accepted newborn care. Many of these regulations were struck down in the courts or revised in response to public comments. It became clear that in terms of life-and-death decisions in the infant intensive care unit, it was impossible to satisfy all parties. None the less, the era of the physician as unilateral decision-maker in the neonatal nursery was ended.

Informed Consent

During the nineteenth and first half of the twentieth centuries, it was generally accepted that it was part of the doctor's responsibility in certain cases to protect patients from bad news and to "keep hope alive," i.e., to provide the patient with "freedom *from* information". In recent decades this has become viewed as "paternalism," and "the right of the patient to know," i.e., freedom *of* information, has become a requirement. An important landmark with regard to informed consent occurred in the case of *Canterbury v Spence* 1972, in which the root premise of a concept fundamental in human jurisprudence was confirmed: "Every human being of adult years and sound mind has a right to determine what shall be done with his [or her] own body...". Judge Spottswood W. Robinson III went on to state:

> Respect for the patient's right of self-determination on particular therapy demands a standard set by law for physicians rather than one which physicians may or may not impose upon themselves.

This concept has been widely accepted and followed in many subsequent jurisdictions [55].

Medicine as a Trade

Before 1975, the courts had maintained that the medical profession should not be subject to the same rules as a trade because it would not enhance medical care and would be demeaning and self-defeating. In 1975, however, there occurred the landmark decision known as *Goldfarb v Virginia State Bar*. The Supreme Court stated that the legal profession—and by extension medicine—*is* a trade because a charge is made for the services provided. This subjected the medical profession to the rules of the Federal Trade Commission (FTC). Thus, the government limited the medical profession's right to enforce rules of medical ethics. Members of the profession were placed in jeopardy of being in restraint of trade unless great care was used in refusing admission to a society, expelling a member, or denying a place on a scientific program based on ethical grounds. In 1982, the FTC redefined medical activities as being "no different from the work being done by commercial enterprises". This ruling was upheld by the US Supreme Court.

Life-and-death Decisions

In March 1976, the New Jersey Supreme Court returned a verdict ordering St Claire's Hospital to disconnect Karen Ann Quinlan from her respirator. This landmark challenge to the use of life-sustaining technologies that were advocated by the hospital and her physicians and opposed by her parents and their legal advocates became a symbol of the country's ambivalence about maintaining life in a persistent vegetative state. The court contended that the questions raised transcended medical authority, and it called for the establishment of hospital ethics committees, intending this mechanism to resolve such future dilemmas. The following month in the case of *Superintendent of Belchertown State School v Saikewicz 1976*, a Massachusetts court ruled that chemotherapy could be withheld from a mentally retarded adult suffering from leukemia. In contrast to the New Jersey court's ruling, the *Saikewicz* decision stated that "questions of life-and-death" should be decided by the judicial branch of government and not be entrusted to ethics committees. Arnold Relman, editor of the *New England Journal of Medicine*, declared that this decision left "no possible doubt of [the court's] total distrust of physicians' judgment in such matters" [56].

The Limits of Confidentiality

In July 1976, the courts broke further new ground in the case of *Tarasoff v Regents of the University of California 1976*. At issue was the conflict between the obligation of confidentiality and the obligation to protect others from harm. A psychologist was faced with the choice of either preserving the confidentiality of a patient who confided he intended to kill a third party or bypassing the principle of confidentiality in warning the young woman that her life was in danger. The court ruled in this case that confidentiality is at first sight and before closer inspection (i.e., *prima facie*) a duty, but not an absolute duty, and a physician must weigh a "peril to the public" against the "disvalue of infringing confidentiality". Although ambiguity persists, it appears that the courts feel that the reporting of contagious diseases, child abuse, and gunshot wounds are among those situations that justify infringement of confidentiality [57].

The Right of Physicians to Advertise

Another important decision diminishing the residual guild and professional aspects of the legal profession—and by extension medicine—was made in 1977 in the case of *Bates v Arizona State Bar Association*. Here the courts stipulated that advertising could not be proscribed unless it was false or misleading. The courts maintained that advertising was a type of free speech and to restrain it would constitute a violation of the First Amendment as well as restraint of trade. The FTC has required, none the less, that advertising be truthful and not false, misleading, or deceptive. However, enforcement of this restriction is difficult. These decisions essentially moved the enforcement of aspects of medical ethics from the medical profession itself to the control of the government.

Criteria for Brain Death

In the nineteenth century, the increasing skill and knowledge of physicians assured the public that death could be diagnosed reliably using cardiopulmonary criteria. The case of Karen Ann Quinlan and similar cases made the public aware of the fact that patients could survive without higher brain functions for months or years through the employment of respirators, antibiotics, and feeding through intravenous or nasogastric tubes. Survival without higher brain function was often possible, in fact, without a respirator. In 1981, the President's Commission for the Study of Ethical Problems in Medicine and Biomedical and Behavioral Research attempted to redefine death. The report stated [58]:

> The President's Commission...regards the cessation of the vital functions of the entire brain—and not merely portions thereof, such as those responsible for cognitive functions—as the only proper neurologic basis for declaring death.

This superseded the report of the Harvard Brain Death Committee, which in 1968 published their conclusions that irreversible coma should be "a new criterion for death". This latter report had defined the criteria for establishing death as two flat EEG readings from a patient not on barbiturates who displayed no reflex activity [59].

Living Wills

Between 1976 and 1988 there were 54 judicial decisions in the state and federal courts involving the right to refuse life-sustaining treatment [60]. In 1990, the US Supreme Court finally addressed the issue in the *Cruzan v Director, Mo. Dept of Health 1990* decision and agreed that competent patients have the right to make their own decisions about life-sustaining treatment. As a result, hospital admission offices are beginning to routinely ask patients for their living wills.

Conclusions

It is far easier to identify the problems that exist in medical ethics today than it is to propose effective solutions for them. But before we can propose solutions, whether for ourselves personally or for medicine generally, we must understand the present status of medical ethics and its challenges and how we got there. Toward these ends, the study of medical history and some knowledge of philosophy is valuable. "Think like a philosopher," physicians are told by the bioethicist [61], but philosophers think in many different ways, and the ethical problems are not only philosophical but also contain legal, political, and socioeconomic aspects. Physicians are generally more accepting of philosophers who advise flexibility, such as Aristotle, and of decisions that are appropriate for particular circumstances such as Joseph Fletcher proposed in his popular book *Situation Ethics* [62], than they are of rigid adherence to universal rules as philosophers such as Spinoza have proposed.

Next we must consider which ideas and ethical values we can endorse, which we can live with, and which we must try to change. The reality of medicine as a patient right, the concept of patient autonomy, the importance of population medicine, and the need to coexist and share responsibility with bioethicists and others who represent patients' interests must be accepted as part of modern medical practice. On the other hand, we can reject the idea that doctors represent only the narrow view of self-interested technicians who are unaware of social values and the common moral judgment of the community at large. Nor are things as bleak as the case presented by those who claim that doctors are "cast as wrong-doers and incompetents who yearly require new laws, regulations, admonitions, court decisions, and exposés to make them more honest, ethical, competent, corrigible and contrite" [63]. Sharing of autonomy and discretion need not be associated with loss of status and authority, as many would have us believe.

As Jonsen eloquently points out [64]:

The new problems...are new in their technical, social, and economic detail. They are old in the ethical outlines that were pre-figured within the traditions: The outlines of limits to competence, finitude of compassion, protection of privilege, and propriety over skills. The new language of bioethics, summed up in the mantra (beneficence, nonmaleficence, autonomy, and justice), becomes under close examination little more than the modern version of the old traditions.

Therefore, the first line of defense is to extend, reinforce, and refine the old ethics of medicine in our struggle with the new science of medicine. One important way to do this, as advised by Sir William Osler and many others, is through familiarity with the humanities—those subjects such as literature, philosophy, and history that are concerned with people and their culture, as distinguished from the sciences. The study of the humanities contributes to producing educated, humane, and compassionate physicians, reinforces social values, and reduces the insularity and isolation of the medical world. The teaching of communication skills that allow doctors to listen and to interview effectively is also important. In addition, both as individuals and as a profession, we must reformulate our principles to deal with the new problems, develop procedures for decision-making that are in our patients' best interests, and seek solutions that go beyond the scope of traditional medical ethics. Only a handful of physicians are seriously involved in the forging of new medical ethics and there is a desperate need for the input of bright minds who have experienced first hand the responsibilities of patient care and who have mastered the new technologies and are aware of the moral, social, and economic problems that beset today's health care delivery.

Finally, from a personal and pragmatic standpoint, we who practice medicine are beholden to two distinct ethical codes. One is a personal code of values that reflects our medical heritage and has been influenced throughout our education, medical training, and professional experience. This is self-enforced. The second ethical code is that imposed on us by our hospitals, professional organizations, terms of licensure and certification, and government regulations and statutes. We must adhere to this latter code, but we must view it critically and with discretion and work to improve it for the benefit of our patients and our profession.

References

1. Rothman DJ. *Strangers at the Bedside*. New York: Harper Collins, 1991: 101.
2. Jonsen AR. *The New Medicine and the Old Ethics*. Cambridge, MA: Harvard University Press, 1992: 8–9.
3. Rothman DJ. *Strangers at the Bedside*. New York: Harper Collins, 1991: 102.
4. Stevens R. *American Medicine and the Public Interest: a History of Specialization*, 2nd edn. Berkeley, CA. University of. California Press, 1998: xi.
5. Jonsen AR. *The New Medicine and the Old Ethics*. Cambridge, MA: Harvard University Press, 1992: 149–50.
6. Osler W. *The Evolution of Modern Medicine*. New Haven, CT: Yale University Press, 1921: 27.
7. Nuland SB. *Doctors. The Biography of Medicine*. New York: Vintage Books, 1988: 4.
8. Jonsen AR. *The New Medicine and the Old Ethics*. Cambridge, MA: Harvard University Press, 1992: 22.
9. Osler W. *The Evolution of Modern Medicine*. New Haven, CT: Yale University Press, 1921: 65.
10. Garrison FH. *An Introduction to the History of Medicine*, 4th edn. Philadelphia: WB Saunders, 1929: 96.
11. Wear A, Geyer-Kordesch J, French R, eds. *Doctors and Ethics: the Earlier Historical Setting of Professional Ethics. The Wellcome Institute Series in the History of Medicine*, Clio Medica, 24. Amsterdam, Netherlands: Rodopi, 1993: 14–25.
12. Rosner F. *Maimonides Medical Writings*. Haifa, Israel: The Maimonides Research Institute, 1984: 4.
13. de Mondeville H. Chirurgie de maitre Henri de Mondeville composée de 1306 a 1320. In: Reiser SJ, Dyke AJ, Curran WJ, eds. *Ethics in Medicine: Historical Perspectives and Contemporary Concerns*. Cambridge, MA: MIT Press, 1977: 15.
14. Jonsen AR. *The New Medicine and the Old Ethics*. Cambridge, MA: Harvard University Press, 1992: 11.
15. Jonsen AR. *The New Medicine and the Old Ethics*. Cambridge, MA: Harvard University Press, 1992: 65.
16. Albert DM, Edwards DD. *The History of Ophthalmology*. Cambridge, MA: Blackwell Science, 1996: 66.
17. Barker E. *Social Contract*. New York: Oxford University Press, 1962: xvi.
18. Numbers R. The third party: health insurance in America. In: Vogel MJ, Rosenberg C, eds. *The Therapeutic Revolution*. Philadelphia: University of Pennsylvania Press, 1979: 177–200.
19. Jonsen AR. *The New Medicine and the Old Ethics*. Cambridge, MA: Harvard University Press, 1992: 100.
20. Jonsen AR. *The New Medicine and the Old Ethics*. Cambridge, MA: Harvard University Press, 1992: 87.
21. Haakonssen L. *Medicine and Morals in the Enlightenment: John Gregory, Thomas Percival. and Benjamin Rush. The Wellcome Institute Series in the History of Medicine*, Clio Medica, 44. Amsterdam, Netherlands: Rodopi, 1997: 55.
22. Gregory J. *Lectures on the Duties and Qualifications of a Physician*. London: W Strahan & T. Cadell, 1772: 19–21.
23. Haakonssen L. *Medicine and Morals in the Enlightenment: John Gregory, Thomas Percival. and Benjamin Rush. The Wellcome Institute Series in the History of Medicine*, Clio Medica, 44. Amsterdam, Netherlands: Rodopi, 1997: 123.
24. Percival T. *Medical Ethics; or, a code of institutes and precepts adapted to the professional conduct of physicians and surgeons*. Manchester: J. Johnson, 1803, 45–6.
25. Leake C, ed. *Percival's Medical Ethics*. Huntington, NY: Krieger, 1976: 71.
26. Jonsen AR. *The New Medicine and the Old Ethics*. Cambridge, MA: Harvard University Press, 1992: 106.
27. Garrison FH. *An Introduction to the History of Medicine*, 4th edn. Philadelphia: WB Saunders, 1929: 379.
28. Haakonssen L. *Medicine and Morals in the Enlightenment: John Gregory, Thomas Percival. and Benjamin Rush. The Wellcome Institute Series in the History of Medicine*, Clio Medica, 44. Amsterdam, Netherlands: Rodopi, 1997: 208.
29. Haakonssen L. *Medicine and Morals in the Enlightenment: John Gregory, Thomas Percival. and Benjamin Rush. The Wellcome Institute Series in the History of Medicine*, Clio Medica, 44. Amsterdam, Netherlands: Rodopi, 1997: 218.
30. Haakonssen L. *Medicine and Morals in the Enlightenment: John Gregory, Thomas Percival. and Benjamin Rush. The Wellcome Institute Series in the History of Medicine*, Clio Medica, 44. Amsterdam, Netherlands: Rodopi, 1997: 224.
31. Stevens R. *American Medicine and the Public Interest: a History of Specialization*, 2nd edn. Berkeley, CA: University of. California Press, 1998: ix.

32. Albert DM. Edward Jackson in 1896. a man and his specialty at a crossroads. *Am J Ophthalmol* 1996; **122**: 469–75.

33. Burns C. Richard Clarke Cabot and reformation in American medical ethics. *Bull Hist Med* 1977; **51**: 353–68.

34. Jonsen AR. *The New Medicine and the Old Ethics*. Cambridge, MA: Harvard University Press, 1992: 64.

35. Jonsen AR. *The New Medicine and the Old Ethics*. Cambridge, MA: Harvard University Press, 1992: 68–9.

36. Jonsen AR. *The New Medicine and the Old Ethics*. Cambridge, MA: Harvard University Press, 1992: 113.

37. Rothman DJ. *Strangers at the Bedside*. New York: Harper Collins, 1991: 24.

38. Rothman DJ. *Strangers at the Bedside*. New York: Harper Collins, 1991: 23.

39. Stevens R. *American Medicine and the Public Interest: a History of Specialization*, 2nd edn. Berkeley, CA: University of California Press, 1998: 11.

40. Bettman JW Sr. Ethics and the American Academy of Ophthalmology in historical perspective. *Ophthalmology* 1996; **103**(suppl 85): 529–39.

41. Haller JS Jr. *American Medicine in Transition*. Urbana, IL: University of. Illinois Press, 1981: 234–79.

42. Rothman DJ. *Strangers at the Bedside*. New York: Harper Collins, 1991: 117.

43. Rothman DJ. *Strangers at the Bedside*. New York: Harper Collins, 1991: 126.

44. Stevens R. *American Medicine and the Public Interest: a History of Specialization*, 2nd edn. Berkeley, CA: University of. California Press, 1998: 66–71.

45. Shaffer RN. *The History of the American Board of Ophthalmology, 1916–91*. Rochester, MN: Johnson Printing Co., 1991, 7–36.

46. Rothman DJ. *Strangers at the Bedside*. New York: Harper Collins, 1991: 133.

47. Rothman DJ. *Strangers at the Bedside*. New York: Harper Collins, 1991: 124.

48. Rothman DJ. *Strangers at the Bedside*. New York: Harper Collins, 1991: 141.

49. Stevens R. *American Medicine and the Public Interest: a History of Specialization*, 2nd edn. Berkeley, CA: University of. California Press, 1998: xxiii.

50. The Institute for Health and Aging, University of California-San Francisco. Chronic care. In: *America: a 21st Century Challenge*. Princeton, NJ: Robert Wood Johnson Foundation, 1996: 8.

51. Jonsen AR. *The New Medicine and the Old Ethics*. Cambridge, MA: Harvard University Press, 1992: 97.

52. Rothman DJ. *Strangers at the Bedside*. New York: Harper Collins, 1991: 132.

53. Wolinsky F. The professional dominance perspective. Revisited. *Milbank Q* 1988; **66**(2): 33–47.

54. Beauchamp TL, Walters L. *Contemporary Issues in Bioethics*, 3rd edn. Belmont, CA: Wadsworth Publishing, 1989: 73–85.

55. Beauchamp TL, Walters L. *Contemporary Issues in Bioethics*, 3rd edn. Belmont, CA: Wadsworth Publishing, 1989: 384.

56. Relman A. The Saikewicz decision: judges and physicians. *N Engl J Med* 1978; 298: 508–9.

57. Beauchamp TL, Walters L. *Contemporary Issues in Bioethics*, 3rd edn. Belmont, CA: Wadsworth Publishing, 1989: 376.

58. President's Commission for the Study of Ethical Problems in Medicine and Biomedical and Behavioral Research. *Defining Death: Medical, legal, and ethical issues in the determining of death*. Washington DC: US Government Printing Office, 1981: 13–20.

59. Ad Hoc Committee to Examine the Definition of Death, Harvard Medical School. A definition of irreversible coma.. *JAMA* 1968; **205**: 337–40.

60. Rothman DJ. *Strangers at the Bedside*. New York: Harper Collins, 1991: 258–9.

61. Rothman DJ. *Strangers at the Bedside*. New York: Harper Collins, 1991: 209.

62. Fletcher J. *Situation Ethics: The new morality*. Philadelphia: Philadelphia Westminster Press, 1966.

63. Radovsky S. US medical practice before Medicare and now—differences and consequences. *N Engl J Med* 1990; **332**: 263–7.

64. Jonsen AR. *The New Medicine and the Old Ethics*. Cambridge, MA: Harvard University Press, 1992: 133.

15

Quality Issues, Outcomes, and Patient Satisfaction

James E. Davis

Introduction

According to the President's Commission on Quality, "Millions of Americans have access to the best quality health care in the world" [1]. It can further be argued that the quality of health care providers, as well as the highly productive and well-financed US health care research agenda, guarantees Americans access to the latest advances that medical science has to offer. However, despite these remarkable advantages, there is increasing concern about the day-to-day quality of care that Americans receive and whether the health care industry is structured to assure that all Americans can consistently get high-quality care. Recently, the Institute of Medicine has reported a shocking rate of "medical errors," prompting responses from the White House, government agencies, and various public and industry organizations. In this chapter, we explore the historical roots of quality in American medicine, trace the evolution of paradigms used for measuring and improving quality, and explore the accreditation and regulatory procedures that have shaped the modern health care landscape.

Terms and Definitions

Defining quality has proven to be one of the greatest challenges of American health care. Most physicians will say they cannot define quality but that they know it when they see it. Most providers, especially physicians in training, have been exposed to this kind of subjective evaluation. Attending physicians and other health care educators will often make judgments about the quality of a learner's presentation, differential diagnosis, initial treatment strategy, or procedural technique. These kinds of judgments can vary greatly from one clinical instructor to another. This subjective approach to quality has made it difficult not only to define, but also to measure and implement, in American health care.

There are a number of accepted definitions of quality health care. In its 1974 monograph, *Advancing the Quality of Health Care*, the Institute of Medicine defined quality in this way [2]:

> The primary goal of the quality assurance system should be to make health care more effective in bettering the health status and satisfaction of a population, within the resources which society and individuals have chosen to spend for that care.

This statement remains an effective working definition of quality in health care and in many ways anticipated many of the current dimensions of quality. First, the definition suggests that both health status and satisfaction of patients should be measurably improved, notions that have been hallmarks of recent health care quality improvement efforts. A second important concept in this definition is the use of the term "population" rather than "individual patient," because we are also seeing the emphasis move from individual patient care toward assessing the care of groups of patients served by a health care organization.

Finally, the definition highlights the need to factor in cost, suggesting that there may be a cost–quality trade-off that must be considered in efforts to improve the quality of care for a given population.

Another definition, from the Joint Commission on Accreditation of Healthcare Organizations (JCAHO), defines quality as follows [3]:

> The degree to which patient care services increase the probability of desired patient outcomes and reduce the probability of undesired outcomes, given the current state of knowledge.

This definition includes several important caveats. First, it suggests that there is a relationship between patient care services and patient outcome, but that it is related by a probability rather than a guarantee. Previous approaches to quality assumed a clear relationship between appropriate care and desired outcomes, which failed to acknowledge the fact that adverse outcomes occur even under the best of circumstances. This definition also includes the notion of trying to reduce errors and undesired outcomes, again recognizing these same limitations.

Brief History

Concerns about the quality of American health care are not new. However, the issues leading to those concerns, the focus of quality efforts, and the methods used have changed dramatically over time. The Flexner report, released in 1910, is often cited as the first systematic effort to improve the quality of American health care. The authors of this report evaluated the quality of undergraduate medical education in the US and Canada; their findings resulted in the closure of 60 of the 155 medical schools in existence by 1920. The goal of this effort was clearly to disband the poorest medical schools and to identify structural and educational characteristics of high-quality institutions. There were also a number of early pioneers in American quality. Ernest Codman, a surgeon at the Massachusetts General Hospital, systematically evaluated his surgical patients 1 year after surgery to determine whether they were benefited, harmed, or unaffected by the surgical procedure. Unfortun-

ately, his efforts were not embraced by the American College of Surgeons, who rejected his proposal to require outcome assessments of all American surgeons.

Despite the rejection of Codman's ideas, the American College of Surgeons (ACS) provided early leadership in the improvement of American health care. In 1917, the ACS created the Hospital Standardization Program. A year later, the ACS conducted on-site inspections of 692 American hospitals, finding that only 89 met the minimum standards of the college. At a now-historic event, ACS leaders burned the list of hospitals after making the inspection numbers public at a meeting held at the Waldorf Astoria Hotel in New York City. ACS standards soon became a driving force in improving the quality of American health care. However, by 1951, the number of hospitals in the US had quintupled, and accreditation was sought from other health care organizations besides the ACS. In 1952, the newly formed Joint Commission on Accreditation of Hospitals (JCAH) began formal voluntary accreditation through a process called the Hospital Accreditation Program (HAP). The JCAH quickly became the industry accreditation leader, deriving its authority from support by major health care organizations, including the American College of Physicians, the American Hospital Association, the American Medical Association, the Canadian Medical Association, and the American College of Surgeons. The JCAH eventually expanded its accreditation activities to other health care institutions, and it is now known as the JCAHO. It continues to be a major accreditation and regulatory force in American health care.

In 1965, Congress enacted Title XVIII and Title XIX legislation, creating the Medicare and Medicaid programs. By 1972, the federal government was suddenly the predominant purchaser of US health care services. Concerns about the escalating costs of these programs led to the creation of the Professional Standards Review Organization (PRSO) Act of 1972. The goal of this landmark legislation was to improve quality and contain health costs for beneficiaries of federally sponsored health care. This program, renamed the Professional Review Organization (PRO), has undergone substantial change with time but remains a major overseer of American health care quality and utilization.

The most recent major entrant into the health care regulation and accreditation landscape has been the National Committee for Quality Assurance (NCQA). First created in 1979 and reorganized in the 1990s, NCQA has become a leading force in developing standards for the accreditation of health care plans and organizations, especially health maintenance organizations (HMOs).

Independent of these developments has been the gradual but highly effective introduction of a voluntary quality-oriented effort stimulated by the Institute for Healthcare Improvement (IHI). This organization has enlisted the support of a variety of health care organizations, including hospitals, health plans, and most recently office practices, to examine ways to improve health care delivery. The IHI's effectiveness is especially impressive because commitment by organizations is devoid of any regulatory or accreditation incentives.

Beyond the evolution of organizations committed to quality, there has also been an evolution in approaches to conceptualizing quality. The early efforts of the ACS were designed mainly to create in hospitals an optimal environment for practicing surgeons. This early emphasis on such structural features as operating rooms and equipment came with several important assumptions. It assumed that surgeons were skilled and that a lack of standardization among hospitals was a major contributor to variations in quality care. Structural issues remain important, but the focus of concerns has shifted with time to other aspects of structure such as access to care and timely access to appointments. With a growing uninsured population, access to care has taken on another structural connotation in that many Americans do not feel they can afford to seek care despite its availability.

As the JCAHO became an established accreditation organization, and PRSOs became a major monitor of quality of health care in the 1970s, there was a shift in emphasis. The original focus of what is now termed "process-oriented quality" had to do with the care provided by individual providers to individual patients. Quality reviews often focused on whether or not the pro-

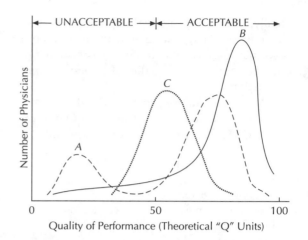

Figure 15-1. Theoretical examples of the distribution of physicians with respect to quality. Source: Greene [4].

vider effectively obtained appropriate historical information, completed key physical examination maneuvers, performed appropriate laboratory tests, and gave treatments consistent with the reported diagnosis. There were two important underlying assumptions to this approach to quality measurement. The first was that the reviewers knew what optimal quality was and that their goal was elimination of suboptimal quality.

A second underlying assumption, first described by Cochrane, was the notion that there may be a distribution of health care providers who provided less than optimal care. As Fig. 15-1 demonstrates, Cochrane suggested that physician quality might be normally distributed, have a bimodal distribution, or some other distribution [5]. Efforts to improve quality were therefore expected to identify suboptimally performing physicians and either rehabilitate them or eliminate them from the health care environment. Quality efforts carried with them the distinct possibility of labeling someone a poor physician. Physicians during this era did not embrace such efforts, partly from a feeling of being coerced by regulations, and partly because of the potential threat to their professional livelihood.

The most recent evolution of quality efforts differs from earlier approaches in several important respects. First, industrial theories of quality improvement began permeating health care in the 1980s. These efforts focused not on individual physicians but on systems of care. This paradigm change was described by Dr Donald Berwick as a shift from the Theory of Bad Apples (e.g., bad doctors) to the concept of continual improvement [6]. Accompanying this change was the important acknowledgment that the doctor was only one piece of the quality equation. Most previous approaches to quality assumed that surgeons could determine the best structure of hospitals, or doctors could determine the best process of patient care. There was little input from other professionals or patients in these more narrowly defined quality approaches. The current movement has a distinctly multidimensional approach that uses the patient, other health care workers, and other customers in making judgments about quality.

The other distinguishing feature of current approaches to quality is in the concept of measuring the quality of care of populations, not individual patients. Although population health is a relatively new science, the emphasis on populations is emerging in the kinds of quality measurements being required by accreditation bodies such as the National Committee for Quality Assurance (NCQA) in the form of health plan enrollee population indicators of quality. We can expect population health to increase in prominence.

Provider Performance in the US

Although the Flexner report prompted the standardization of American medical schools, and specialty societies defined the prerequisites for board certification, physicians were traditionally given wide latitude in the way they organized and practiced medicine. Professionalism and physician autonomy were among the driving influences in American medicine. However, increasing concerns about variations in the quality of care, the belief that there were substandard physicians, and a widely held belief that physicians were resistant to change led some to pose fundamental questions about American health care education. This is ironic in a nation that prides itself on not only the best health care in the world, but also the best health care education.

A number of factors contribute to these concerns. First, although the science of medicine and the development of a factual database about health care can be standardized, the practice of medicine permits a great deal of variation, e.g., it was reported in one study that patients of the same age, sex, and other co-morbidities had hospital stays that differed by more than 6 days, depending on whether they had their cholecystectomy performed in Syracuse, New York, or Sacramento, California. In each case, the patient presented with symptoms consistent with the need for an operation, a board-certified surgeon completed the operation, and the patients were cared for in hospitals accredited by the JCAHO. One theory is that medical practice has local norms and patterns. Given the high cost of hospitalization, this example demonstrates that education should cover not only basic science, but also health care processes, to promote efficient care in all settings.

Medical education in the US has several limitations. First, physicians are introduced to new technologies and therapies without careful guidance on how they fit into today's resource-conscious health care settings. New research data are seldom assessed for their applicability to real-world practice. A second problem with current approaches is the model of cumulative experience. Clinical teachers will often state, "In my experience...," without providing enough data to justify a given approach. Finally, the traditional reliance on expert opinion to set goals for health care quality may lead to unrealistic expectations or exorbitant health care costs without any evidence of measurable improvement in health status.

Many other things prevent physicians from learning to provide optimal health care. Unlike some industrialized countries, the US lacks a data warehouse with which to assess health care delivery. Dr Paul Ellwood has argued that such a data warehouse should be a national priority if we are to more effectively improve the health care of Americans [7]. A second barrier to optimal health care delivery is the fact that physicians often lack feedback on care. In retrospect, Codman's proposed 1-year follow-up evaluation of surgical patients may have been an excellent contribution to current health care science.

What this all means is that we should understand how educational methods influence physician behavior. Eisenberg demonstrated that physicians who are taught medical information will use it, but they will not continue to do so without feedback [8]. In another study by Pinkerton *et al.* resident physicians given a didactic curriculum on dental hygiene were given pre- and post-tests to assess whether they had learned from the curriculum [9]. Medical records of patients cared for by the same residents were reviewed before and after the intervention to assess the impact of the curriculum on practice. The resident physicians demonstrated significant increases in cognitive knowledge, but their practice performance did not change. Therefore, a second educational principle is that cognitive knowledge is required, but taken alone it does not guarantee a change in clinical practice behavior.

Beyond the educational influences on physician performance, there are environmental influences. Physicians are often influenced by the practices of their colleagues. As mentioned previously, they often operate without much feedback about their effectiveness. And fear of lawsuits may drive physician behavior to some degree.

Beyond those influences discussed to this point, what else may enhance physician performance? One current notion is that medical students and physicians in training should be introduced to concepts of quality and population health early in their training rather than after they have completed all of their formal medical education. This idea is not new to nursing education, in which an initial assessment of patients and the setting of goals for health care improvement are fundamental tenets. Medical education, on the other hand, has traditionally assumed that a set curriculum of cognitive information and a required series of clinical experiences will guarantee high-quality physician performance.

Another suggestion is to increase the emphasis on teaching physicians how to function as part of a health care team, rather than as autonomous managers of care. As health care becomes increasingly complex, physician education needs to be broadened to cover patient management within systems of care.

Current Approaches to Managing and Improving Quality

Peer Review

A traditional concept in organized medicine's approach to quality has been peer review. As a profession, organized medicine has consistently argued that only physicians can review the quality of care provided by their colleagues. This notion has also been embraced by key specialty societies, and it was a hallmark of the early accreditation and hospital standards programs. In fact, as the initial JCAH standards evolved, a major emphasis of their quality program was on developing methodologies with which peers could systematically review quality of care. Physicians were required to develop ways to monitor patient care so that cases falling outside accepted standards could be subjected to a retrospective peer review process.

There have been many approaches to peer review. The most common has been implicit review, i.e., a case is identified as an outlier, because of length of stay, an adverse event, or some other quality indicator, and a physician colleague of that specialty provider is asked to review the medical record and make a judgment as to whether the care was acceptable. The advantages of implicit review are that it can be timely, it is conducted by a professional colleague, and it allows for dialogue if there are differences in opinion. The disadvantages are that it is subjective, not rule based, and traditionally has led to a tendency to err on the side of finding cases acceptable. A second disadvantage of peer review is that it is cost and labor intensive.

Explicit review requires professional colleagues to agree on standards, criteria, or indicators of quality that can be applied to medical records or patient care by other personnel. The advantages of explicit criteria for peer review are that it tends to be more objective, practitioners are aware of the standards in advance, and fewer expensive personnel can be trained to abstract medical records to assess quality.

With the advent of quality improvement strategies, clinical practice guidelines, interest in outcomes, and continued frustration with the perceived inefficiency and ineffectiveness of peer review, most accreditation organizations have maintained peer review but have limited its role in requirements for quality programs. As an example, the JCAHO maintains peer review as an important aspect of the hospital quality program, but it has been de-emphasized. Most accreditation organizations now use peer review only to review outlier cases or issues that have been detected through complaints or adverse events, a significant change from its earlier central role in monitoring the majority of care.

Clinical Practice Guidelines

In the early 1980s, rising health care costs led to the introduction of the prospective payment system and a general emphasis on containment of health care costs. A number of strategies emerged to link quality initiatives with efforts to contain health care costs. Quality improvement was embraced as one such strategy, because implicit in quality improvement techniques was the recognition that cost and the customer–supplier relationship were intrinsic to any process or product improvement. Another approach was championed most notably by Dr David Eddy, who authored a series of now-classic articles on practice policies and guidelines in the *Journal of the American Medical Association* in 1990 [10–15]. The concept of practice guidelines or practice policies is not new. However, researchers, clinicians, and other policymakers now see practice guidelines as a way to reduce variation while factoring in quality and cost of care.

Most of the precursors of practice guidelines, such as practice protocols and algorithms, had met with significant physician resistance and concerns about "cookbook medicine." Eddy portrayed them as an array of flexible strategies. He defined *standards* as rules for which there is no dispute; he stated that exceptions to standards should be rare and that violations of standards should be considered a breach of practice. A familiar example for anyone who has cared for patients in hospital is the requirement for a hospital admission history and physical examination. This is a recognized standard of care; the provider need not agonize about whether it should be part of the admission process.

Unlike standards, practice guidelines are designed to be more flexible and to provide a general template for health care providers, policy-makers, and health care purchasers. Practice guidelines should be based on scientific evidence, but they should recognize when that evidence lacks clarity. They have been embraced by most specialty societies, and the development of practice guidelines has been made a research and policy priority of the US Public Health Service. Methods for guideline development have been created and promoted by various specialty societies, and many guidelines have been distributed nationally for such conditions as depression and low back pain.

Although guideline development has grown in popularity, and many guidelines have been promulgated, the implementation and use of guidelines in clinical practice have been less successful. One concern about clinical practice guidelines is whether or not they will achieve their intended goal, i.e., although guidelines are based on scientific evidence, expert opinion, and the collective judgments of people invested in creating high-quality recommendations, their impact has been open to debate. However, it is clear that practice guidelines are needed, and that efforts to decrease unnecessary practice variation will be a part of the health care landscape for the foreseeable future.

Industrial Models of Quality Improvement

Many paradigms have been applied to monitoring and improving health care, but they have often tended to oversimplify the health care environment and have required a great deal of effort for little apparent gain. Wennberg identified variation in care delivery as a substantial contributor to differences in resource use and also observed that these variations seemed to occur within geographic locales [16,17].

Industrial quality management had a substantial impact on the resurgence of Japanese manufacturing after the Second World War. Two leaders in the development of industrial quality management, Deming and Juran [18], used statistical methods to analyze variation in industrial processes and they created principles, tools,

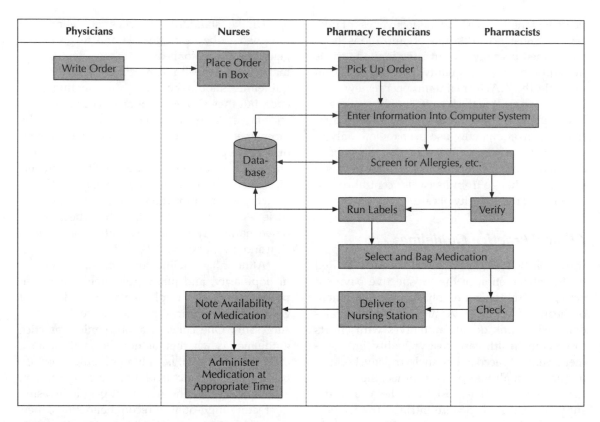

Figure 15-2. Flowchart: dispensing medications at Brigham and Women's Hospital, Massachusetts. Source: Laffel and Blumenthal [19].

and techniques for improving efficiency and product quality. Although there was some reluctance to apply this approach to health care there was clearly a need for techniques that could be applied to complex health care processes. Laffel and Blumenthal [19] presented an example of the complexity of health care processes and compared traditional health care quality approaches to industrial quality improvement techniques. As Fig. 15-2 demonstrates, when physicians write orders for a medication a number of steps must occur before the patient finally receives the appropriate medication at the appropriate dosage by the appropriate administration technique. Previous approaches to quality would have focused on the physician as the sole source of variation in quality. This example demonstrates that flaws at any step could result in a medical error. Industrial quality improvement techniques provided tools for flowcharting these complex processes into methods for understanding processes from the perspective of everyone

involved and statistical tools to help determine the most significant causes of either errors or unnecessary steps. One of the statistical rules of thumb is that two or three steps in a process are often responsible for 85% or more of the variation in quality. It is important to identify the two or three key flawed process steps and fix the first rather than changing many steps or the entire process.

Industrial quality improvement has several important tenets. First, quality is measured in terms of customer satisfaction. Customers are defined broadly to mean not just patients but other recipients of health care services, e.g., the emergency room physician is a customer of the radiologist and the laboratory. When requested radiographs or laboratory tests are delayed, the emergency room physician may be unable to provide high-quality service. Second, as stated previously, all health care work is done through processes, i.e., health care delivery must be viewed as a system providing services and care

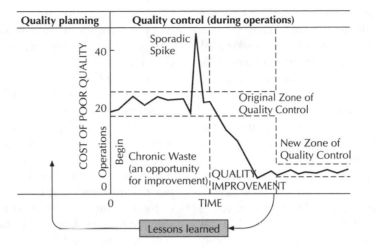

Figure 15-3. Quality trilogy. Source: Juran [18].

through an orchestrated and orderly series of steps or processes. A third key tenet of quality improvement is that the main source of poor quality is process errors. These errors can occur at any step in the process, and their elimination is the primary focus of quality improvement. These errors are also considered systemic errors, meaning they are likely to recur. This also distinguishes quality improvement from other approaches to quality, which primarily looked for random errors and which tended to take a punitive approach.

Another key tenet of quality improvement is that poor quality is costly, in terms of both inefficiency and unnecessary steps in care. Fifth, quality improvement is based on a scientific method and can be articulated in a logical, scientific manner with clearly articulated principles. Many of these methods and principles are fundamental to engineering fields such as industrial engineering and health systems engineering, but they were foreign to American health care workers. Finally, and possibly most significant, leadership involvement and cultural change within the organization are crucial to the effective implementation of quality improvement strategies, i.e., it is everyone's job to provide quality; it is not something that is done by a select few to meet accreditation or regulatory requirements.

A second key rule of industrial quality improvement is that quality can forever improve.

Previous approaches to quality presumed the existence of a known standard; providers either performed at that level or they were providing substandard care. Quality improvement, on the other hand, holds that, after flawed steps are revised, a process should continue to be refined over time. This latter concept is best described by the quality trilogy presented in Fig. 15-3, which demonstrates that initial quality is defined, key flaws in processes are identified and eliminated, and then quality is again analyzed and the process repeats itself.

The quality improvement model achieves quality by evolution, not revolution. Quality management science is also predicated on the belief that processes tend to be complex, and that they often include steps that create waste or errors without contributing anything positive to the process.

A final tenet of quality management is that everyone contributes to quality improvement efforts and that everyone in the organization must have the same level of knowledge and skill to participate on quality improvement teams. This is fundamentally different from traditional approaches to health care quality, in which organizations identified a few quality champions and a small cadre of workers who were responsible for the entire quality program.

Among those groups that now embrace quality improvement techniques are the JCAHO, which emphasizes organizational and clinical performance improvement, and NCQA, which requires statistically significant improvement in clinical and service quality of plans seeking accreditation. Physicians also tend to embrace the quality improvement model, because it recognizes that health care processes are complex and that physicians are not solely responsible for quality. Physicians need not feel that they are the targets of quality concerns, and quality improvement efforts often improve processes that previously caused them frustration.

Quality improvement has limitations as well. Training everyone in quality improvement (QI) is expensive in both time and cost. Also, because the application of QI to health care is rather recent, QI teams often take a long time to understand and/or improve systems.

Report Cards, Dashboards and Storyboards, and Other Methods to Display Quality Information

Organized medicine has always taken the stance that performance reviews should be done by peers and that the results should remain confidential. This has been one of the hallmarks of professionalism in medicine, and the concept of confidential peer review was deemed necessary both to ensure acceptance by physicians and to allay anxiety about public embarrassment or potential litigation. Confidentiality also became a hallmark of JCAHO accreditation hospital surveys. The survey results were provided to the hospital or organization requesting accreditation, and it was the option of the organization to make the accreditation decision public. Details of the accreditation decision were always protected from public view.

However, with increasing requests for public accountability came increasing demands for public knowledge about accreditation and clinical performance of both physicians and health care organizations. During the last decade, there has been a proliferation of "report cards" on quality from sources including *Consumer Reports*, *US News* and *World Report*, NCQA, and others. These have been promoted to give the public a systematic way to assess quality, acceptability, and accessibility of care. Although data are collected to help improve the performance of health plans and other health care organizations, this comparative information is also used by large purchasers of health care in their purchasing decisions.

Despite the apparent merits of report cards, they have significant limitations. The data are often limited to what is available across a number of health plans. There are also factors that can make the raw numbers misleading to unsophisticated readers, e.g., an organization that cares for a population with economic or other barriers to health care access may demonstrate lower levels of performance despite making valiant efforts to provide optimal care. Nevertheless, large health care purchasers and the public have increasingly demanded accountability. Large employers are faced with rising budgets for employee health benefits, and they are frustrated when they cannot learn the value of what they are purchasing. Interestingly, several recent articles suggest that report cards may be more influential to large purchasers of health care than they are to individual patients.

Report cards are typically created to compare hospitals, health plans, or other provider groups. They are usually requested by an external organization, and that organization determines what data will be included. Report cards are generally intended for consumption by external audiences rather than by the organizations providing the data.

Another kind of report card, often termed a "dashboard" or "instrument panel," is based on a health care organization's own need to monitor progress in quality improvement and customer satisfaction. These dashboards are designed to provide a longitudinal reporting mechanism to help health care leaders to ascertain whether their organization is achieving quality goals.

Another form of internal report, which can also be used for external reporting, is a storyboard to display quality improvement projects and to celebrate successes. Storyboards have been used in quality improvement in other industries, and they have only recently been adopted in health care as a way to communicate quality efforts.

Communication of quality performance will be a continuing theme in health care for the foreseeable future, e.g., there are local, regional, and national efforts to establish report cards on performance by surgeons and other specialists. This kind of performance reporting, once kept within the medical community, will increasingly be part of the data that will be available to patients and health care purchasers.

The Important Role of Quality in the Hospital Setting

With the introduction of the Joint Commission on Accreditation of Hospitals (JCAH) in 1952, American health care underwent dramatic change. By 1960, nearly 3000 hospitals were accredited by the JCAH, and currently more than 5000 American hospitals are part of the JCAHO accreditation process. For medical students and physicians in training, the benefits of the JCAHO may not be readily apparent. However, as physicians move from one hospital to another, they can expect to find a familiar structure and organization in each. This standardization allows them to function effectively and also helps to ensure an optimal patient experience. The JCAHO publishes an annual update of an *Accreditation Manual for Hospitals*, which is now also available online. The manual contains standards and expectations for every hospital, including the performance and makeup of the medical staff, the nursing staff, and all other professionals who provide services. The manual also outlines physical requirements for the facility, expectations for patient and employee safety, standards for patient care, and expectations for monitoring and improving quality. In every hospital the physician will find a medical record that is organized with predictable features, including a written record of orders, physicians' daily progress notes, and copies of relevant tests, radiographs, and procedures, among others.

The Credentialing and Privileging Process

All hospitals require physicians seeking to join their medical staff to undergo a rigorous application process. This process, which includes such things as the verification of medical training from the primary source, ensures high-quality medical staff. The process of obtaining hospital privileges has a similar set of standards and, again, ensures that physicians practicing at the hospital can demonstrate both training and current competence. Hospital privileges include the ability to manage different kinds of patients, to care for patients in intensive care settings, and to perform procedures such as obstetrical deliveries or invasive procedures such as a thoracocentesis, paracentesis, or cholecystectomy.

The hospital medical staff commonly has a defined leader and a set of rules, or "hospital by-laws," that establish expectations for staff members. These by-laws have their origins in standards developed by the JCAHO and other regulatory and accreditation bodies.

The JCAHO has not always enjoyed a positive image in American health care. Initially, JCAHO accreditation was largely voluntary, and it was considered important in improving the public image and desirability of hospitals for both patients and physicians. However, the JCAHO developed a reputation for being overly dogmatic in its standards. Further hurting its image in the early 1980s was a critical exposé published by Walter Bugdanich citing examples of accredited hospitals that were later discovered to be providing substandard care [20]. The Joint Commission underwent a leadership change during this time, with the appointment of Dr Dennis O'Leary as president of the organization. He helped establish a new course for the JCAHO, termed "The Agenda for Change." This major undertaking led to fundamental changes in JCAHO accreditation standards.

Key among these changes was an energetic effort to develop external indicators, or benchmarks, of clinical quality. Before "The Agenda for Change" initiative, the JCAHO depended on hospitals to judge the quality of their own services. The JCAHO had no external mechanisms to assess the accuracy of the quality data reported or to compare it with other comparable organizations. The addition of the external indicator program was important for quieting critics who felt that the survey and accreditation process was too subjective and without any relationship to measurable benchmarks of hospital performance. The net result of the external indicator program has been the development of a set of indicators that hospitals are now required to report to the JCAHO as part of the accreditation and survey process.

Another important, and unique, dimension of "The Agenda for Change" was the development of organization and management indicators. For years the Joint Commission assumed that, if the appropriate committees were in place, the organization could monitor and improve the quality of care. The organization and management indicators now enable the JCAHO to assess whether, in fact, an organization does provide high-quality health care. The indicators also demonstrate the JCAHO's recognition that leadership effectiveness is critical to the effectiveness of the quality program.

A third important element of "The Agenda for Change" was the continuation of its previous approaches to monitoring and evaluating the quality of care delivered by individual providers within a health care organization. Although the JCAHO made a substantial shift toward monitoring overall hospital systems, it recognized the need to continue monitoring the performance of individual providers. Each clinical department must identify ongoing indicators for monitoring and improving quality, so that the department can assure the hospital leadership of both the quality and continuing competence of providers on the medical staff.

Two other key elements of "The Agenda for Change" included the development of risk adjustment methods so that hospitals of comparable size, case mix, and case severity could be compared, and the introduction of a newly revised survey process. Each of these requirements may change annually as the JCAHO updates the *Accreditation Manual* in response to feedback from its member organizations and as it learns more about the effectiveness of these new accreditation and survey changes.

Measuring Quality in the Ambulatory Setting

Unlike the long tradition of hospital quality efforts and the evolution of hospital accreditation, ambulatory care has substantially less history of quality-oriented activities. Although there

has been research and specialty society interest in measuring and improving ambulatory quality, systematic efforts to accredit ambulatory care had been limited until the last decade.

There are some limitations unique to ambulatory care that have delayed the development of quality-oriented activities. In ambulatory practice there is often not an easily definable episode of illness or a specific diagnosis for a given clinical encounter. Hospitalized patients typically have a definable date of admission and discharge, and a more specific final discharge diagnosis. Second, the severity of conditions treated in ambulatory practice covers a broad range, and there are significant differences among ambulatory settings. As there was no uniform accreditation process in ambulatory care, some of the advantages of hospital practice, such as uniform medical records and organized systems of care, had not been a priority in the ambulatory environment.

Despite these limitations, with the evolution of prospective payment, escalating hospital care costs, and less use of expensive hospital resources, ambulatory practice has become an increasing priority. Beyond these pressures, there has also been a substantial commitment of resources to ambulatory practice, both for the management of acute and chronic diseases and for the delivery of preventive health care services. With the advent of managed care and other forms of organized health care delivery systems, there was a growing need to monitor quality of care for patients who were cared for in outpatient settings. Unlike the movement to regulate hospital quality and accreditation, NCQA has among its supporters major corporations and health care purchaser groups, not just health care organizations.

NCQA accreditation resembles JCAHO accreditation in several ways. There is a health plan requirement for the credentialing of providers, as well as a process for reappointment. There is a similar patient rights' requirement. However, there are also some differences. First, NCQA accreditation places heavy emphasis on reporting quality indicators, including aspects of preventive care and chronic diseases. These indicators, termed the "Health Employer Data Information Set" (HEDIS), were created by the insurance and employer purchaser groups to help them determine which health plans provided the best care for their enrollees. Not only do health plans have to report on these indicators, but also their accreditation depends on how well they perform in each area.

Second, NCQA accreditation requires organizations to demonstrate statistically significant improvement in two clinical and two service areas. Although the HEDIS indicators are defined by NCQA, and the methods for capturing the data are prescribed, each health care organization can choose its own areas for improvement.

A final distinction of NCQA accreditation is the active role of the patient in assessing quality and determining accreditation status. Patients should be able to make clinic appointments within a defined time frame, telephones should be answered promptly, and clinic staff and providers should offer service and care that meets NCQA quality standards. This customer service focus is important to employer and health care purchaser groups, who want their enrollees not only to be satisfied with care but also to receive a high level of quality care. All plans are required annually to survey patients about their satisfaction with the plan. This instrument, the CAHPS Survey, has been tested for validity and reliability and is now the required questionnaire for health plans seeking NCQA accreditation.

PSROs, PROs, and the Role of the US Government in Health Care Quality

Before 1965, the federal government had little involvement in financing or overseeing health care in the US. In 1965 the government spent less than $3 billion purchasing health care goods and services. However, in 1965 Titles XVIII, XIX, and V created a new and major purchaser of US health care services. In 1970, projected costs for Medicare alone were double the initial congressional expectations for that year, and Congress recognized that the structure for federal reimbursement of health care services had to be revised. After a complex series of negotiations among Congress, the American Medical Association, and other key constituencies, Public Law

92–603, the Professional Standards Review Organization Act, created a new and significant federal agenda in monitoring both the utilization and quality of health care services provided to federal beneficiaries. The act created more than 200 local and regional organizations that were chartered to monitor health care utilization and quality. Although this was a laudable effort, the PSRO Act may have been ill-fated even before its implementation. To gain both congressional passage and AMA acceptance, the final legislation appeared to be different things to different people. Congress was looking for a cost containment strategy, and organized medicine was looking for the maintenance of professional peer review to improve quality.

By 1980, the costs of the PSRO program had escalated, and there was little evidence of its effectiveness. The Peer Review Improvement Act of 1982 disbanded the previous PSRO organizations and instead created 54 peer review organizations (PROs) with a mandate to focus primarily on quality-of-care review. In 1983, the prospective payment system (PPS) was introduced to help contain health care costs through the creation of payment based on diagnostic related groups (DRGs). This act permitted PROs to focus on quality, whereas DRGs and prospective payment were designed to help control escalating costs.

In 1990, the PROs found themselves under escalating criticism. A report by the Institute of Medicine (IOM) identified a number of limitations of the PRO program, including its continued emphasis on utilization review rather than quality, its undue focus on outliers or substandard providers, the use of sanctions rather than positive incentives, a continued emphasis almost exclusively on inpatient care, and lack of evidence that it had provided any leadership for improving quality of health care. In 1992 the Health Care Quality Improvement Initiative (HCQII) shifted the emphasis of the PRO program toward education and more interaction and cooperation with providers and health care organizations. The PRO movement has gained momentum in the area of measuring and improving quality. The current PRO initiatives, described as the Sixth Scope of Work, include both inpatient and outpatient quality initiatives and continued commitment to collaboration with other health care organizations to improve patient care.

Measuring Outcomes and the Changing Role of the Patient in Health Care Quality

Perhaps the most dramatic change in measuring and improving health care quality has been the development of techniques to obtain patients' views about their health care. Although this may not seem novel today, the patient traditionally was a passive recipient of care under almost every quality-of-care paradigm. The initial efforts of the American College of Surgeons sought only the opinions of surgeons. As peer review evolved, quality of care was defined only through the eyes of providers. Eventually, several factors led to the need to include patient input. For one, patients have become much more active in becoming informed about health care. Second, patients are not only more informed, they are also more discriminating in their health care choices. A third influence has been the rising power of aggregate purchasers of health care, who have increasingly wanted information about not only the quality of care but their employees' satisfaction with that care.

Involving the patient in quality-of-care assessment has a number of potential benefits. First, obtaining patient perspectives may help us to better understand patient expectations for care. Second, as proposed by Codman, it is important to find ways to determine whether or not services that we have provided to patients have actually benefited them. Finally, as new technologies emerge, we need to be able to make decisions about priorities, effectiveness, and acceptability of alternative therapies.

Measuring and defining outcomes is not easy. Outcomes could be defined as short-term measures, as, for example, a patient being improved after a brief hospitalization for a self-limited problem such as pneumonia. More important for quality assessment is a knowledge of long-term outcomes, e.g., we have excellent data supporting the untoward effects of not treating sustained moderate or severe hypertension and the benefits in terms of improved morbidity and mortality from its effective treatment. Beyond defining outcomes, it is often difficult to determine the cause-and-effect relationship between some interventions and the outcome of care. Outcomes may also result from multiple factors.

Despite these limitations, the measurement of outcomes has become a major new quality strategy. Initial attempts at measuring and improving outcomes came from many different fields. Rutstein *et al.* first proposed examining preventable deaths in children as a way to improve their care [21]. Others have looked at outcomes through the use of valid and reliable instruments that allow the measurement of health function and health status. Utilization of these instruments may be especially important in monitoring the effects of interventions and treatments for chronic conditions such as arthritis, for which there are many subjective as well as objective consequences.

Although it may sound difficult to apply outcomes measurement to health care, a number of simple systems have been used to interpret patient health status over time, the most simple of which has been the traditional use of a pain scale ranging from 0 for no pain to 10 for unbearable pain. Other systems for classifying patient function that have had long-term application in health care include the New York Heart Association classification system for patients with coronary artery disease and the Dripps – American Society of Anesthesiology (ASA) system classification of patients undergoing risk evaluation for surgery. In each case, these simple measurements can help determine whether or not the patient has been improved by a health care intervention or treatment.

Outcomes research has become a major agenda item, and the concept of outcomes management as a quality and health care improvement strategy has been championed by Dr Paul Ellwood. Although this outcome measurement technology has been available to researchers, it has only recently been applied in selected health care settings. However, measurement of outcomes appears to have gained momentum and will most likely end up being a more commonplace approach to measuring and improving quality in the future.

References

1. The President's Advisory Commission on Consumer Protection and Quality in the Health Care Industry. The state of health care quality. How Good Is Care? In: *Quality First: Better health care for all Americans.* Washington, DC: US Government Printing Office 1998: 21.

2. Institute of Medicine. *Advancing the Quality of Health Care. Key issues and fundamental principles. A policy statement.* Washington, DC: National Academy of Sciences, 1974, 1.

3. JCAHO. Definition of quality patient care. *Modern Healthcare* 1988, December 16.

4. Greene R. *Assuring Quality in Medical Care: The state of the art.* Cambridge, MA: Ballinger; 1976: 7.

5. Cochrane AL. *Effectiveness and Efficiency: Reflections of health services.* London: Nuffield Provincial Hospitals Trust; 1971.

6. Berwick DM. Continuous improvement as an ideal in health care. *N Engl J Med* 1989; **320**: 53–6.

7. Ellwood PM. Shattuck lecture—outcomes management. A technology of patient experience. *N Engl J Med* 1988; **318**: 1549–56.

8. Eisenberg JM. An educational program to modify laboratory use by house staff. *J Med Educ* 1977; **52**: 578–81.

9. Pinkerton RE, Tinanoff N, Willms JL, Tapp JT. Resident physician performance in a continuing education format: Does newly acquired knowledge improve patient care? *JAMA* 1980; **244**: 2183–5.

10. Eddy DM. Clinical policies and the quality of clinical practice. *N Engl J Med* 1982; **307**: 343–7.

11. Eddy DM. Clinical decision making: From theory to practice. Designing a practice policy. Standards, Guidelines, Options. *JAMA* 1990; **263**: 3077, 3081, 3084.

12. Eddy DM. Clinical decision making: From theory to practice. Practice policies—what are they? *JAMA* 1990; **263**: 1839–41.

13. Eddy. Connecting value & cost—Whom do we ask, and what do we ask them? *JAMA* 1990; **264**: 1737–9.

14. Eddy DM. The challenge. *JAMA* 1990; **263**: 287–90.

15. Eddy DM. Practice policies. Where do they come from? *JAMA* 1990; **263**: 1265–75.

16. Wennberg JE, Gittelsohn A. Small area variations in health care delivery. *Science* 1973; **142**: 1102–008.

17. Wennberg JE, McAndre WM, eds. *The Dartmouth Atlas of Health Care in the United States.* Chicago: American Hospital Publishing 1998.

18. Juran JM. *Juran on Leadership for Quality.* New York: The Free Press, 1989: 29.

19. Laffel G, Blumenthal D. The case for using industrial quality management science in health care organizations. *JAMA* 1989; **262**: 2869–73.

20. Bugdanich W. Small comfort: Prized by hospitals, accreditation hides perils patients face. *Wall Street J* 1988; October 12: 1.

21. Rutstein DD, Berenberg W, Chalmers TC, Child CG, Fishman AP, Perrin EB. Measuring the quality of medical care: a clinical method. *N Engl J Med* 1976; **294**: 582–8.

16

Technology Assessment for Physician Executives

Dennis G. Fryback

A Conceptual Model for Technology Assessment

The Purposes of Technology Assessment

Modern medicine offers a wide smorgasbord of technological tools for the diagnosis and treatment of patients as well as for preventive interventions. And new options are being introduced almost daily. The purpose of health care technology assessment is driven by the purpose of the technology: to improve the health prospects of people either affected by disease or at risk of being affected. Physicians know that the benefits of many interventions are not "for sure;" they know that most interventions carry with them some risk, and that potential benefits must be weighed against potential risks. Physician *managers* know this; they are also acutely aware that *all* interventions have costs.

Many actors have a stake in decisions about the use of medical interventions. Patients and their families have an obvious interest in the benefits and risks with respect to their circumstances. If their health care is paid for by a third party, patients may not be concerned about the direct costs of their medical care, but they still may be affected by out-of-pocket ancillary costs, time costs from lost activities, and other, non-financial "costs" of complying with the medical regimen, such as personal or family and caregiver stress. The third-party payers have an obvious interest in the costs of care. Employers and government entities who pay the third-party

payers may examine benefits and costs from yet another point of view.

Physician managers are squarely in the middle of this. As *physicians*, they are concerned about the medical benefits and risks to their patients. But as physician *managers* they must also be concerned about the health of the organization they manage and its ability to provide health services to the patients who depend on it.

It is a simple fact that resources are constrained. Although the constraints may be elastic to some extent, they eventually do constrain. When constraints are felt, higher-level decisions must be made that weigh the relative net benefits and costs of using one intervention against another. Modern health technology assessment (HTA) is the process of weighing the potential benefits, the potential harms, and the potential costs of health care interventions. As a result of the many actors involved, the multiple and competing interests of these parties, and because the data about benefits and risks or even about costs are often weak, the HTA process is complex, ambiguous, and at times seems to be built on an infinite set of assumptions.

What does HTA have to offer the physician executive caught in the middle?

The author believes that HTA offers three things:

1. First, it offers an organizing principle for thinking about managing the portfolio of technologies and resources an organization has to

apply to the health care problems of the population for which it is responsible.

2. Second, it provides a template for bringing together information about a specific technology and recognizing what information is missing.

3. Third, it can help to structure communication between the physician executive and others in the organization who wish to use a specific technology, and it provides pointers to measures that might be used for quality assurance and improvement with respect to the use of the technology.

In this chapter the major ideas behind HTA are outlined, resources in the literature for further elaboration pointed to, and a brief amplification made on each of the three main benefits just described.

Principles Underlying HTA

The Goal of Investment in Health Technology is to Produce Health

Cynics might think the sole purpose of the health care business is to make money for investors. But physicians, with their grounding in patient care, should understand better than most executives that the core business of health care is to produce health. This should be distinguished from the view that the business of health care is to provide health *services*. Certainly the choice between these two views may be controversial. The latter view is neutral with respect to the value of the services. We could amplify on what we consider to be services worthy of providing, e.g., services that are safe, services that we believe to be effective, and services that we consider legitimately the domain of health and medical care. The ethical compass of medicine should guide this elaboration. And we would end in the same place: the purpose of health technology is to produce health.

Another premise behind HTA is that health technology is to produce health in the context of constrained budgets, and so the goal is to produce as much health as possible as efficiently as possible. The pointed question asked by HTA about a specific technology is: How much health is produced per dollar invested in applying this technology? Or turning this around: what is the price of a unit of health obtained using this technology?

The implication behind this question is that there may be other ways to invest that are more productive. A bit of thought in this direction leads to the realization that we must consider more than just devices or high-cost technology when thinking about HTA. In fact, all forms of intervention, including devices, drugs, tests, clinical examinations, counseling, and even the decision *not* to intervene but to wait and/or observe, fall under the rubric of health technology. Such a broad definition is needed to encompass all the potential ways for a health care organization to produce health for the population that depends on it.

To summarize, HTA weighs the potential benefits, harms, and costs of a health care intervention in order to compare the cost of producing health using that intervention to the cost of producing health with alternative interventions (or not intervening), with the broad purpose being to choose a portfolio of services that produces the most health possible for the served population subject to the resources available.

To date the author has never seen this accomplished in any comprehensive, quantitative way. It is, after all, an ambitious goal! Many technologies have been analyzed, but assembling these into a portfolio of services is as yet a dream on the horizon. The reader who wishes to get a sense of what the portfolio might include is referred to a recent demonstration for the selection of a portfolio of preventive services [1]. The author recognizes that health care organizations have other goals as well, and there will be trade-offs between high-level goals. But the principles are useful for organizing our thinking about how health care organizations decide what services to offer.

When applied to a particular health technology, e.g., using accelerated thrombolysis with tissue plasminogen activator (t-PA) compared with using streptokinase (in patients meeting specified criteria)—HTA will lead us to quantify the incremental price per unit of health produced on average by using t-PA versus using streptokinase. All that remains is to define what we mean by "a unit of health" and to specify how to compute and compare the costs of the interventions.

Table 16-1. Estimated incremental costs and effectiveness of guaiac testing for fecal occult blood using protocols with varying numbers of stool smears; calculations in 1975 by Newhauser and Lewicki [2].

No. of smears in protocol	No. of cancers found on average in cohort of 10,000	Average total costs of screening and follow-up ($)	Incremental total costs (Δ$)	Incremental cancers found (Δ cases)	Cost effectiveness ratio: (Δ$/Δ cases)
1	65.95	77,511	77,511	65.95	1175
2	71.44	107,690	30,179	5.50	5492
3	71.90	130,199	22,509	0.46	49,150
4	71.938	148,116	17,917	0.038	469,534
5	71.9417	163,141	15,024	0.0032	4,724,695
6	71.9420	176,331	13,190	0.0003	47,107,214

Incremental Cost per QALY

The broad concept of health now used in HTA did not come about all at once. Often, in the early literature, one will encounter assessments of cost per case found, or cost per patient treated, e.g., in the classic paper "What do we learn from the sixth stool guaiac?" [2], Newhauser and Lewicki estimated the cost of fecal occult blood testing to screen for colon cancer with protocols using varying numbers of stool smears to constitute the screen. They computed the cost per colon cancer found to screen 10,000 people with a one-smear protocol, a two-smear protocol, etc. up to the now-familiar six-smear protocol. Table 16-1 shows their main result: although the nominal cost of a stool guaiac test is small—they estimated $4 for the mail-in card with a window for the first smear and associated time to instruct the patient, and to conduct, read, and report the test; then $1 additional cost for each additional stool smear in the screen—the costs of finding a colon cancer increase rapidly. Certainly a six-sample protocol is slightly more effective than a five-sample protocol. But it is also slightly more costly when we account for the direct costs of the guaiac testing and for induced costs of (in 1975) barium enemas to follow up positive guaiac results. The additional cost on average to screen a cohort of 10,000 people aged 50 was estimated to be approximately $13,000; the result of this investment was, on average, finding 0.0003 additional cancers among the 10,000 people. Of course we do not find fractional cancers; so if the number needed to be screened were scaled up to find one additional cancer, it would be approximately

30 million. Calculating the investment to find this cancer on a per-cancer basis, the result is about $47 million per cancer found. Although for the 10,000-person cohort this would be an investment of only $13,000, it begs the question whether there are more productive ways to produce health for these people with an investment in a different technology than investing this $13,000 in putting the sixth smear on the screen at an effective marginal rate of $47 million per colon cancer found.

"Cost per colon cancer found" is not a very transportable number. It can be used to compare various methods of screening for colon cancer. But we cannot compare the relative "health productivity" of screening for colon cancer with a six-guaiac protocol versus, say, investing in reducing serum cholesterol using a particular statin, because the two interventions produce health in different ways. Realizing this, researchers conducting HTAs began to use a more generalizable outcome measure: number of life-years gained. The HTA results were reported as incremental costs per life-year saved (see [3]). This allowed comparison of life-extending interventions, both preventive and therapeutic.

Present-day medicine is often concerned with increasing patients' ability to function and decreasing their pain and distress as well as extending life. Many interventions have unintended side effects that may affect patients' quality of life. Increasing concern with quality as well as quantity of life has led to the formulation of the quality-adjusted life-year (QALY) as the measure of health, and HTA now is concerned with calculating the aggregate net effects on patients'

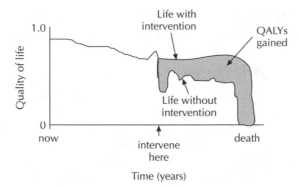

Figure 16-1. Health-related quality of life is shown as a function of time for a hypothetical person. Quality of life shows a gradual decline to the future when a serious health event (e.g., a nonfatal stroke) occurs, after which the person experiences reduced quality until death. A hypothetical intervention is made to reduce the drop in quality of life as a result of the acute event; this intervention has a stabilizing effect on quality of life as well as a salutary effect on length of life. The incremental area between the two curves is the gain in quality-adjusted life-years (QALYs) associated with the intervention. This figure shows an ideal outcome, both higher quality and longer life. Other, less ideal, combinations of quality and life extension are possible.

quality and quantity of life by computing incremental cost per incremental QALY associated with the use of a particular medical technology.

Health-related quality of life is represented at a given point in time by a number, Q, ranging from 1.0 (perfect health) to 0.0 (dead), or perhaps even less than 0 to represent states of health judged worse than death. Conceptually we can think of an individual's Q weight plotted over time from the present into the future until that person's death, and medical interventions applied at a given time deflect this graph in one way or another (Fig. 16-1) [4]. The area under this curve, which will have units of quality × years, can be thought of as the accumulation of health by the person from the present time onward. (If all years were weighted 1, the number would be the number of additional years of life accumulated.).

It is this concept of accumulated QALYs that underpins the comprehensive analysis of health produced by health technologies. To transform the Newhauser and Lewicki sixth-stool guaiac result into cost per QALY units, we would need

to compute the average QALYs experienced by a person with a colon cancer found with fecal occult blood screening and the average QALYs experienced by a person whose colon cancer surfaces symptomatically rather than being found by screening. As there are no data in which quality of life is observed periodically for people with screen-detected colon cancer and people with clinically detected colon cancer, these calculations would use mathematical modeling to estimate the QALY gain from screening, perhaps using quality-of-life weights elicited from patients with various colon cancer-related health states (e.g., Ness *et al.* [5]), and life expectancies from secondary analyses of data from colon cancer screening studies such as the Minnesota study [6]. Although such modeling can be complicated, it can be done in an informative manner, and the results of many such models are published in the medical literature every year [7].

Overview of Methodological Issues in HTA

The process of completing a technology assessment can be daunting. Physician managers, and the organizations in which they work, are more likely to be consumers than producers of HTAs. As such they should know that the quality of published assessments can vary widely. The purpose of this section is to review briefly the elements a good assessment should adhere to. This discussion relies heavily on two recent books on the topic. The first is *Methods for the Economic Evaluation of Health Care Programmes* by Drummond *et al.* [8]. This fine book, in an extensively revised second edition, guides the reader step by step through the process of understanding and critiquing HTAs as well as conducting them. The second book can be described as an advanced seminar on the methods: *Cost Effectiveness in Health and Medicine*, edited by Gold *et al.* [9], was commissioned by the US Public Health Service to be the definitive statement about methodological choices in conducting valid analyses.

Selecting a Point of View

The point of view of the analysis specifies whose benefits and whose costs are to be counted. We noted earlier that many parties have a stake in the application of a particular technology. Gold *et al.* specify the societal point of view as the preferred one [9]. Costs from this point of view include those to private payers and third-party payers (insurance companies, state and federal governments). They also include costs borne by patients, their families, and caregivers such as direct out-of-pocket expenses, travel costs, child care, and wages forgone while being treated or as a result of being treated. The benefits generally are accrued by patients, but may also accrue to families and care-givers.

Other points of view include:

• the patient
• patient's family and friends
• the clinician
• third-party payers
• government
• hospital
• health-care provider organization.

A very common misrepresentation of an analysis reported in the literature occurs when the authors state that they are using the societal point of view and then count health outcomes from the patient's point of view and costs from the point of view of a federal payer.

Physician managers may ask why they should be interested in the societal point of view, e.g., if their health maintenance organization (HMO) invests in a preventive service whose benefits may not be realized until years hence, it is quite likely that some other payer will reap the benefit. Russell *et al.* note that many managers say [10, p. 449]:

> ...let's be realistic. No one makes decisions from [the societal] point of view, and decision makers need and want information that reflects their own point of view. The societal perspective is irrelevant in the real world. Real-world perspectives are those of the patient, the clinician, the HMO, and the third-party payer, but not "society".

But they note as well that the societal perspective encompasses all the other points of view, so at the very least a physician manager will understand the strengths of the competing motivations of the various parties.

Assessing Costs

The sixth-stool guaiac example hints at an important point: the cost of a test is not just the apparent cost of the test alone, because the use of the test commits the clinician and patient to following up the results. So, if a test has a nonnegligible false-positive rate, a decision to use the test entrains the costs of follow-up for those patients who test positive. That follow-up may lead to even more downstream costs. This is true not only of tests, but almost of any health technology. Treatments create side effects in some proportion of patients who will need further treatment. Almost any action (or inaction, for that matter) can have further consequences for some fraction of the patients. These costs all have to be counted, albeit weighted by their probabilities of occurrence (a decision tree model is often used to keep track of all the subgroups and to compute their probabilities [11]).

A crucial distinction is that between cost and price. HTAs try to assess costs in economists' terms, which denote the value of the resources actually consumed in producing the service. Assessing true costs can be very difficult (e.g., see Eisenberg [12] for a complete treatment very accessible to clinicians). Often analysts will use Medicare reimbursement rates as proxies for the costs of medical treatments and tests and the *Red Book* average wholesale prices as proxies for the costs of drugs. The cost of diagnostic imaging is a subject unto itself, and analyses often use stated prices as a fallback position, even though over 50% of the price can be assigned to overhead, which can vary greatly from one institution to another.

Out-of-pocket costs to patients and their families—travel to and from a clinic or hospital, child care necessitated by parents' clinic visits, time taken from work that may not be reimbursed to hourly wage-earners—are not often counted, perhaps because they are rarely observed by the medical system and must be obtained by ad-hoc questionnaires or direct observation in systematic studies. This does not diminish their importance to a comprehensive analysis; it just means that they are hard to incorporate, and many published studies are deficient in this regard.

Assessing Effectiveness

The purpose of technology is to produce health; earlier this was described as the incremental QALYs accrued to patients for whom the technology is applied compared with those who do not have it applied. The ideal data from which to make this calculation would seem to be those collected in a prospective, randomized controlled trial (RCT) of the technology. But only rarely are such data available. Furthermore, it may be that we are interested in evaluating variations on a basic intervention—different screening intervals from those studied in the trial, or applying the intervention to people slightly older or younger than those in the trial—in which case it will be necessary to develop a mathematical model of the effect. This model will certainly be informed by what RCT data are available, but it may go considerably beyond it and/or incorporate other types of data. The ramifications of various approaches to determining effectiveness are discussed at length in Mandelblatt *et al*. [7].

Considerable debate surrounds the QALY concept [4]. Given that we accept it as underpinning the model of effectiveness (as the author does), there is still room for debate about how to assign the *Q* weights to represent health-related quality of life. Unlike costs, where we have useful fictions such as the Medicare reimbursement rates and the average wholesale price of drugs in the *Red Book*, no standard set of health quality weights exists (although there have been some beginnings at this—see Fryback *et al*. [13] and Gold *et al*. [14]. There even is debate about *whose* perception of health quality should be used: patients or members of the community at large [4].

Again, the existence of debate should not detract from the underlying model. The concepts are useful for organizing thinking. We need to incorporate health-related quality of life in the computations, because much of medical care is directed at improving this rather than contributing to longevity. But the applied science of eliciting numerical representations of quality of life in the HTA setting is still nascent. Ignoring

quality-of-life measurement because we do not know how to do it well may be less helpful than going forward with what we *can* do.

This section cannot close without noting the strong links from HTA to evidence-based practice. At the core of HTA is the notion that health care organizations should provide services that are effective. Physician managers should look to HTA to understand both the evidence for effectiveness and the costs of a technology. The movement toward assessing the evidential basis of medical practices in the last decade and the exponential growth of HTA have been complementary, if not two aspects of the same phenomenon. It is beyond the scope of this chapter to review this development. Three recent articles provide perspective on the relationship between evidence-based medicine and HTA, and the reader is referred to them [15–17].

Discounting

Physician managers will be familiar with the time value of money. Investments that have different patterns of payments and receipts over a course of time cannot be compared directly without bringing all the cash flows to one point in time. This is known as considering the *present value* of each potential investment. The computations are usually treated as discrete cash flows at points in time in the medical literature on cost-effectiveness analysis [8,11,12], but those interested can find extensive analysis of continuous discounting in business school texts such as Kellison's [18].

If all HTAs considered only dollar cash flows, there would be little controversy about discounting these to present value to consider different investments. The unique aspect of HTA is that there are nonmonetary benefits—QALYs—as well as monetary cash flows. Analysts almost universally agree that these benefits must be discounted to present value *at the same discount rate* as the monetary cash flows. Although this may be nonintuitive, the arguments are strong. The state-of-the-art recommendation for analyses performed since 1996 is to discount all dollars and QALYs in an assessment to present value at a rate of 3% [19], although results may be reported in both discounted and undiscounted forms [20]. Older literature used a discount rate of 5%. If both benefits and costs are not discounted to present value, substantial differences in the timing of resource expenditures and the receipt of benefits between alternatives may invalidate comparisons.

Sensitivity Analyses

A quantitative HTA is a composite model using information from many different sources about the costs and effectiveness of medical interventions. A well-reported analysis will tabulate every parameter in the analysis and its source(s). The "base case" analysis uses the best estimates available for the parameters. Often a few of these parameters have a great deal of influence on the results, and small changes in the assumed values because these may produce substantial changes in the results. A sensitivity analysis may vary parameters away from the base case one at a time (one-way sensitivity analysis), two at a time (two-way sensitivity analysis), or in higher-order combinations. Resulting changes in the conclusions are often displayed graphically to give readers a sense of how secure they may be in the base-case analysis. Some analysts report probabilistic sensitivity analyses [21], in which each parameter is given a probability distribution to represent our uncertainty about its value, and sets of parameter values are repeatedly chosen at random according to these distributions and the resulting cost-effectiveness ratios are recorded for each set. This process (termed "Monte Carlo simulation") produces a distribution over the final results to reflect the uncertainty in the parametric assumptions underlying the analysis.

Other variations on sensitivity analysis may be encountered in the literature [22]. Although there is not one "correct" way to do sensitivity analysis, it is agreed that some form of sensitivity analysis will be present in a high-quality HTA [20].

The Incremental Nature of Analyses

Among the most important aspects of HTA is that analyses should consider *incremental* costs and benefits of an intervention compared with the medically reasonable alternative. This is demonstrated well in Table 16-1. The average

total cost of a six-smear screen protocol ($176,331) divided by its average total number of cancers found (71.9420) is $2451 per cancer found—a considerably different result from the incremental ratio of some $47 million per cancer found. Why the difference?

The first figure effectively compares the six-smear protocol to doing no screening at all, and it is prompted by the question: "Should we screen for colorectal cancer using the standard six-smear guaiac test?" The second figure is the incremental comparison of the costs and benefits of using a six-smear protocol versus a five-smear protocol; it asks whether the investment to go from a five-smear protocol to a six-smear protocol is reasonable. In 1975, it might well have been reasonable to ask the former question, because it was not until the 1990s that prospective trials had proved the benefit of fecal occult blood screening. Once it is accepted that screening with guaiac testing is appropriate, we may well ask how to optimize that screening given that we have different screening intervals (1 year, 2 years, or longer), different variations on the guaiac test itself (e.g., rehydrated slides or not), and potential variations on the protocol in terms of the number of smears to be collected per screen (with implications about sensitivity and specificity of the screening panel of smears as a whole). We might also inquire about other modes of screening altogether, such as flexible sigmoidoscopy, helical computed tomography ("virtual colography"), or colonoscopy, and each of these has variants with cost and consequences implications.

For the reason that we can represent the HTA result for six-smear guaiac testing as $2451 per cancer found or $47,107,214 per cancer found, it is important to consider what is the appropriate comparison being made and to conduct the analysis incrementally in light of this decision.

The equivalent questions for, say, the current technology of using coronary artery stents might be to compare use of stent with angioplasty versus angioplasty alone. Given that this increment seems cost-effective, we could reasonably consider variations on the stent to optimize this choice.

In all events, an appropriately framed HTA question and analysis asks about the effectiveness and costs of a particular intervention *compared with an appropriately chosen, realistic alternative* (often this is the current treatment or management course for the condition being addressed) and does an incremental comparison of these alternatives. Further elaboration on this important methodological point can be found in [8,9,12].

What price per QALY is "Cost-effective"?

The label "cost-effective" has often been misused. Doubilet *et al.* note that it is commonly used to mean cost *saving* [23]. New technologies may or may not be cost saving compared with the interventions they replace. Russell argues— convincingly—that preventive interventions are often perceived as being cost saving, but in fact may not be [24]. In fact, most new technologies add costs to the health care system. Why do we put up with this? The answer is easy: they add value in the sense that they gain us incremental QALYs compared with the alternatives they replace.

The question becomes, then, what is a good price for additional QALYs? Below what threshold dollar-per-QALY result should we consider a new technology to be "cost-effective"? This is a hotly debated question in whatever serves as the equivalent of congressional cloakrooms for cost-effectiveness analysts. The default answer used in print is $50,000. In the discussion section of the majority of cost-effectiveness analysis reports, the authors compare their results to this magic threshold, with results falling under this implying that the technology being assessed is cost-effective and results above this amount implying that it is a questionable investment.

Strangely, this is a threshold without parents. No one claims authorship. This author traces it to a discussion of the relative cost-effectiveness of population-based strategies to lower serum cholesterol in the US population versus screening for and treating high cholesterol [25]. In that paper, Goldman *et al.* note that interventions that are generally unquestioned and in broad use in medical care have cost-effectiveness ratios of less than $40,000, those in the $60,000–80,000 per QALY range begin to raise eyebrows, and those

above $100,000 per QALY are often considered to be very expensive. In no way did these authors endorse a threshold under which an intervention is considered to be cost-effective. However, following the publication of this paper there seems to be a substantial rise in analyses using an explicit or implied threshold of $50,000. No stronger basis for the use of the $50,000 per QALY threshold than this appears in the literature to the author's knowledge—in spite of its widespread tacit use.

In theory, the threshold should be that amount above which society has more productive ways in which to produce well-being. Tengs *et al.* have collected the dollars per life-year calculated for 587 life-saving interventions across medicine and regulations regarding residential safety, transportation, occupational safety and health, and the environment [26]. The observed dollar-cost-per-life-year-saved values range from less than 0 (i.e., the intervention is cost-saving) to more than $10 billion per life-year saved. Overall the median was $42,000 per life-year saved, with the median medical intervention weighing in at $19,000 per life-year saved.

Informal discussions that the author has had with other analysts at national meetings seem to reflect the following ideas. First, there is no defendable threshold. Second, if there were, in 1999 from observing the technologies that seem to get adopted rather easily by the medical establishment we would guess that it would be in the neighborhood of $50,000–100,000 per QALY; above $100,000 per QALY still seems expensive. Third, whatever the threshold, it will probably increase with growth in our economy and with inflation. Fourth, there are other strategic considerations that health care organizations care about that will lead to individual exceptions to any rule (e.g., for competitive reasons they may offer a technologic "loss leader"). Fifth, not only is dollar cost per QALY important, the total dollar cost to the organization or to society is a consideration as well.

The Special Case of Diagnostic Tests

Diagnostic tests are meant to provide information to guide patient management decisions.

Evaluation of diagnostic tests often focuses on their information content without taking the next step to link increases in information to increases in desirable patient outcomes. Fryback and Thornbury have discussed a six-tiered hierarchy to classify evaluations of diagnostic imaging that generalizes directly to all diagnostic testing [27].

Most published assessments of diagnostic tests involve direct evaluation of the sensitivity and specificity of the test for diagnosing a particular entity in a particular clinical setting. The major analytic tool for doing this is the receiver operating characteristic (ROC) curve [11,28]. ROC curve analysis has been directly linked to cost-effectiveness analysis through the use of decision trees as shown by Phelps and Mushlin [29]. Hunink *et al.* recently published a particularly nice example of this methodology asking what conditions a new technology for noninvasive imaging of coronary arteries must meet in order to meet reasonable criteria for being cost-effective [30].

HTA for Physician Managers

In this section the author returns to the bulleted points of the introductory section, where it was said that HTA offers managers three things:

1. an organizing principle for thinking about managing the portfolio of health services maintained by an organization
2. a template for bringing together information
3. a way to structure communication between the physician executive and others in the organization who wish to use a specific technology.

HTA is not the only basis for making decisions about technologies. It is also a substantial step from asking "Is [name a technology] worth it?" to framing the question such as: "When it is compared to the marginal productivity of the portfolio of services we now offer our service population, is the incremental cost per unit of health produced by [this technology] consistent with our strategic goals and objectives and with good stewardship of health care resources for society as a whole?" In this step we have linked a model for thinking about costs and

effectiveness of health care services to goals and objectives of the organization and the society within which it resides.

The second point is important, too. This model of HTA acknowledges that the assessment of a proposed or current technology will draw information from many sources. The modeling process gives a structured way to bring this diverse information together and to give it appropriate weight.

Finally, the HTA process gives a structure for communication and advocacy. When pressing for investment in a new technology, the advocates should prepare a structured argument. This should include the health objective of the technology—what exactly is the health problem it addresses and how is it expected to improve the quality or quantity of patients' lives—and what is the empirical evidence that it can/does have this effect? What current treatment or process of care is it incremental to or replacing? What are not only the direct costs but also the entrained costs expected to be, and why? To whom do the costs accrue? What is the time flow for accrued costs and benefits? And so forth. A structure such as this helps to organize communication and appraisal of proposals for technology acquisition.

Resources for Technology Assessment

Cost-effectiveness analyses are becoming common in the medical literature. However, there is no guarantee that the right one will appear at the time it is needed for an organizational decision. Actually doing a comprehensive analysis is a formidable task—this author's experience is that devoting even six analyst-months is not unusual. There are consulting firms that contract to perform technology assessments, but the author's experience with these is slight, and he cannot recommend one over another.

Short courses are available to which organizations can send people. Perhaps the best known are conducted through the Harvard School of Public Health under the direction of Professor Milton Weinstein. Professional societies such as the Society for Medical Decision Making, the

Society for General Internal Medicine, and the International Society for Pharmacoeconomics and Outcomes Research conduct short courses in association with their annual meetings. Information about all of these can generally be found on their Internet web pages.

Throughout this chapter books and journal articles have been cited that provide step-by-step entry to the methods. These are worth reiterating. For step-by-step methods, the book by Drummond *et al.* is excellent [8]. An excellent companion for methodology in medical decision analysis is the book by Sox and colleagues [11]. The edited volume from the US Public Health Service's Panel on Cost-Effectiveness in Health and Medicine [9] provides a prescriptive methodological template for doing cost-effectiveness analyses and also has two appendices reporting analyses in a "think aloud" manner, where the authors reflect on the methodological steps and how they accomplished them. Finally, for assessing preventive interventions especially but also for general methods, an edited book by staff at the Centers for Disease Control and Prevention offers discussion of methods and a number of examples [31].

References

1. Wang LY, Haddix AC, Teutsch SM, Caldwell B. The role of resource allocation models in selecting clinical preventive services. *Am J Managed Care* 1999; **5**: 445–54.
2. Newhauser D, Lewicki AM. What do we gain from the sixth stool guaiac? *N Engl J Med* 1975; **293**: 226–8.
3. Wright JC, Weinstein MC. Gains in life expectancy from medical interventions—standardizing data on outcomes. *N Engl J Med* 1998; **339**: 380–6.
4. Gold MR, Patrick DL, Torrance GW *et al.* Identifying and valuing outcomes. In: Gold MR, Siegel JE, Russell LB, Weinstein MC, eds. *Cost-Effectiveness in Health and Medicine*. New York: Oxford University Press, 1996: 82–134.
5. Ness RM, Holmes AM, Klein R, Dittus R. Utility valuations for outcomes states of colorectal cancer. *Am J Gastroenterol* 1999; **94**: 1650–7.
6. Mandel JS, Church TR, Ederer F, Bond JH. Colorectal cancer mortality. effectiveness of biennial screening for fecal occult blood. *J Natl Cancer Inst* 1999; **91**: 434–7.

7. Mandelblatt J, Fryback D, Weinstein M, Russell LB, Gold MR. Assessing the effectiveness of health interventions for cost-effectiveness analysis. Panel on cost-effectiveness in health and medicine. *J Gen Intern Med* 1997; **12**: 551–8.
8. Drummond MF, O'Brien B, Stoddart GL, Torrance GW. *Methods for the Economic Evaluation of Health Care Programmes*. Oxford: Oxford University Press, 1997.
9. Gold MR, Siegel JE, Russell LB, Weinstein MC. *Cost-Effectiveness in Health and Medicine*. New York: Oxford University Press, 1996.
10. Russell LB, Fryback DG, Sonnenberg FA. Is the societal perspective in cost-effectiveness analysis useful for decision makers? *The Joint Commission J Quality Improvement* 1999; **25**: 447–54.
11. Sox HCJ, Blatt MA, Higgins MC, Marton KI. *Medical Decision Making*. Boston: Butterworths, 1988.
12. Eisenberg JM. Clinical economics. A guide to the economic analysis of clinical practices. *JAMA* 1989; **262**: 2879–86.
13. Fryback DG, Lawrence WF, Martin PA, Klein BEK, Klein R. Longitudinal population estimates of age-specific, quality-adjusted life-expectancy: Results from the Beaver Dam health outcomes study [abstract]. *Med Decision Making* 1994; **14**: 430.
14. Gold MR, Franks P, McCoy KI, Fryback DG. Toward consistency in cost-utility analyzes. Using national measures to create condition-specific values. *Med Care* 1998; **36**: 778–92.
15. Eisenberg JM. Ten lessons for evidence-based technology assessment. *JAMA* 1999; **282**: 1865–9.
16. Perry S, Thamer M. Medical innovation and the critical role of health technology assessment. *JAMA* 1999; **282**: 1869–72.
17. Woolf SH. The need for perspective in evidence-based medicine. *JAMA* 1999; **282**: 2358–65.
18. Kellison SG. *The Theory of Interest*. 2nd edn. Homewood, Il: Irwin, 1991.
19. Lipscomb J, Weinstein MC, Torrance GW. Time preference. In: Gold MR, Siegel JE, Russell LB, Weinstein MC, eds. *Cost-Effectiveness in Health and Medicine*. New York: Oxford University Press, 1996: 214–46.
20. Siegel J, Weinstein M, Russell L, Gold MR. Recommendations for reporting cost-effectiveness analyzes. Panel on cost-effectiveness in health and medicine. *JAMA* 1997; **276**: 1339–41.
21. Doubilet P, Begg CB, Weinstein MC, Braun P, McNeil BJ. Probabilistic sensitivity analysis using Monte Carlo simulation. *Med Decision Making* 1985; **5**: 157–77.

22. Manning WG, Fryback DG, Weinstein MC. Reflecting uncertainty in cost-effectiveness analysis. In: Gold MR, Siegel JE, Russell LB, Weinstein MC, eds. *Cost-Effectiveness in Health and Medicine*. New York: Oxford University Press, 1996: 247–303.
23. Doubilet P, Weinstein MC, McNeil BJ. Use and misuse of the term "cost effective" in medicine. *N Engl J Med* 1986; **314**: 253–5.
24. Russell LB. *Is Prevention Better Than Cure?* Washington, DC: The Brookings Institution, 1986.
25. Goldman L, Gordon DJ, Rifkind BM *et al*. Cost and health implications of cholesterol lowering. *Circulation* 1992; **85**: 1960–8.
26. Tengs TO, Adams ME, Pliskin JS *et al*. Five-hundred life-saving interventions and their cost-effectiveness. *Risk Anal* 1995; **15**: 369–90.
27. Fryback DG, Thornbury JR. Efficacy of diagnostic imaging. *Med Decision Making* 1991; **11**: 88–94.
28. Hanley JA, McNeil BJ. The meaning and use of the area under a receiver operating characteristic (ROC) curve. *Radiology* 1982; **143**: 29–36.
29. Phelps CE, Mushlin AI. Focusing technology assessment using medical decision theory. *Med Decision Making* 1988; **8**: 279–89.
30. Hunink MG, Kuntz KM, Fleischmann KE, Brady TJ. Noninvasive imaging for the diagnosis of coronary artery disease. Focusing Development of New Diagnostic Technology. *Ann Intern Med* 1999; **131**: 673–80.
31. Haddix AC, Teutsch SM, Shaffer PA, Dunet DO. Prevention effectiveness. *A Guide to Decision Analysis and Economic Evaluation*. New York: Oxford University Press, 1996.

17

Medical Informatics

Richard Friedman

Introduction

Medical informatics is the use of technology to organize and apply information in all aspects of medicine. Experts in medical informatics must be familiar with topics in biomedicine, decision science/statistics/research, computer science/technology assessment, psychology, health policy/social issues/ethics, and operational research/management. Applications of medical informatics in medicine include electronic patient records, artificial intelligence in biomedicine, decision support systems, networking, telemedicine, instructional technology, multimedia, imaging, information retrieval, hospital information systems, and databases.

Health Care Information Systems

A computerized health care information system (HCIS) is composed of a set of functional modules. These modules can exist in the form of a single integrated system from a single vendor, or they may be individual units purchased from a variety of vendors. The integration of these disparate modules then becomes the responsibility of the system information services unit. The purchase of a single integrated system has many advantages for ease of implementation. However, for a variety of reasons, most systems in use today consist of modules from a number of vendors.

The major functional modules of the HCIS are usually divided into the administrative, financial, clinical, practice management, and managed-care areas. The administrative modules include admission/transfer/discharge, scheduling, medical records, utilization review, QA/QR, outcome management, human resources, and materials management. The financial modules include accounting (patient billing, accounts receivable, accounts payable, general ledger, budgeting) and decision support (financial profile of providers, reimbursement modeling, case rate analysis, market analysis, budgeting). Clinical modules include computer-based patient records (charting, order entry, results reporting, care planning, physician profiling), clinical laboratories, pharmacy, radiology, and surgery scheduling. Practice management includes patient information, electronic billing, claims tracking, risk management, managed-care requirement (HEDIS), medical equipment purchasing, practice marketing, and time management. The managed-care module includes information on the plan members, providers, payers, health plan, and home health. Major players in the HCIS field are Shared Medical Systems (SMS), BDM International, Cerner Corporation, HBOC, Hewlett Packard Healthcare, Marquette Medical Systems, Sybase, and Darca Inc.

Admission/Transfer/Discharge

This module tracks admissions, discharges, and transfers (ATD). It is the core of any hospital information system. It establishes the patient record and details such information as bed availability, call lists, scheduling, collection of demographic information, referral data, reason for admission, precertification, verification of benefit plan and ability to pay, preadmission orders, and presurgery preparation procedures.

This module is usually integrated with the accounts receivable and medical records modules. Patient types are user-defined and can include inpatient, swing bed, outpatient, emergency room, observation, or series outpatient (patient with an ongoing scheduled treatment plan). This module usually contains some form of patient master index (PMI), which provides most information required for admission. PMI records can be created during admission. Patient classes are used to provide defaults based on patient type and insurance coverage. UB–92 and HCFA-1500 information can be reviewed at the time of admission. Admission cover sheets can be printed as part of the admission process. Online lookup is available for quick access to information. Programs in this module track admissions by user-defined codes such as referral sources, room type, race codes, and nurse's stations. The hospital can set up a user-defined insurance code file to maintain information on third-party payers. Patients are easily transferred between rooms or to different patient types or classes. Discharge programs allow easy entry or editing of discharge date, time, and status. Reports can be prepared to include patient profile, room chart, patient census, period-to-date transactions, preadmission, patient days, and file lists.

Accounting

The core elements of the accounting module include charge capture, utilization review, professional and technical billing, proration of revenue, corrections and late charges, adjustments and payments, account aging, category of patient, date of encounter, date of payment, collections, charge master, and handling of delinquent accounts. The general ledger program is the centerpiece of the accounting software. It can create income statements and balance sheets, and it usually includes complete budgeting capabilities, including comparative budget reports. It should be able to maintain the current budget while creating a budget for the new year. In a typical system, charges are entered in batches for easy verification of data. Detail and/or summary bills are available for each patient. They can be printed, verified, edited, and reprinted if necessary. UB-92 forms and

HCFA-1500 forms can be created and edited before they are printed. This module interfaces with accounts receivable to establish payers (guarantors) and record patient bills. It also interfaces with medical records and admission, discharge, and transfer.

Online lookup is usually available for quick, easy access to charge codes, patient number, and other information. The charge code file (charge master file) lists the charge for each supply item, test, or procedure and provides for exceptions by insurance code for price and coverage. A different price can be set for each insurance code. Interim billing is supported for patient bills, UB-92 and HCFA-1500 forms. Journal entries are generated and can be merged to the general ledger, if desired. If the general ledger is not being used, a billing report is available for the accountant. Charge code labels can be printed to assist in inventory control. Billing interfaces with inventory for charge code price updates and item disbursement. Reports available include outstanding charges, billing journal, revenue reports by charge code/financial class, department/financial class, and department/patient type. Statistical entries can be created from statistical general ledger account numbers in the charge code master. These can then be merged to the general ledger for statistical reports. Room charges can be billed automatically or entered manually. Inpatients can be automatically billed X days after discharge to allow for late charges.

Order Entry

At a minimum, all orders must be entered either in batch mode or interactively on the units to facilitate charge capture. When fully functional, this module includes order capture, urgency, frequency and scheduling of procedure, performer, ordering physician, order verification, order sets, activation of preorders, check for inappropriate orders, and credential verification.

Resulting Reporting

This module's functions include reporting of results, completion of procedure, ability to cancel procedures, entry of results, billing, entry of normal or abnormal results, check for data accuracy, flowcharts, graphing, and data calculations.

Specialized Functions

Clinical Laboratories

This module typically includes a set of tools to manage work flow, data, and decision-making processes. It includes flexible patient reporting, billing, and workload systems. It must be compliant with CLIA regulations, and it must include comprehensive quality control and interfaces to all major analyzers. It must have a reference laboratory–HL7 interface.

Specimen information can be added to the computer-assigned accession number. This information includes an ordering physician, facility ordering the test, type of sample, date of collection, and receipt initials of the technologist collecting the sample. Tests and profiles are ordered via the mouse or a few keystrokes. The module prints labels, eliminating writing on the tubes to be drawn. Usually several label formats are available, including barcodes. The patient's charges are on the daily charges' list. The patient's name and identification data appear on all daily logs. Results are automatically sent to the computer on completion. This module provides quality control and workload reporting reports. It supports remote report printing, batch results entry, batch printing, security system, direct database access, daily billing summary with CPTs, single patient charges summary, and the ability to fax reports directly from the program.

Radiology

The radiology module handles procedure scheduling, report generation and transmission, generation of patient instructions and preparation, order entry, file room management, and picture archiving and communication systems (PACS). A PACS is an electronic filmless information system for acquiring, sorting, transporting, storing, and electronically displaying medical images. Its benefits include the elimination of expensive silver-based film, improved access to new and old films, reduction in the physical storage requirement of bulky films, and lower personnel costs. The important elements of the PACS are the image acquisition, data management, display substation, and network communications. Images may be acquired directly from the capture device (computed tomography [CT], magnetic resonance imaging [MRI], etc.) via phosphor cassettes or by digitization of X-ray films. A computer that acquires the images from the capture computer, archives the images, distributes the images to the display workstations, processes image retrieval requests, and handles data management. The display system is a high-resolution device that is primarily oriented toward the rapid display of images. The PACS encompasses a digital communication network for the transmission of images and image-related data.

PACS and teleradiology existed before the Internet, but they are being completely transformed by it. Traditionally, the PACS was considered a departmental network dominated by a single vendor. Teleradiology was a small-scale system that compromised diagnostic quality in exchange for tolerable communication costs. Wavelet compression technology has effectively eliminated this compromise by combining the high-quality image distribution required of a PACS with the low communication costs essential to teleradiology. The merging of PACS and teleradiology provides clear benefits for cost-justifying the shift to filmless clinical practice.

Pharmacy

This module handles the tracking of drug inventory location, drug expiration dates, and drug costs. It tracks patient allergies, drug interactions, medication history, and diagnoses. It can handle multiple formularies and provide drug alerts and patient information sheets. It can also facilitate automatic dose dispensing and usage cost and billing.

Medical Records

This program establishes and maintains the patient master index (PMI). The PMI includes the following information for each patient at the facility: the patient's name, address, phone number, social security number, Medicare number, mother's maiden name, demographic information, allergies, blood type, insurance information, tetanus immunization, and employment information. Features include a medical record number maintained for each patient through all episodes of care. DRG (diagnostic related groups) Grouper with integrated ICD-9-CM and CPT-4 coding module has a flexible reporting capability, allowing ad-hoc reports to be created according to the hospital's specifications and saved for perpetual use.

Each patient care episode is recorded along with pertinent data, including: multiple diagnosis and procedure codes; tests run for this episode, including results; patient class; financial class; LOS data for admission; and service categories. Procedures can be flagged for automatic review. Chart deficiencies may be easily identified and reported under user-defined criteria. Complete chart control allows the user to identify a medical records borrower, new temporary location, and expected return time, and to report on delinquencies. Indicators can be established to track quality performance and provide systematic review. This module usually includes automatic reordering and flagging of critical diagnoses and procedures.

Materials Management

This program tracks the vendors of, the charges for, and the current number of items in your inventory and generates purchase orders. Inventory items can be assigned to any category desired, multiple vendors, and vendor numbers can be assigned to each inventory item, and packaged units are converted to dispensing units within the system. List price, last cost, and average cost are kept for each item, and the module maintains minimum and maximum stock levels. It also maintains purchase history, quantity on hand and quantity on order, and quantities and dollars dispensed on a month-to-date and year-to-date basis, including cost data, multiple markup factors, and customer receipts.

Data Warehouse

A data warehouse provides the base infrastructure and analytic capabilities needed to understand and manage costs, quality, and performance. It helps users to import, integrate, and manage data from a variety of disparate sources (regardless of where the data originate). The data warehouse provides users with a variety of administrative tools to manage, secure, and consolidate both detailed and summarized data

into an integrated source of information. The analytical tool provided within the data warehouse helps organizations to manage overall risk by enabling users to perform efficient, data-driven, business evaluations.

The depth of information in the data warehouse and the flexibility of the analytical tool work together to help users to analyze key business drivers, such as performance, cost, quality, market share, and revenue. The analytic tool focuses on specific user-defined data sets so that users can spend more time analyzing and sharing the information and less time looking for it. To extend their decision support analyses, it enables users to cut, copy, and paste data into a variety of formats. It also permits integration with SPSS third-party software for statistical process control. This gives users a range of presentation options, such as graphics and text, for both summarized and detailed analyses.

Managed Care

The managed care module includes information on the plan members, providers, payers, health plan, and home health. For plan members it includes identity of plan members, plan benefits, co-payments, and scheduling. For providers it coordinates referral tracking, claims submission, capitation, utilization management, and HEDIS reporting. With regard to payers it tracks plan members, plan providers, prior approval of services, referral tracking, IBNR, processing and adjudication of claims, case management, member recruitment, provider recruitment, case management, trend tracking, and capitation. For individual health plans it must track member eligibility, authorization, claims reporting, premium billing, member services, membership reporting, capitation, administration of risk sharing, contract management, outcomes management, utilization review, and case management. The home health module must deal with scheduling, clinical care, billing, productivity, and clinical charting.

Coding of Data

The creation of a health care information infrastructure requires the integration of existing and new architectures, application systems, and services. To make these diverse components work together, health care information standards are needed.

Patient Identification

Although the Social Security Number (SSN) is being considered for use as a patient identifier in the US today, critics point out that it is not an ideal identifier. Not everyone has an SSN; several people may use the same SSN, and the SSN is so widely used for other purposes that it presents a threat to confidentiality. On the other hand, it may be some time before funding is available to develop, disseminate, and maintain a more ideal patient identifier. A number of groups, including the American Society for Testing and Materials (ASTM) and the Computer-Based Patient Record Institute (CPRI), are working on this problem.

The Health Care Financing Administration (HCFA) has created a widely used provider identifier known as the Universal Physician Identifier Number (UPIN). The UPIN is assigned only to physicians who handle Medicare patients. To address this limitation, HCFA developed the National Provider File (NPF). It created a new provider identifier for Medicare, which includes all caregivers and sites of care.

Two site-of-care identifier systems are widely used. One is the Health Industry Number (HIN), issued by the Health Industry Business Communications Council (HIBCC). The HIN is an identifier for health care facilities, practitioners, and retail pharmacies. HCFA has also defined provider-of-service identifiers for Medicare usage.

Three product and supply labeling identifiers are widely accepted. The Labeler Identification Code (LIC) identifies the manufacturer or distributor and is issued by HIBCC. The LIC is used both with and without bar codes for products and supplies distributed within a health care facility. The Universal Product Code (UPC) is maintained by the Uniform Code Council and is typically used to label products that are sold in retail settings. The National Drug Code (NDC) also serves as an identifier and is described later in the Clinical Data Representations section.

Data Transfer Standards

Standards have been developed for the transfer of clinically related information between elec-

tronic devices. The ASTM develops many of these standards. This group has developed standards for the transmission of laboratory results representing medical logic (Arden Syntax), and transmitting digital neurophysical data (electroencephalograms and electromyograms).

The Digital Imaging and Communications (DICOM) standard governs radiological data transmission. This standard was developed by the American College of Radiology—National Electrical Manufacturers' Association (ACR-NEMA). It defines the message formats and communications standards for diagnostic and therapeutic images. Most radiology PACS vendors support DICOM. It has also been incorporated into the European MEDICOM (Medical Image Communication) standard and the Japanese "second common" standard for medical communications over networks.

Health Level Seven (HL7) defines transactions for transmitting data about patient registration, admission, discharge and transfers, insurance, charges and payers, orders and results for laboratory tests, image studies, nursing and physician observations, diet orders, pharmacy orders, supply orders, and master files. The HL7 standard is supported by most system vendors and used in most large US hospitals today. It is also used in many foreign countries. HL7 is also developing transactions to exchange information about appointment scheduling, problem lists, clinical trial enrollments, patient permissions, voice dictation, advanced directives, and physiological signals. Furthermore, task forces in HL7 are developing prototype transactions with new object-oriented technologies such as CORBA and Microsoft's OLE objects.

The Engineering in Medicine and Biology Society (EMB) of the Institute of Electrical and Electronic Engineers, Inc. (IEEE) is developing the MEDIX standards for the exchange of data between hospital computer systems. It is based on the International Standards Organization (ISO) standards for all seven layers of the OSI reference model. MEDIX is working on a framework model to guide the development and evolution of a compatible set of standards.

The National Council for Prescription Drug Programs (NCPDP) has developed standards for the communication of billing and eligibility information between community pharmacies and third-party payers. They have been in use since 1985 and now serve the vast majority of the nation's community pharmacies.

Data Codes

Clinical data representations have been widely used to document diagnoses and procedures. There are over 150 known code systems. The codes with the widest acceptance in the US include ICD-9-CM, CPT, SNOMED, DSM, DRG, NDC, and ULMS.

The *International Classification of Diseases* (ICD) codes are now in their tenth edition (ICD-10). These codes are maintained by the World Health Organization (WHO) and are accepted worldwide. In the US, HCFA and the National Center for Health Statistics (NCHS) have supported the development of a clinical modification of the ICD codes (ICD-9-CM). The ICD-9-CM codes were first introduced in 1977 and are updated on a regular basis by HCFA. The UHDDS, UB-82 and UB-92 forms all use the ICD-9-CM codes. WHO has been developing ICD-10 and HCFA has formed a voluntary technical panel to assist with the development of the ICD-10 procedure coding system (ICD-10-PCS). Payers require the use of ICD-9-CM codes for reimbursement purposes, but they have limited value for clinical and research purposes as a result of their lack of clinical specificity.

The Current Procedural Terminology (CPT) codes are maintained by the American Medical Association (AMA) and are widely used in the US for reimbursement and utilization review purposes. The codes are derived from medical specialty nomenclatures and are updated annually. CPT-4 was introduced in 1996.

The Systematized Nomenclature of Human and Veterinary Medicine (SNOMED) International code structure is maintained by the College of American Pathologists (CAP) and is widely accepted for describing pathological test results. It has a multiaxial (11 fields) coding structure that gives it greater clinical specificity than the ICD and CPT codes, and it has considerable value for clinical purposes. The CAP has begun to coordinate SNOMED development with the message standards organizations HL7 and ACR-NEMA. SNOMED is a leading candidate to become the

standardized nomenclature for computer-based patient record systems.

The *Diagnostic and Statistical Manual of Mental Disorders* (DSM) code is now in its fourth edition (DSM-IV). The American Psychiatric Association (APA) maintains this code structure. It sets forth a standard set of codes and descriptions for their use in diagnoses, prescriptions, research, education, and administration.

Diagnostic related groups (DRGs) codes are maintained by HCFA. They are derivatives of ICD-9-CM codes and are used to facilitate reimbursement and case-mix analysis.

The National Drug Code (NDC) code is maintained by the Food and Drug Administration (FDA) and is required for reimbursement by Medicare, Medicaid, and insurance companies.

The National Library of Medicine (NLM) maintains the Unified Medical Language System (UMLS). It contains a metathesaurus that links biomedical terminology, semantics, and formats of the major clinical coding and reference systems. It links various medical coding systems to the NLM's medical index subject headings (MeSH codes) and to each other. The UMLS also contains a specialist lexicon, a semantic network, and an information sources map.

Indicators, Data Sets, and Guidelines

Although there is no single universally accredited standard to measure health care quality, several quality indicators, data sets, and guidelines are gaining acceptance. They include the following:

- The Joint Commission on Accreditation of Health Care Organizations (JCAHO) has been developing and testing the Indicator Measurement System (IMSystem). The IMSystem includes indicators that address obstetrics, perioperative, oncology, trauma, and cardiovascular care.
- The Health Plan Employer Data and Information Set (HEDIS) has been developed with the support of the National Committee for Quality Assurance (NCQA). It identifies data to support performance measurement in the areas of quality (e.g., preventive medicine, prenatal care, acute and chronic disease, and mental

health), access and patient satisfaction, membership and utilization, and finance.

- The Uniform Hospital Discharge Data Set (UHDDS) was conceived in 1972 as a uniform but minimal data set. Since 1974 DHEW has mandated that all hospitals report inpatient admissions using this data set. It contains 14 core data elements.
- The Uniform Hospital Bill (UB-92) data set was introduced in 1992 and includes all the UHDDS elements. It has more than 90 data entry fields. All Medicare fiscal intermediaries are required to submit this form electronically to HCFA.

Computer-based Patient Records

The 1996 Institute of Medicine report defined the computer-based patient record system as:

The set of components that form the mechanism by which patient records are created, used, stored, and retrieved. It includes people, data, rules and procedures, processing and storage devices, and communication and support facilities.

A computer-based patient record is electronically maintained information about an individual's lifetime health status and health care. The computer-based patient record replaces the paper medical record as the primary record of care, meeting all clinical, legal, and administrative requirements. However, the computer-based patient record is also more than today's medical record. Information technology permits much more data to be captured, processed, and integrated, thereby providing meaningful information and contributing to the knowledge of authorized users for legitimate uses.

In order for computer-based patient record systems to accomplish their clinical, legal, and administrative requirements, an information infrastructure must be in place to support: data capture, storage, processing, communication, security, and presentation functions.

Data Capture Functions

Data capture refers to the collection and entry of data into a computer system. The data may come from patient-monitoring devices, from telemedicine applications, directly from the patient, or from others such as relatives, friends, and public health agencies. The data may be captured by such means as key entry, medical device transmission, and pattern recognition (voice, handwriting, or biological characteristics).

Data capture includes the use of controlled vocabularies and code systems to ensure common meanings for terminology. Data capture also encompasses authentication to identify the author of an entry. Authentication may also include the validation of data accuracy. Computer-based patient record system rules and procedures determine how authentication may be interpreted.

Storage Functions

Storage refers to the physical location of data. In computer-based patient record systems, health data are distributed across multiple systems at different sites. As a result of this, there must be common access protocols, retention schedules, and universal identification. Access protocols make data available to authorized users for legitimate uses. The systems must have backup and recovery mechanisms in the event of failure. Retention schedules address the maintenance of the data in active and inactive form and the permanence of the storage medium. A person's identity can be determined by many types of data in addition to common identifiers such as name and number. Universal identifiers or other methods are required for integrating health data across multiple systems at different sites.

Information Processing

Application functions provide for the effective retrieval and processing of data into useful information. These include decision support tools, such as alerts and alarms for drug–drug interactions, laboratory–drug interactions, allergies, and abnormal results. Reminders can be provided for appointments, critical path actions, medication administration, and other activities. The systems may also provide access to consensus- and evidence-driven diagnostic and treatment guidelines and protocols. The caregiver could integrate a standard guideline or protocol into a specific person's computer-based patient record, modify it to meet unique circumstances, and use it as a basis for managing and documenting care. Outcomes data communicated from various caregivers and health care recipients may also be analyzed and used for continual improvement of the guidelines and protocols.

Communication

Information communication refers to the interoperability of systems and linkages for the exchange of data across disparate systems. To integrate health data across multiple systems at different sites, identifier systems (unique numbers or other methodology) for health care recipients, caregivers, providers, payers, and sites are essential. Infrastructures that connect all participants under standard data communication protocols are key to the linkage function. Hundreds of types of transactions or messages must be defined and agreed to by the participating stakeholders. Computer-based patient record systems must provide access to point-of-care information databases and knowledge sources, such as pharmaceutical formularies, referral databases, and reference literature.

Security

Computer-based patient record systems provide better protection of confidential health information than paper-based systems, because only authorized users with legitimate uses have access to health information. Security functions address both the confidentiality of private health information and the integrity of the data. Security functions must be designed to ensure compliance with applicable laws, regulations, and standards. They must limit access to those who are both authorized to use the data and have legitimate purposes for its use. Security functions must also provide a way to audit for inappropriate access.

Information Presentation

The wealth of information available through computer-based patient record systems must be managed to ensure that authorized caregivers and others with legitimate uses have the information that they need in their preferred presenta-

tion form. Caregivers, for instance, may wish to have tailored views of data by source, caregiver, encounter, problem, dates, or other variables. Data may need to be presented in detail or summary form. Tables, graphs, narrative, and other forms of information presentation must be accommodated. Some users may need only to know of the presence or absence of certain data, not the nature of the data itself, e.g., a life insurance company may not need health data for potentially high-risk people if computer-based patient records could be probed to determine whether a criteria set has been met. This would help to protect the confidentiality of private health information.

Current System Costs

The cost of these systems ranges from $5000 to $50,000 for single-provider, multiple-workstation environments, to $50,000 to $300,000 for single-location, eight-physician, 40-workstation systems. For practices with multiple sites and 20 or more practitioners with over 100 workstations, prices range from $150,000 to $1,000,000. Most vendors support problem-oriented medical records, several coding systems, and graphical user interfaces. They have extensive search capabilities, easy access to data, and email interfaces. The vendors all have training programs with many supporting online help screens. All major systems have password protection, although few require regular password changes and almost none can generate passwords automatically. Most systems maintain data accuracy and integrity using multiple methodologies. Many can limit who enters the data, provide redundant data storage, and track who enters the data and who makes changes.

Many systems can compile patient profiles based on demographic data, disease states, and other variables. Record- and case-management elements are included in all the systems. Most systems can generate appointment reminders; many allow patients to access their own records in the clinic, and a few permit access from the patients' homes. The better systems include the ability to print educational materials, and some include catalogs and inventories of previously developed material. An increasing number have integrated web browsers.

Data Security

Security is the protection of information systems against unauthorized access and against the denial of service to authorized users. Computer-based patient record systems must include a variety of security features to preserve the privacy and property rights of patients, providers (individual caregivers and enterprises), and others who interact with the patient record. The essential features of a secure system and network include authentication, authorization, integrity, audit trails, disaster prevention/recovery, and secure data storage and transmission.

Authentication

Authentication is assuring the identity of a subject or object, e.g., ensuring that a user is whom he or she claims to be, or confirming that the source of data is as claimed. Authentication can be accomplished through biometric identifiers (e.g., fingerprint, retinal scan, voice print); the use of a smart card, token, or other physical thing one possesses; a password; or a combination of these. One of the most prevalent means of authentication is passwords. Passwords stored on the system must be encrypted, and they should expire at routine intervals.

The opportunity for unauthenticated users to utilize another's access can be minimized through the use of automatic logoff after a stated period of inactivity or when the authenticated user accesses the system from another terminal. The logon and logoff processes should be quick and efficient so that users will comply with the requirement that they log off after completing their activity.

Authorization

Authorization is the granting of rights, which includes granting of access based on access rights. Authorization enables authenticated users to have access to the functions, information, and privileges that they request from the system. Authorization includes both authorization to

connect to the system and authorization to gain access to resources in the system. It also provides evidence of action on data.

Integrity

Integrity means that information is changed only in a specified and authorized manner. Data integrity, program integrity, system integrity, and network integrity are all part of this. Data integrity refers to the accuracy, consistency, and completeness of data. Data errors can lead to erroneous actions by caregivers, so data integrity measures ensure that data have not been changed or destroyed in an unauthorized manner. Program integrity refers to the quality of software design and protection against modification. Software "bugs" and software design complexity can contribute to corruption or loss of information. Effective software development tools must be used to design application systems. System integrity is the ability of an automated system to perform in an unimpaired manner, free from deliberate or accidental manipulation. Hardware and software features should be used to periodically validate the correct operation of the system hardware. In addition, sound backup and recovery procedures are needed for quick and secure recovery in the event of a system failure. Network integrity extends system integrity to interconnected local and wide area networks.

Audit Trails

An audit trail is a chronological record of activities occurring in the system. Audit trails can be examined to detect and investigate breaches in security, to determine compliance with established procedures, and to reconstruct a sequence of events affecting the information. Audit trail records contain the identification of the user, data source (for automated devices), person about whom the health information is recorded, provider facility, and other participant users if applicable. Audit trail records also contain the date/time and location of the activity and the nature of the activity.

Disaster Prevention/Recovery

Disaster recovery is the process whereby an enterprise would restore any loss of data in the event of fire, vandalism, natural disaster, or system failure. To ensure the safety of and prevent the potential loss of data, the computer-based patient record system needs to support the organization's disaster recovery plan. This includes measures to protect health information from damage, minimize disruption, ensure stability, and provide for orderly recovery in the event of a disaster. There should be redundant system components such as processors, network links, and databases. The system must back up information without impairing its functions, and it must be able to recreate information from backups.

Data Storage and Transmission

Data storage refers to the physical location and maintenance of data. Transmission of data is the exchange of data between person and program, or program and program, when the sender and receiver are remote from each other. Physical location considerations include physical security for processors, storage media, cables, and workstations. Other data storage issues include the permanence and durability of the storage media, system maintenance, precautions against sabotage, and preventing obsolescence. Retention—the preservation of information in some form for a given period of time—is a data storage issue that is often governed by legal and regulatory requirements as well as provider policy.

Data transmission is critical to the implementation of a computer-based patient record system. Today's health care environment requires the use of information from disparate sources. Data may be accessed via remote workstations, the Internet, and complex networks supporting one or more organizations, potentially within a national information infrastructure.

Encryption should be considered for protecting information when it is impossible to control the physical storage media or the transmission network. When properly implemented, encryption can provide cost-effective protection of health care information from both unauthorized disclosure and unauthorized changes during transit. Essential to encryption is a numeric value called the *key* that becomes part of the encryption. Many different types of encryption

algorithms are available, but the most widely used are DES, a *symmetric* or *secret* key algorithm, and RSA, an *asymmetric* or *public* key algorithm. Currently most encrypted transactions use symmetric keys to encrypt and decrypt the text or transaction. That encrypted text is sent to the other party along with the secret key, which itself is encrypted and decrypted using asymmetric RSA encryption.

This combined method of encryption not only assures data privacy; it also enables an authentication mechanism called the *digital signature*. Public keys are generally authenticated with *digital certificates*, which accompany transactions and are signed by a *certificate authority*, which officially links a public key to the user.

Connecting a network to different network systems requires the implementation of a *firewall* to serve as a control point and filter. A firewall is simply a barrier between two networks – in most cases an internal network, often called the trusted network, and an external network, the so-called untrusted network (in many cases the Internet). Firewalls examine incoming and outgoing packets and, according to a set of rules defined by the administrator, either let them through or block them.

Security Requirements

In 1995 the Medical Records Confidentiality Act came before Congress. It established the concept of a *health information trustee* and set up provisions for inspecting, copying, correcting, or amending medical records. It also placed time limits on the disclosure of information, established who was authorized/accountable for disclosure, and set up stiff sanctions for access. The bill was not passed by Congress.

In 1996 the Health Insurance Portability and Accountability Act (HIPAA–Kennedy–Kassenbaum Act) was passed. It called for the establishment of an electronic patient record and rules for privacy. It called for federal efforts to standardize health data, including unique health identifiers for every individual, employer, health plan, and health care provider. A National Committee on Vital and Health Statistics was established with the purpose of reporting to the Secretary of HHS on data standards, security and confidentiality provisions, and the implementation of unique identifiers. The committee has now reported to the Secretary, and full implementation awaits her final recommendations.

The JCAHO is responsible for accrediting hospitals for Medicare and Medicaid programs. It has a number of standards on information confidentiality, security, and integrity.

Decision Support Systems

Decision support systems can help clinicians and administrators to assess the quality of care delivered at their institutions. A few systems can help to make diagnoses. Systems for assessing quality of care usually try to normalize the acuity of the patients seen at the institution in order to compare it with some recognized national standard. The most widely used systems of this type are the MedisGroups, Acuity Index, Apache II, Computerized Severity Index System, and PRAGmatic System. The MedisGroups are based on the normative risk of organ failure and change in clinical status. They involve normative criteria for 260 key clinical findings. They identify admission severity, in-house morbidity, and discharge status. The Acuity Index is based on UHDDS and UB-82 data. It uses ICD-9-CM procedures and diagnosis. It is based on a large data set from California and assigns a severity scale to each DRG. It provides adjusted LOS, charges and mortality for each DRG. The Apache II index predicts mortality in an intensive care setting. It uses physiological data and a coefficient assigned to the principal diagnosis. It depends heavily on the assigned diagnosis. The Computerized Severity Index System uses DRGs and normative criteria for all diagnoses created by physician panels. It uses a four-point scale for each diagnosis and is useful for concurrent or retrospective consideration of care. The PRAGmatic System creates patient risk-adjusted groups (PRAGS). It uses UB-82 data and has 882 risk categories. Diagnostic support systems include Dxplain, Iliad, and Quick Medical Reference (QMR). These programs accept patient historical, clinical, and laboratory findings as input and then produce a list of possible diagnostic classifications. They have not proven to be very useful clinically and have not been widely accepted.

Health Care on the Internet

The Internet health care industry comprises five segment areas: (1) health information services; (2) health care services; (3) community health sites; (4) connectivity/communications; and (5) e-commerce.

The most successful commercial Internet portals to date have been those providing health information to physicians, patients, and other interested consumers. These sites update and aggregate expert information from a variety of sites. Providers are better able to stay current through customized literature searches and electronic continuing medical education. Effective portals produce better-informed consumers who can avoid unnecessary use of providers while making the actual visits more productive. Commercial content sites such as Healtheon/WebMD and DrKoop are funded via commercial advertising on their sites. Content sites maintained by hospitals, clinics, and drug companies serve as extensions of their advertising and name recognition campaigns. Sites maintained by governmental units, universities, clinics, and nonprofit groups try to further their own educational mission through these sites.

In addition to pure content, the best portals feature communities of users who actively engage in discussion with others who share similar experiences and interests. These "user groups" lend support to people with particular diseases, providers looking to their colleagues for answers to clinical and health services questions, and special-interest groups looking to rally people with a common health goal. In the future we can expect interactive applications, such as disease management and risk profiling, which will seek to modify the behavior of these health care communities. Pioneering programs in the online management of patients with congestive heart failure and diabetes mellitus are already demonstrating their value in reducing emergency room visits, lowering hospitalization rates, and improving the overall quality of life.

The health care industry is one of the least advanced commercial segments in the adoption of information technology to improve information exchange. The Internet's wide reach and connectivity has the potential to bring together all health care participants. Easy and timely access to the Internet can produce a marked decrease in administrative costs. Leading vendors of health care information systems are already moving to Internet-capable applications for electronically delivering medical records, claims submissions, referrals, eligibility verifications, laboratory reports, prescriptions, email, and other clinical and administrative data.

The online consumer health care market (e-commerce) includes prescription pharmacies, over-the-counter drugs, nutraceuticals, and personal care products. Health-related e-commerce also encompasses other products, including health insurance and business-to-business services.

Despite the tremendous potential for Internet health care, some consumers and practitioners remain wary of placing sensitive information online. The Health Insurance Portability and Accountability Act of 1996 mandates security provisions to assure data confidentiality. Still, the technology to allay these fears and fulfill the HIPAA requirements already exists in the form of firewalls, secured socket layers that support key lengths of 128 bits or greater, and digital certificates for authenticating users.

Email

The use of electronic mail in clinical care has the potential to change the nature of interactions between patients and their providers, increase patient satisfaction, and improve patient education. Email has been in use in some form for more than 25 years, but in recent years its use has grown exponentially. However, a recent survey of physicians conducted by Healtheon indicates that only 3% of physicians routinely use email with their patients, although a larger percentage has used email with their patients at some point, and the overall use has risen since an earlier survey. Healtheon's survey identifies four areas that physicians view as barriers to using email in practice: lack of patient use, security concerns, liability fears, and increased office workload.

Community Health Care Networks

A community health care network (CHIN) is an integrated collection of computer and telecommunications capabilities that facilitates the communication of patient, clinical, and financial information among multiple parties within a targeted geographic area. It eases the administrative and bureaucratic burden borne by hospitals, payers, and their staff. It streamlines the delivery of health care.

The constituents of the CHINs are physicians, hospitals, employers, banks, government, laboratories, pharmacies, and payers. There are three levels of CHIN services. Level I involves administrative and financial transactions, such as health plan verification, claims processing, payment processing, clinical applications, and supply transactions. Level II involves augmented transactions, such as data storage, data analysis, data access, and cost, outcomes, and utilization analysis. Level III involves interactive transactions, such as appointment reservations, concurrent utilization management, remote patient monitoring and imaging, and multimedia applications. The early enthusiasm for CHINs has now markedly decreased as a result of the growth of the Internet and the fact that most functions of CHINs can be conducted over the Internet more easily and at a lower cost.

Telemedicine

Telemedicine uses technology to deliver medical services to the point of need. In its report on the evaluation of the clinical applications of telemedicine, a committee of the Institute of Medicine defined telemedicine as "the use of electronic information and communications technologies to provide and support health care when distance separates the participants."

Telemedicine covers a range of technologies, including telephone, radio, facsimile, modem, and video. It may or may not be conducted in real time. Robotics and virtual reality interfaces have been introduced into some experimental applications.

Telemedicine uses various terrestrial and space-based (satellite) transmission media. The medium that is used is important, because its capacity limits the type of technology that may be used. Narrow-bandwidth systems, such as ordinary telephone lines, are inexpensive but lack the capacity for full-motion video. They may be adequate, however, for transmitting still images, voice, text, or data. Interactive video may work on relatively narrow bandwidths if data compression is used, but the images are sometimes too jerky to permit resolution of detail or subtle movement. The minimum data rate for full-motion video (30 frames/s) at the present time is 384 kilobytes/s (kb/s), which requires three ISDN lines. Broad-bandwidth networks permit interactive, full-motion video, but these networks are costly because transmission charges are directly related to bandwidth. Certain rural health care providers may be eligible for telecommunications subsidies.

Most of the early telemedicine programs used interactive video to bring patients, referring providers, and consultants together. From 1959 to the 1970s, telemedicine was tested in medical schools, state psychiatric hospitals, municipal airports, jails, nursing homes, Native American reservations, and other settings. Most of these early programs proved too costly to be self-sustaining and were terminated when external funding ran out.

The clinical applications of telemedicine are even more varied than the technologies, although considerable attention has been focused on the use of interactive video for specialty and subspecialty consultation in rural areas. The generic interactive video telemedicine system typically uses fixed, studio-type video equipment to link a rural facility with an urban tertiary care center. Consultants communicate with patients and often with their primary care providers in an interactive situation. The precise configuration of these networks varies, ranging from a single source of referrals (e.g., a rural community hospital) and a single source of consultants (e.g., an academic medical center) to complex "hub-and-spoke" networks involving many referring and consulting facilities.

Almost every clinical specialty has used telemedicine in some way, although some have used it more than others have, e.g., radiologists have embraced the technology on a large scale. Cardiologists, dermatologists, and psychiatrists have been the clinical specialists most actively involved in telemedicine. The reasons for this are unclear, but this distribution may represent a kind of "founder's effect," because physicians practicing these specialties were among the first to use telemedicine.

Although the early 1990s saw the proliferation of telemedicine systems that provided real-time, broad-bandwidth, synchronous consultations, the focus has shifted toward more personal computer-based "store-and-forward" telemedicine. Store-and-forward technology can be used to forward medical records, laboratory results, and radiographs and other diagnostic images to a consultant. The data can be reviewed, and a report of diagnostic impressions can be emailed to the referring physician.

With a few exceptions (teleradiology, some telepathology, and some cardiologic data and facsimile transmission applications), Medicare reimbursement of fee-for-service telemedicine is generally not available. The reasons for this are complex, but the most immediate impediment to the coverage of telemedicine is that it does not meet the requirements of the Health Care Financing Administration (HCFA) for in-person, face-to-face contact between providers and patients. Thus, most medical consultation through telecommunications technology is ineligible for payment. Moreover, HCFA has expressed concern about the lack of solid cost data, but it is studying the issue and is funding demonstration projects. Other payers have been slow to set policies of their own, although, in several states, some commercial insurance companies, Blue Cross/Blue Shield, and Medicaid pay for telemedicine services.

Lack of reimbursement for telemedicine services is only one of several factors impeding its expansion, e.g., licensure is regulated by individual states, and bills have been introduced or passed in some states that severely limit the interstate practice of medicine through telemedicine. A second difficulty concerns liability and malpractice. Some providers are concerned that the use of telemedicine may increase their risk, e.g., a technical failure or inferior image could lead to an adverse patient outcome. Some are concerned that if telemedicine permits high-quality care, they might be liable for failure to use it. It is not yet possible to assess the validity of these concerns. Finally, the issue of confidentiality remains contentious.

Chief Information Officer

Historically the management of information technology resided at a department-level leadership position. Usually the person in this position was called the vice-president for medical information systems, data-processing manager, or medical information technology director. The person reported to the chief financial officer. The position usually was operations rather than strategy oriented and concentrated on technical rather than enterprise issues. As the need for information management has increased in most health care organizations, this position has become more prominent. It is often an enterprise-level executive called a chief information officer (CIO) who is involved in strategy and tactical decisions. Individuals in this position have varied backgrounds and usually have advanced degrees in management, computer science, medical informatics, and/or many years of hands-on experience.

The CIO is usually an executive team member who is involved in information technology (IT) planning, development, trend analysis, forecasting, and capital building. This person exercises leadership in financial, strategic, and operational planning. He or she is involved in the education of senior management in all areas of IT.

The CIO typically spends 30% of his or her time on planning, 30% on coordination, 20% on implementation, 10% on operations, and 10% on maintenance. Planning activities include developing the hospital business plan, strategic IT plan development, hospital and information technology budgeting, and security and disaster recovery planning. Coordination includes serving on IT committees, developing IT policies and procedures, evaluation and selection of

software, and integration with hospital operations. Implementation involves developing IT guidelines, executing plans, and vendor relations. Operations involve the setting of policies and procedures and the oversight of IT managers. Maintenance involves establishing user training and support functions, monitoring systems functionality, and establishing a program of regular system updates.

Vendor Selection

A major function of the CIO will be vendor selection and system development. IT vendors can be segmented into five areas: software; hardware; services; telecommunications and network services; and system integration. Software vendors can be divided into those that provide comprehensive integrated systems and those that supply niche markets. The field is constantly changing through mergers, acquisitions, and alliances. The track record and viability of a software vendor must be a consideration in any software purchase. Hardware vendors are increasingly made up of a few dominant players, including IBM, Dell, SUN, and Silicon Graphics. Telecommunications and network suppliers make up the fastest-growing segment of the hardware and software market. Most do not have systems that are specifically geared toward health care. AT & T and Cisco are major players in this area. System integration vendors are usually consultant groups. Typically they help to connect disparate elements of the IT enterprise. Major players in this area are the big five consulting firms (such as Anderson Consulting) as well as Hewlett Packard Health Systems and Perot.

In selecting a health care information system, one has two major choices: buy a packaged, integrated system or build a customized system. The integrated system is the most common route and involves the least risk for the purchaser. The vendor has already dealt with the interface problems between the various elements of the system. Installing such a system does not require the high level of expertise needed to build a customized system. These systems' major drawbacks include a higher initial price and the fact that the system may not have universally excellent elements. The customized option permits the purchaser to "cherry pick" the best programs in each application area. However, system integration may be difficult, and such systems tend to require a longer development period.

In selecting a vendor, one typically uses a request for information (RFI) and a request for proposal (RFP). The RFI is usually sent first and asks for information about the vendor, such as basic sales and marketing literature. The RFP describes the purchaser's organization and its requirements. It asks for the history and financial condition of the vendor, its user base, references, training, support, and competitive features. It then presents a very detailed list of questions for the vendor to respond to in a set period of time. It also asks for a firm price and delivery date. Once the RFPs have been received and the top two or three are selected, it is best to visit operational sites. The vendor should be asked to provide a list of possible sites, with the purchaser making the final selection.

18

Medical Risk Management and Contracting (the Business of Medicine)

Michael E. Bernstein

Managed Care Defined

The term "managed care" is often used without definition, yet it is an extremely versatile descriptor. We might be referring to the health maintenance organization (HMO) industry, the act of utilization management, the exclusive nature of the provider network, or a rules-based approach to providing medical care. In this chapter the term "managed care" is intended to refer to all insurance products that feature a limited provider network, risk assumption (usually capitation) by the providers, and a comprehensive level of benefits. The terms "utilization management" or "medical management" will refer to the act of reviewing and controlling the delivery of medical surgical care, whether conducted internally by the provider or externally by the insurer.

Managed-care programs are ubiquitous. Although there are still parts of the country where HMO offerings are limited, most population centers feature robust local, regional, and even national HMO plans. Even the rural markets have witnessed the growth of managed-care plans, despite the absence of competition among providers in rural communities, which is often the impetus for HMO development. Given the significant penetration of managed-care programs in most markets, it is common for a physician practice to include a significant number of managed-care patients. If the physician works within a large multispecialty medical group or for an integrated health system, it is not unusual for the percentage of managed-care patients to approach 50% of that physician's total patient roster.

Even as external medical management (utilization management that is conducted by the insurer or its specialized subcontractor) is under siege in the political arena, the risk inherent in capitated managed-care programs practically requires providers to do their own self-focused medical management programs. As large managed-care organizations such as United Healthcare announce their intention to reduce or eliminate their active and aggressive medical management of physicians, the risk of overutilization, duplication, and other wasteful practices will fall even more heavily on the capitated physician groups. Rather than reducing the likelihood that physicians will face medical management, this move by the national insurance companies to reduce scrutiny may actually cause the number of utilization management programs to grow as provider organizations take on the role of managing risk. In fact, the diversity of providers doing their own medical management may increase the complexity, administrative demands, and inconsistencies that cause medical management to draw fire from critics.

Types of Risk Arrangements

There are a variety of risk arrangements that physician groups and medical systems routinely undertake. These range from the relatively simple withholds (see below) to complex and high-risk global capitation. Component capitation, in which the provider organization is capitated for a specific type or category of care, is perhaps the most common form of risk sharing. The term "capitation" is derived from "per capita". In practice, capitation is a prepaid amount, commonly calculated on a per-member per-month (hereafter referred to as pmpm) basis, which is intended to be payment in full for all services provided to the identified population within defined health care guidelines. If a physician organization is globally capitated for a given population, it is responsible for either providing all care covered by the HMO policy or paying for such care when it is provided by others. Although some globally capitated physician groups get into trouble when required to provide more care than anticipated, it is far more common to be unexpectedly harmed by the obligation to pay other participating providers out of the group's capitation. Often, the HMO administers the program by paying claims on behalf of the capitated provider but reporting the outside utilization of care and claims payments retrospectively. These purchased-service payments are then offset against future capitation payments to the capitated physician group, causing a reduction in the group's cash flow. This negative cash flow phenomenon is seldom encountered by provider organizations that are capitated for only the care that they render, without financial risk for services provided by other participating providers.

In contrast to capitation, the most primitive risk arrangement is the simple withhold. A withhold is a defined percentage of each fee-for-service payment made to a provider that is retained by the payer for the purpose of reserving against risk fund deficits. A risk fund deficit results when the HMO pays out more in claims for the designated members than is budgeted for that purpose. Usually, in a withhold contract, the risk-bearing provider's loss is limited to the amount of the withhold. If the risk fund deficit is smaller than the amount withheld, the surplus withhold is customarily paid to the risk-bearing provider. As withholds represent payment reductions in advance of any need, whereas risk fund performance reporting occurs after the fact, and often with dubious accuracy, providers are apt to treat these arrangements as discounts rather than risk sharing. In other words, they do not budget or otherwise anticipate a return of with-

hold funds. Although the withhold was intended to reward efficient behavior, once the provider treats the withhold as a discount, the financial incentive is gone. It is because of the passive nature of the withhold that HMOs have favored the higher risk and more complicated capitation methods that are so common today.

Capitation contracts, in addition to defining the scope of the care that must be provided, also define the amount of the pmpm payment. The pmpm capitation payments may be arrayed by the age and sex of each member, e.g., the provider organization may be paid $15 pmpm for a 14- to 18-year-old boy and $25 pmpm for a 14- to 18-year-old girl, as a result of the actuarially determined levels of care normally required by different demographic groups. The amount of the pmpm payment may be a predetermined dollar figure or a defined percentage of the premium paid by the enrollee. Although a percent-of-premium capitation allows the capitated provider to be more closely aligned with the HMO, sharing the benefits of disciplined rate setting, it also puts the provider squarely at risk for undisciplined or predatory pricing behavior that sometimes occurs in hyper-competitive markets. For this reason, percent-of-premium capitation arrangements occur most often when there is an ownership link between the HMO and the provider organization.

The Health Care Market Forces Providers to Assume Risk

The author has noted at least four unique market influences that have accelerated the demands on providers to assume risk. The first, and most prominent, is governmental action. States, with the approval of the federal government, have instituted managed-care initiatives for their Medicaid populations all over the country. The institution of a Medicaid HMO initiative often forces large numbers of government-funded patients to select a private HMO to manage their care. As a consequence, in markets where the development of commercial HMOs has been slow or otherwise hampered by provider reluctance, providers must now agree to contract with the HMOs in order to maintain their Medicaid patient load. Even in affluent communities, physician practices can rarely flourish without these government-funded patients.

More recently, the federal government has encouraged the development of Medicare risk programs. Unlike Medicaid HMO programs, which often force Medicaid enrollees to select an HMO if two or more are offered in the marketplace, Medicare HMO enrollment is always voluntary. In the mid- and late 1990s, the rates that the federal government was willing to pay commercial HMOs in the most densely populated senior communities were so substantial that the managed-care companies expanded rapidly in these markets. Competition forced the HMOs to offer increasingly attractive plans to the senior patients, including inducements such as low or no premium to the member and prescription drug coverage. As with the Medicaid initiatives, the rapid movement of senior patients into commercial HMOs forced otherwise reluctant providers to contract with the HMOs that were now able to control access to the hugely important Medicare patients.

The second major market phenomenon that increased the pace at which providers were required to assume risk was the expansion of the publicly traded HMOs, such as United Healthcare, Humana, Oxford, and Aetna/US Healthcare. These well-financed, aggressive companies entered new markets and expanded in their existing markets through acquisition and facile marketing programs. In the mid-1990s, as the equity markets were rewarding these companies with high stock valuations, the growth in HMO membership was quite dramatic. As a result of their ability to use their stock as acquisition currency, the most prominent publicly traded HMOs were acquiring regional and local HMOs, often provider owned, thereby entering smaller markets that had escaped the attention of the national insurers and managed-care companies.

The publicly traded HMOs were not content to simply acquire other HMOs. In fact, the trend in the late 1990s was to acquire indemnity insurers, with the intention to convert these indemnity or fee-for-service populations into HMO members. One variation on this theme was the acquisition of the US Healthcare HMO operation by Aetna. Here a powerful, largely indemnity insurer intended to convert its huge fee-for-service membership to a risk-based HMO by acquiring that critical mass and expertise from the eastern HMO market leader.

When the equity markets began to lose enthusiasm for the health care sector, and particularly HMO stocks, the pace of acquisition activity slowed considerably. Smaller transactions occur infrequently, but it is still common to see the publicly traded HMOs acquire insured populations from the old-line insurers that have decided to exit the challenging and erratic health insurance business.

Aggressive and creative product development is the third factor that contributed to the rapid expansion of risk taking in the provider world. As "freedom of choice," the term used to describe less restrictive benefit plans, became a popular subject and object of desire, the HMO industry reacted by developing point of service (POS) products. These new POS plans usually looked like HMOs but, rather than providing no coverage for members seeking care outside a provider network, the POS plan simply reduced coverage. In effect, the POS product operated like the familiar major medical indemnity policies that offered substantial, though not complete, coverage (usually 80% of the cost of care), but rewarded the use of specified providers with far more complete coverage (often 100%). Although these "open-panel HMOs" were forced to assume some risk themselves in these programs, they continued to capitate providers for much of the care that was expected to be obtained from within the HMO network. In some cases, providers were expected to share or even assume the risk for the amount of care that their patients sought outside the network.

The fourth phenomenon that has contributed to the expansion of provider risk-taking is consolidation in the provider community. The 1990s saw the rise of the large, integrated health systems. Initially, consolidation of provider organizations was driven by the hospital industry. Hospital systems, both for profit and, more recently, not for profit, have been expanding through acquisition and mergers at unprecedented rates. These well-capitalized operations began acquiring physician practices, forming what has been termed "integrated delivery systems". In fact, these large, vertically integrated provider organizations often fail to achieve anything more than consolidation of ownership. They are often characterized by complex governance, multiple incompatible computer systems, and incompatible cultures.

Later, partly in response to the rise of hospital-led consolidation, multispecialty physician groups began to consolidate into large physician-led organizations. The development of these large, or even giant, clinics was often explained as necessary in order to preserve leverage when dealing with the sophisticated HMO or hospital industries. Although these large physician groups could presumably generate efficiencies from scale, this has seldom been the focus or outcome of these consolidations. It is common, however, for the largest physician groups to have a more substantial share of their revenue derived from capitated programs.

Contracting Strategies

Vertical Integration

As described previously, a common global strategy for addressing the increased risk inherent in this age of managed care is vertical integration. This strategy entails forming a health care organization that can offer a comprehensive scope of care, from primary care in the office to specialty and tertiary care in the inpatient setting and follow-up care in the home. These integrated delivery systems often incorporate long-term care options as well, such as skilled nursing facilities. These organizations are perfectly poised to accept global capitation, given that most or all of the care required by HMO members can be provided within the enterprise.

It is still uncertain whether the vertical integration model will succeed. There have been some notorious failures, such as Allegany, but others continue to develop and may prove successful. The challenge of integrating the vastly divergent cultures of the physicians and hospitals and managing the enormously complex infrastructure of health care, and the barriers presented by the regulatory environment are just a few of the reasons that this strategy may not be practical. Although the antitrust regulators were quite liberal with health care provider mergers

in the early and mid-1990s, there seems to be a heightened level of scrutiny today.

Horizontal Integration

Horizontal integration is another global strategy for addressing the increased risk created by the managed-care environment. Structurally, this approach is far less complicated. It involves merging similar health care entities into larger organizations. Rather than pursuing the comprehensive scope of care that characterizes vertically integrated organizations, horizontally integrated entities are merely trying to achieve larger scale. The premise is that a multihospital system, if appropriately constituted, can serve all, or at least some, of the needs of any given HMO.

Horizontal integration is usually justified by the economies of scale that can be realized. Although the obvious cultural barriers inherent in combining physician and hospital organizations are not present, there are still notable cultural challenges in horizontally integrated combinations. The health care market has distinct sectors, even among like provider types. For-profit hospitals and physician groups operate very differently from their not-for-profit counterparts. Academic hospitals and physician organizations are likewise uniquely different than their community-based equivalents. Horizontal integration efforts often try to bridge these differences by merging providers from different sectors. Strategically, these mergers usually make sense because of the practical or competitive market opportunities that are inferred by their combination. The cultural differences, however, often prevent these horizontal combinations from ever reaching their full potential.

Niche Strategy

A final global strategy for weathering the challenges of managed-care contracting is developing a niche profile. This strategy is usually employed by highly specialized providers or those more conventional organizations that are blessed with unique market characteristics (e.g., the only hospital or clinic in town). A niche strategy calls for going it alone.

A highly specialized niche provider, such as a hospice or home care organization, may represent such a small component of health care costs that the HMO industry will not demand that they be capitated. Although this allows the niche provider to avoid the risk of this form of reimbursement, it also denies them the obvious economic benefits of providing the most efficient level of care. Likewise, a hospital that controls the inpatient niche for a given community can often demand its own terms from an interested HMO. These negotiations are often characterized by brinkmanship, because the HMO may threaten to move the care of its members to another nearby community, although solo community hospitals and clinics usually have the upper hand because of patient loyalty.

Obviously, a successful niche strategy depends on being able to protect and maintain one's niche. Competition, in the form of either other niche providers or integrated delivery systems expanding to incorporate your niche, can usurp the fragile benefit of this strategy. Niche providers must make an objective assessment of the barriers to entry that face new entrants into their markets.

Management of Risk

Quality versus Utilization Management

Medical management activities often have two distinct goals, quality improvement and economically focused utilization management. Quite often, the same management staff are responsible for both quite dissimilar activities. In the mid-1990s the effort to accredit HMOs as quality-focused organizations picked up steam. It is very common today for large and even modest-sized HMOs to be NCQA (National Commission for Quality Assurance) accredited. Interestingly, the NCQA review is not as concerned with the quality of the care or clinical outcomes that members receive from a given HMO as it is with the existence of a constant and consistent process for reviewing, reacting to, and improving quality measures.

Unlike utilization management, which tries to enforce the most efficient delivery of care in order to avoid unnecessary medical costs, quality management has little or no economic

motive. Quality assurance activities are normally embraced by the rank-and-file providers in a medical group. Utilization management efforts, by their nature, are often invasive, annoying, and cumbersome. Physicians tend to dismiss this activity as pure harassment. With the advent of global capitation risk, many provider organizations have begun to undertake these medical management responsibilities that were formerly the function of managed-care organizations and insurance companies. This poses interesting cultural challenges as the medical group itself begins to monitor and enforce efficient clinical practice by its physicians.

Information Needs

The greatest technological challenge in assuming managed-care risk and medical management activity is data collection and dissemination. Although every managed-care organization and provider collects data, few can boast that they have done a good job of informing their physicians about critical measures of their performance. The problem is one of fragmentation. Inpatient, outpatient, ambulatory, laboratory, imaging, and pharmacy encounters are often billed or paid from separate computer systems, even when provided by or paid by the same organization. Although systems integration is becoming more common, it is usually incomplete. Without the ability to link separate but related clinical activities to a single episode of care, it is difficult to achieve an acceptable level of management and efficiency. Clinicians, as scientists, are sometimes reluctant to change their practice patterns or even accept oversight without data to support findings and recommendations.

Although information technology is advancing rapidly, the cost of implementing state-of-the-art information systems is enormous. HMOs and provider organizations alike are already so dependent on computer systems for their business vitality that the act of converting to new, more capable systems represents a daunting challenge. It is not unusual for a complicated computer conversion to take six to nine months or more to complete. Hence, the technology is improving far more quickly than new systems can be put into operation.

Gatekeeper Strategies

Among the most popular strategies for managing the risk inherent to capitated HMOs is the primary care gatekeeper system. A gatekeeper HMO will require that its members select a primary care physician (PCP) as that patient's key point of access into the health care system. Generally, members are required to get all their care from that PCP or obtain a written referral from the PCP to see a specialist. This strategy presumes that the most cost-effective location for most care will be the PCP's office. Although this approach may encourage unnecessary visits to the PCP, this type of care is far less costly than hospital-based care or even a specialty office visit.

As the gatekeeper model matured, provider groups, integrated delivery systems, and hospitals all raced to develop PCP networks, at great expense. Some of the notorious provider system bankruptcies of the late 1990s have been blamed on the huge losses that resulted from the inability to manage these acquired physician practices with a reasonable return. This phenomenon has also spurred a return to less restrictive access to specialists by many HMOs. Nevertheless, the gatekeeper model is still extremely common, providing a low-tech approach to coordination of care. As the patient must contact his or her PCP before accessing most types of medical treatment, the PCP is at least nominally aware of the scope and scale of care that each patient is receiving. Theoretically, even a casually involved PCP will have the opportunity to intervene if it appears that an inappropriate level of care is being provided.

Critical Pathways and Clinical Guidelines

Many organizations have been developing protocols for the treatment of chronic diseases and conditions. This approach to medicine has been dubbed evidence-based medicine. The protocols are most commonly referred to as critical pathways or clinical guidelines. It is widely understood that there is enormous variability in how different practitioners treat the same condition.

The premise of evidence-based medicine is that it is possible to record the best practices, from both an efficiency and outcome perspective, and distribute these records as guidelines for others to follow in treating similar conditions.

Many organizations have tried to tackle the project of compiling these clinical guidelines, including large medical groups such as the Mayo Clinic, actuarial firms such as Milliman & Robertson, and business enterprises such as InterQual. In addition, many medical groups and integrated delivery systems have tried to develop their own internally focused clinical guidelines. Perhaps the most common use of the commercially available clinical guidelines is as utilization management templates for HMOs and insurance companies. These managed-care organizations require that certain types of care be preauthorized by the medical management department, which then compares the proposed plan of care to the applicable published protocol to test appropriateness.

Currently, most provider organizations that use clinical guidelines do so on a voluntary basis. In effect, the guidelines are offered to physicians and other clinical staff for informational purposes with the hope that these tools might persuade the practitioners to adopt the documented and efficient approach to care.

Conclusion

Physicians often express frustration at having to interrupt their clinical work to attend to the business of medicine. Most clinicians were not trained or educated in finance, law, government affairs, public relations, or any of the myriad skills that are required by the demands of managed care. It should be abundantly clear, however, that the complexion of the typical practice environment has been dramatically changed and that managed care is an unavoidable challenge. A willingness to learn the concepts, understand the tactics, and embrace the most beneficial components of the business of medicine will improve a new physician's chances immeasurably.

19

Marketing Issues in Managed Care

Elizabeth M. Zaher

Marketing has emerged as an important strategic function in many health care organizations. Just as the health care industry has witnessed significant change over the past 20 years, so has health care marketing. In the mid-1970s, marketing was primarily a promotional function designed to increase volume. More was better.

Today's health care market involves large delivery systems serving populations of managed-care patients, which means that there is no longer a financial advantage to providing more physician services and longer hospital stays. To survive, health care organizations must attract more patients and gain an increasing market share. Direct provider contracting with large employer coalitions means employers are now an important target market along with patients and families.

The high costs of medical buildings, medical technology, and information systems are requiring physicians to merge into multispecialty group practices. Consolidations of physician groups and hospitals mean that former health care competitors are now working together. In addition, regional and national players with tremendous resources, such as Mayo Clinic, Kaiser Permanente, United Health Care, and Aetna, are entering local markets.

The health care industry is also facing consumers empowered by today's service economy. As consumers demand and receive personalized service from their banks, hairdressers, and car repair shops, they expect the same from their health care providers. Unprecedented access to clinical and medical information on the Internet means that patients are also asking tough ques-

tions and expecting more from their health care providers.

These changes have required health care marketing to become increasingly similar to marketing in consumer industries. Instead of simply conducting promotional campaigns designed to increase volume, health care marketing involves research, customer feedback, pricing sensitivity, and distribution strategies as well as promotional efforts. Effective health care marketing requires thorough understanding of the environment in which an organization exists, clear articulation of organizational goals, being as knowledgeable as possible about competitors, and identifying target markets and their expectations for service.

This chapter familiarizes you with basic marketing concepts and how they may someday affect you in your professional practice.

Marketing Defined

The American Marketing Association (AMA) defines marketing as the process of planning and executing the conception, pricing, promotion, and distribution of ideas, goods, and services to create exchanges that satisfy individual and organizational objectives.

This definition implies that marketing is both a strategic and a tactical function. To be effective, the marketing plan must be part of an organization's strategic planning process. However, plans are nothing without effective implementation. The AMA definition also implies that an organization must be preoccupied with identifying its customers, understanding their needs, and making a commitment to meet or, ideally, exceed those needs.

Health care organizations typically provide services, not tangible products. Marketing a service such as health care creates some unique challenges. Health care services cannot be separated from the providers who deliver the care. Services within the same organization can vary depending on who is providing the care, when it is being provided, where it happens, and what else happens during the service delivery process. The challenge is to reduce variation in order to provide a consistent patient care experience at all clinical sites. Health care marketers need to feel confident that they can fulfill promises made to consumers about the type of care an organization delivers. They need to motivate their organizations to maximize every patient care experience [1].

"Moments of truth" is a phrase that describes the nuances of a consumer's experience with a product, service, or organization. A moment of truth is any experience, observation, or interaction that makes an impression about an organization in the consumer's mind. Implicit in this concept is the adage, "when expectations are met, no one notices" [2].

Organizations such as Disney, Midwest Express, Nordstrom, Ritz Carlton, and Wal-Mart are expert at managing moments of truth. Effective health care marketers concern themselves with all aspects of the care delivery experience in order to retain existing patients, attract new patients, and maximize their organization's effectiveness. From the awareness and reputation of the organization to the way in which telephones are answered and the ease of getting an appointment, health care marketers should ensure that their organizations are maximizing their moments of truth in order to build long-term customer loyalty. Keeping a current customer satisfied is easier (and cheaper) than attracting a new customer.

Health care marketers need to understand their customers and help their organizations to continually reinvent themselves to meet customer needs. If patients complain that it is inconvenient to schedule physician office visits between 9am and 4pm, organizations will have to adjust. If patients want to communicate with their physicians via email, physicians will have to comply. A "one size fits all" strategy no longer works. Patients have options and they know it [3]. The health care organization that fails to analyze and redirect itself to serve patients as customers will eventually lose patients and market share when competitors begin to innovate. In the end, the innovative organization will win.

Consumer behavior data show that the average business never hears from 96% of its unhappy clients. In addition, each complaint received represents another 26 clients with similar problems who have not come forward. Of those complaints, at least six concerns are serious. Additional data show that a dissatisfied patient will tell 9–10 other people about his or her dissatisfaction. Conversely, patients who have a positive experience will tell only three or four others [4]. Bad news travels fast and can have a strong impact on how the public perceives the service quality of a health care organization.

The Strategic Plan

An organization's strategic plan should drive its business plan. The strategic plan is global, often with at least a 3-year outlook. The business plan is usually updated annually. As marketing is both a strategic and tactical function, it should be included in both long-term strategic and annual business planning.

Strategic planning is "the set of processes used in an organization to understand the situation and develop decision-making guidelines (the strategy) for the organization" [5]. Some strategic planners add the concept of measurement to the definition to track the effectiveness of organizational efforts.

Strategic planning can be described as a process designed to answer three key questions:

1. Where are we now?
2. Where should we be going?
3. How do we get there?

Strategic planning is a disciplined, systematic way for organizations to monitor and interpret trends in their environment. Understanding the market in which it operates allows an organization to modify its mission, strategies, and objectives in order to adjust to changing environmental conditions, take advantage of new market opportunities, and avoid potential threats. Strategic planning is necessary given the simple fact that the future is not an extension of the past and that current strategies and tactics may not continue to be effective.

Situation Analysis

Strategic planning begins with a situation analysis. This section of the strategic plan answers the question: "Where are we now?" The situation analysis focuses on two items: an external assessment and an internal assessment. The external assessment includes a review of the local, regional, and national health care environments. It discusses general health care trends, regulatory and legislative concerns, managed-care issues, technological trends, and competitive concerns. The external assessment culminates in a discussion of external opportunities and threats facing the organization.

The internal assessment describes the current state of an organization. It covers such key functional areas as clinical operations, medical management, administration, business office, finance, information systems, compliance, human resources, and marketing. The internal assessment should focus on the strengths and weaknesses of the organization's operations. Ultimately, the internal assessment should describe the distinctive competencies that differentiate the organization from its competitors. Some strategic planners refer to the situation analysis as the SWOT analysis, named because it describes the organization's *strengths* and *weaknesses* as well as environmental *opportunities* and *threats*.

The situation analysis also defines and profiles customers. Health care organizations must serve multiple customers. It is critical that they answer the question: "Who are our customers and what are their wants and needs from our organization?" For example, a health care organization's customers may include:

- Patients
- Health plans/managed-care organizations
- Employers
- Physicians
- Employees
- Insurance companies and other payers
- Community
- Regulators
- Legislators
- Governmental agencies
- Hospitals.

The SWOT analysis should be applied to each of the key customer groups to identify the organization's strengths and weaknesses in serving each customer. Customer trends that may represent opportunities and threats should also be addressed.

Strategic Direction

The next section of the plan answers the question "where should we be going?" by establishing a strategic direction for the organization. This section begins with general statements about what an organization is trying to accomplish. It reviews and may even propose changes to an organization's mission, vision, and values.

Mission refers to the organization's fundamental purpose for existing. Mission statements are written to set the tone for the organization and to provide management with a broad set of directions for developing further business strategies [6], e.g., one community hospital describes its mission in this way: "Provides high quality health care services in a cost efficient manner to all who are in need; sponsors programs and activities for the benefit of the communities we serve; and fosters gifts and contributions on behalf of these activities. We are committed to providing these services for charitable, educational and scientific purposes."

The *vision* statement articulates the organization's vision for what it intends to become. It often speaks in terms of a 5-year horizon, e.g., one hospital describes its vision as "providing a seamless system of continuous, connected care and services that exceed the expectations of the people we serve."

Values describe organizational philosophies and guiding principles, including the code of behavior that guides an organization's operations. The following is an excerpt from the value statements of a multispecialty physician practice:

> We believe every patient is a unique person deserving respect, dignity and genuine concern. We strive to provide them individual, high quality care, rendered in a timely, courteous and understanding fashion. We consider our patients to be full partners in a joint effort to sustain their own good health and to assure the effectiveness of their medical treatment....

After establishing a high-level direction, the strategic plan lays out goals and objectives. The goals and objectives may be identified for central administrative departments, such as marketing, human resources, and finance, as well as clinical departments, sites, and programs. SMART is a mnemonic device that can be used in developing organizational and departmental goal statements. Effective goal statements should be:

Specific
Measurable
Actionable
Reasonable
Time-limited.

For example, a health plan's sales goal for the year could be to "increase health plan membership among employers with 500 or more employees by 10% next year". A human resource department goal could be to "reduce employee turnover by 15% next year". A multispecialty physician group's goal may be to "increase the number of patients served by 10%". Quantifying goal statements and describing a time frame for completion make them specific and easy to measure. Being "actionable" refers to a manager's ability to break apart goals into smaller steps, e.g., the goal of reducing employee turnover can be broken down into several actionable steps, including developing an employee work satisfaction survey, conducting exit interviews, and hosting monthly brown bag employee opinion discussions.

Tactical Planning

The final section of a strategic plan involves tactical implementation. The action plan describes the steps an organization will take to achieve its goals and answers the question "how do we get there?" The action plan establishes priorities, describes necessary resources (staff and financial), and lays out a time frame for completion.

The benefits of strategic planning are many. An organized, well-articulated strategic plan serves as an organizational road map, providing a clear direction, not only for management, but for all employees to follow. Disciplined planning should result in proactive behavior, forcing staff to better understand the organization and what is needed for future success. Finally, strategic planning should increase organizational performance as resources are thoughtfully allocated, performance standards are developed, and staff are engaged in achieving clear goals.

The Marketing Plan

The well-known architectural adage "form follows function" translates into the marketing application, "structure follows strategy". This means that the marketing plan should follow the direction described in an organization's strategic plan. The marketing plan typically concentrates on three strategic areas: target markets, competitive positioning, and the marketing mix.

Target Markets

Although the strategic plan describes multiple customers who interact with an organization, target markets include the *key* set of customers the organization currently serves or wishes to serve. Target markets are sets of people defined in various ways, such as geographically, by type of employer, or in other ways, e.g., people within a target market can be defined by their age, sex, income level, presence of children, lifestyle characteristics, health profile, insurance coverage, or geographic location.

The target market for a hospital obstetrics unit may be insured women, aged 18–45, who live in a certain geographic area. Clearly, identifying the target market provides direction for the creative approach used in advertising and public relations activities as well as the media used to deliver the messages, e.g., the local newspaper's sports section would be an unlikely place for the obstetrics unit to advertise, whereas the lifestyle section would be ideal.

Market Positioning

Many health care organizations are selling intangibles, meaning their products cannot be seen or held before they are purchased. A patient who needs surgery cannot know the outcome before the procedure. The surgeon will likely try to increase tangibility by describing the procedure's benefits and outcomes. If the surgeon is part of a larger organization, the organization may also work to increase the tangibility of its services by developing an image or reputation, often referred to as a *brand name* and a *market positioning* strategy.

Originally used to market and sell tangible products, a *brand* is the collective information and experience about a product, service, or organization communicated through a name, logo, tagline, and direct personal experience with the organization (a "moment of truth"). Brands are created to distinguish one product, service, or organization from another.

Although catchy advertising slogans and logos help create a brand, successful brands are much more than that. They represent an enduring promise of what an organization will deliver to its customers. It's this promise that builds trust and creates long-term, lasting customer relationships.

Branding is a strategic effort that involves identifying what makes an organization unique, what promises it intends to make to patients, and how it intends to live up to those promises. Ultimately, the brand is a summary of every experience a person has with an organization that affects the perception and value of that brand, e.g., a person's experience and perception of a brand could involve an advertisement, a medical procedure, or even a conversation with a friend.

Health care organizations can shape patients' perceptions of their brand before, during, and after an encounter. A brand's success depends on how well an organization delivers services in relation to patient expectations. All members of a health care organization—physicians, nurses, administration, even the janitorial staff—must perform as expected, or the brand is at risk [7].

One executive tells a story about his recent surgical procedure. The scheduling process, admission, hospital stay, and discharge process went smoothly, meeting his expectations for service quality. One aspect of his experience went beyond his expectations. His surgeon placed several follow-up calls to check on his recovery. One day, the surgeon was unable to reach the executive at his office or home, so he tried his cellular phone. The executive was shocked to be standing in O'Hare Airport, 120 miles from home, and receiving a follow-up call from his surgeon. This was a memorable moment of truth for this satisfied and loyal patient.

Fortunately, there is such a thing as a second chance in brand management. If a mistake is made, organizations can use this as an opportunity to demonstrate their commitment to service. In fact, customer loyalty actually can increase if mistakes are quickly and sensitively resolved [8].

Campbell's Soup, McDonald's, Coca-Cola, and Disney all represent strong, enduring consumer brands with powerful market advantages:

- Strong brands differentiate a product/organization from its competitors.
- Strong brands create long-term customer relationships.
- Strong brands make it easier for prospective customers to switch their purchase patterns.
- Strong brands enhance customer retention.

Mayo is probably the number one brand in health care. When it was a single-location organization in Rochester, Minnesota, word-of-mouth marketing built the Mayo Clinic brand. Patients told family members and friends about their experiences. Today, with its multiple health care ventures, Mayo uses a sophisticated brand management program to monitor perceptions of its brand, to conduct research to identify opportunities for brand extensions, to educate all Mayo entities about the value of its brand, and to support branding projects throughout the Mayo enterprise.

Although branding describes product attributes and promises, *positioning* occurs in the minds of consumers, e.g., 7-Up is a brand with specific attributes—clear, carbonated beverage with a refreshing taste. The tagline "The Uncola" is a positioning statement designed to establish a place for 7-Up in consumers' minds compared with its soft drink competitors.

Probably without realizing it, hospitals have been positioning themselves for years, e.g., some hospitals are commonly known as "heart hospitals," "cancer hospitals," "children's hospitals," or "transplant hospitals". The marketing plan should articulate an organization's branding and positioning strategy and reinforce the advantages of consistently implementing the strategy. Branding (building awareness of product/service attributes) and positioning (carving out a unique place in the market compared with competitors) should be the core of the marketing plan. The plan should also translate your brand strategy into interrelated tactical actions, e.g., advertising, direct mail, brochures, and Internet sites all need to communicate the same messages with a unified look and feel.

Typically, the development of a branding and positioning strategy begins with market research. Health care organizations need to get out and talk with people who have experience with their organizations. Research should include both statistically valid quantitative research and focus groups, personal interviews, or other qualitative methods.

Marketing Mix

One of the basic marketing concepts is the four Ps: *product*, *price*, *placement*, and *promotion*. Health care *products* can range from services delivered to patients to prepaid health insurance plans offered by health maintenance organizations. *Pricing* focuses on what customers must pay for services, whether the service is cosmetic surgery or a health plan premium. *Placement* refers to the way goods or services are distributed to consumers. Placement strategies may involve decisions about the location of a walk-in urgent care clinic. A placement, or distribution strategy, may also identify the health plans, preferred provider organizations, and insurance carriers

that a health care provider intends to contract with. Finally, *promotion* represents any way of educating the market about the products or services an organization makes available. Although many people think advertising is the primary form of promotion, news stories, community health fairs, and sponsorships of local fitness or athletic events are also considered promotional activities.

Health care marketing plans typically include recommendations about at least some of the four Ps, especially promotion or "marketing communications" as it is often called. Often, a placement strategy is fixed (you cannot easily relocate a clinic site) or other departments are involved in decision-making (few finance executives will leave pricing decisions to the marketer). Health care promotional activities typically include:

- Advertising
- Public/community relations (including community service)
- Media relations
- Health fairs and other special events
- Internal and external publications
- Brochures and other informational/educational materials
- Internet sites
- Charitable giving programs
- Giveaways.

All marketing communications efforts should begin with a description of the target audience and a definition of the objectives of the communications initiative. The challenge is to send messages tailored to the audience's needs that also meet the organization's communications objectives.

Objectives appropriate for a consumer audience include:

- to increase awareness of the organization
- to differentiate services from those of competitors
- to increase value in order to drive preference and choice.

Before launching any external marketing communications initiatives, a comprehensive internal campaign should be launched. This internal communications effort should include a description of the branding strategy, the organization's positioning *vis-à-vis* competitors, promises the organization intends to make to patients, and how it plans to live up to those promises. The goal is to educate employees about the organization's marketing objectives and motivate them to support the effort.

A budget should be developed to describe the costs associated with the creative concept development, production, and media vehicles (television, radio, newspaper, Internet sites, etc.).

Tracking and measuring the results of the marketing communications efforts are critical for evaluating performance and making future investment decisions. Measures may include: amount of positive editorial coverage (measured in column inches and minutes of TV or radio time); changes in patient satisfaction levels; changes in physician referrals; number of new patients; and increase in market share.

In summary, marketing is both a strategic and tactical organizational function that requires a great deal of coordinated planning. Simply running an advertisement for an organization is not a comprehensive marketing strategy. Marketing is a disciplined effort that identifies an organization's unique attributes, the promises it intends to make to patients, and how it intends to deliver on those promises. Ultimately, the organization's reputation is created through every experience a person has with it. It is the job of the chief executive officer, in concert with marketing and operations staff, to ensure that there is alignment between the expectations patients have of an organization and the organization's ability to live up to or, ideally, to surpass those expectations.

References

1. Kotler P, Clarke R. *Marketing for Health Care Organizations*. Englewood Cliffs, NJ: Prentice Hall, 1987.
2. The Alliance for Healthcare Strategy and Marketing. *The Moment of Truth. The Alliance Report—Strategies for the Healthcare Marketplace*. The Alliance for Healthcare Strategy and Marketing, November 1998: 1–3.
3. Miller K, Eliastram M. Time for physicians to reconfigure. *Med Network Strategy Report* June 1999; **8**: 6.
4. Luecke RW, Roselli VR, Moss JM. The economic ramification of "client" dissatisfaction. *Group Prac J* 1991; **40**: 8–18.
5. Duncan WJ, Ginter PM, Swayne LE. *Strategic Management of Health Care Organizations*. Boston, MA: PWS-Kent, 1995.
6. Berkowitz E. *Essentials of Health Care Marketing*. Gaithersburg, MD: Aspen Publishers, 1996.
7. Petromilli M, Michalczyk D. Your most valuable asset (increasing the value of your hospital through its brand). *Marketing Health Services*. American Marketing Association, Summer 1999: 5–9.
8. Rogers D. Branding the customer's expectations. *The Alliance Report*. The Alliance for Healthcare Strategy and Marketing, July 1999: 1–11.

Index